Nutrition for Serious Athletes

Dan Benardot, PhD, RD
The Laboratory for Elite Athlete Performance
Georgia State University

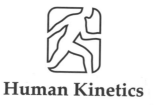

Human Kinetics

Library of Congress Cataloging-in-Publication Data

Benardot, Dan, 1949-
    Nutrition for serious athletes / Dan Benardot.
        p. cm.
    Includes bibliographical references and index.
    ISBN 0-88011-833-4
    1. Athletes--Nutrition. I. Title

    TX361.A8 B45 1999
    613.2'024'796--dc21

                                                                99-046572

ISBN 0-88011-833-4

Acquisitions Editor: Martin Barnard; **Developmental Editor:** Cassandra Mitchell; **Assistant Editors:** Laura Ward Majersky and Wendy McLaughlin; **Copyeditor:** Harbour Hodder; **Proofreader:** Erin Cler; **Indexer:** Sharon Duffy; **Permissions Manager:** Cheri Banks; **Graphic Designer:** Nancy Rasmus; **Graphic Artist:** Dawn Sills; **Photo Editor:** Clark Brooks; **Cover Designer:** Jack W. Davis; **Photographer (interior):** Tom Roberts, unless otherwise noted; **Illustrator:** Kim Maxey; **Printer:** United Graphics

Human Kinetics books are available at special discounts for bulk purchase. Special editions or book excerpts can also be created to specification. For details, contact the Special Sales Manager at Human Kinetics.

Printed in the United States of America   10 9 8 7 6 5 4

Human Kinetics
Web site: www.HumanKinetics.com

United States: Human Kinetics
P.O. Box 5076
Champaign, IL 61825-5076
800-747-4457
e-mail: humank@hkusa.com

Canada: Human Kinetics
475 Devonshire Road, Unit 100
Windsor, ON N8Y 2L5
800-465-7301 (in Canada only)
e-mail: orders@hkcanada.com

Europe: Human Kinetics
107 Bradford Road
Stanningley
Leeds LS28 6AT, United Kingdom
+44 (0)113 255 5665
e-mail: hk@hkeurope.com

Australia: Human Kinetics
57A Price Avenue
Lower Mitcham, South Australia 5062
08 8277 1555
e-mail: liahka@senet.com.au

New Zealand: Human Kinetics
P.O. Box 105-231, Auckland Central
09-523-3462
e-mail: hkp@ihug.co.nz

My family is simply wonderful. I love them and appreciate all the big and little things they do for each other and for me. Deborah, Jacob, and Leah—this book is for you.

Contents

Foreword

Rarely is a book written by an author who has the academic training *and* practical experience necessary to be called a real expert. Dr. Dan Benardot is the exception. From his early days of toiling in nutrition and exercise laboratories to his more recent successes on the floor of the gymnastics venue during the Olympic Games, Dr. Benardot has proven to be the world's foremost authority on sports nutrition. From chapter 1 to the final appendix, athletes, coaches, students, and teachers will find this book to be the authority on sports nutrition.

On this dawn of a new millennium, scholars will look back on the 20th century as a time of great advances. During the last half of the century, astronauts took off into space and even walked on the moon. The Berlin Wall crumbled and with it so did Communism. We saw the breakup of the Soviet Union. We saw the Atlanta Braves win a World Series. We experienced a gold medal performance by the United States Women's Artistic Gymnastics Team during the 1996 Atlanta Olympic Games. Advances in the diagnosis and treatment of disease are far too many to list here. One thing that has not changed, however, is the way athletes continue to search for a winning training program, which includes nutrition.

There is much confusion about proper nutrition and how important it is to the successful athlete. It seems that there is a daily introduction to the market of some new endurance-producing, power-enhancing mega-nutrient that will transform an average athlete into a superstar. This book makes no such claims. Instead, the reader is introduced first to the science of nutrition and what we know about the value of vitamins, minerals, and a balanced diet. Each chapter concludes with either practical applications or recommendations. You will see no commercials here marketing a single product claiming to enhance performance. You are introduced, however, to the real story (based on scientific fact as we know it today) of successful nutrition.

As an added bonus, Dr. Benardot includes in the appendixes a section he labels "Sample Meal Plans." This section alone is worth the price of the book! It is a must read for the serious athlete.

For the better part of four decades (my professional life and that segment I was called an "athlete"), I have had an interest in the relationship between physical activity and nutrition. As a professor, I have been asked numerous times to recommend a good text that was readable, understandable, and could answer the tough questions. This is the book that I can finally recommend without any hesitation.

Walter R. Thompson, PhD, FACSM, FAACVPR
Professor of Kinesiology and Health
Professor of Nutrition
Director, Center for Sports Medicine, Science & Technology
Georgia State University
Atlanta, GA

Preface

This book is meant for all athletes who take their sport seriously and those who work with them. The number of people involved in organized sports is swelling, and the age at which people are involved at the elite levels of sport is expanding at both ends of the age continuum. As this involvement grows, so does the quantity of *misinformation* about what should be done to assure that nutritional needs are met for both athletic performance and health. You don't have to look too far to find "nutritional" products that are marketed with the idea that their consumption will lead to improved performance. The sports medicine literature is filled with cases of athletes who have used some of these products with disastrous (at times fatal) results. To compound the potential for problems, there is a tendency for many beginning athletes to try to achieve too much too quickly, with training paradigms that mimic those of the most highly trained and seasoned professionals. Elite gymnasts often reach their performance peak at around age 16, and 5-year-old boys are in full football uniform being cheered on by equally serious 5-year-old girls. Women's soccer in the United States, following the recent gold medal of the popular U.S. Women's team at the 1999 World Cup, is likely to create a soccer boom for girls of all ages and may even increase the involvement of boys in soccer programs. The 1998 Hawaii Ironman Triathlon competition had athletes in their 60s and 70s who were serious age-group competitors. This would have been unheard of several years ago, and the rapidity with which this phenomenon has occurred has created a need for information in sports nutrition for these diverse populations that would not have existed just a few short years ago.

There certainly is more information available for athletes, but the reliability of much of this information is in question. It is difficult for an athlete interested in optimizing performance to be completely rational in determining what constitutes information and what constitutes misinformation. Walking into a "nutrition" center that sells vitamins and other health products can leave a person more confused (certainly more financially strained) than before they walked in. When there's a money motive, you can be virtually certain you're not getting an unbiased account of what's right. When you're told that the active football player needs more protein, you're likely to believe it because it's become common knowledge that there is a relationship between high protein intake and high achievement in sport. The next leap of judgment is simple. If more protein is needed, then why not the building blocks of protein, amino acids. And then it's a short leap to hearing, "The amino acids I sell are better than the amino acids *they* sell...." The truth is, the commonly held beliefs about protein are big myths, and most of the money spent on protein and amino acid pills is making someone richer but probably isn't making the athlete any better.

Part of the problem is that sports nutrition information is expanding so rapidly that what we may have assumed to be fact a few short years ago we now know to be fiction. A review of position papers from the American Dietetic Association and the American College of Sports Medicine underscores this point. A few short years ago these organizations properly recommended (it was the state of the art at the time) that sports beverages should have an energy concentration that did not exceed 2.5 percent. These same organizations, given more and better information, now both recommend that sports beverages should have an energy concentration that does not exceed 8 percent (a threefold increase in energy concentration!). The first recommendation was based on gastric emptying time (the standard technique used in the past), while the current recommendation is based on intestinal absorption time (the current and better means of determining this issue). To compound the confusion, many athletes tolerate higher concentrations of energy in sports beverages than the current recommendations, and many have difficulties consuming the recommended level. The recommendations given are typically based on the common response to a substance or protocol, but there is a huge individual difference around that common response. Therefore, when general recommendations are provided in this book and others, they should be considered the starting point in determining what's right for you or the athlete you're working with. All too often these general recommendations are taken as set-in-concrete fact.

Relying on the lay media as the sole source of information may also be dangerous to your health. This is not because the information provided is necessarily wrong, but it may not relate specifically to you. It is common for the media to provide a case study of what a single successful athlete does to stay healthy and strong, but transferring that information to others may be a big mistake. Here's that athlete who has trained for six hours each day for years, has a terrific coach, and takes a nutrient supplement. We are, of course, led to believe that this success is attributable to the nutrient supplement. I'll put my money on an excellent training regimen, a favorable genetic makeup, and what must also be a pretty terrific food intake.

Despite a boom in sports nutrition information in recent years, there still are many questions that are not easily answered. Are 15-year-old elite gymnasts likely to experience the same problems as the 19-year-olds who have been competing longer? Are they at the same or different developmental stages? Should adolescent females fear not achieving menses until they reach the age of 16, 17, or 18? Is it appropriate for a 5-year-old to consume a sports beverage during a game, just like the big boys? Is there a problem with the energy restrictions high school wrestlers undergo to make weight, when many of these same wrestlers are in what should be their adolescent growth spurt? What happens to the bones of a young skater when she eats just enough to satisfy her immediate needs, but not enough to satisfy her developmental needs? Does the high protein intake common in bodybuilding, weight-lifting, and football represent a potential for premature kidney failure, since there is an inevitable increase in the amount of nitrogenous waste that must be excreted? Or does it just represent another source of energy that is burned without short- or long-term difficulty? Where do runners, who go out for their morning run *before* breakfast, get the fuel to make their muscles work?

These questions should not lead you to misunderstand the thrust of this book. Exercise and involvement in sport can be, should be, and usually are wonderful things. The philosophical basis for this book is that sport involvement should lead to an enhancement of lifetime health rather than a lifetime of problems, and that what is done nutritionally can make a tremendous difference in seeing to it that this is what happens. Doing things right nutritionally will also make an enormously positive difference in a serious athlete's ability to train and compete. The aim here is to provide you with information that can make you more assured that nutrition is not a limiting factor in performance and health and to provide you with a framework for making the right nutritional decisions.

Acknowledgments

The longer I stay in academe the more I have come to realize that nothing I do is done alone, even if it has only my name on it. I have many colleagues who are always there with good science, innovative ideas, solutions to problems, and experiences that complement my own.

Dr. David Martin, with whom I codirect the *Laboratory for Elite Athlete Performance*, has an encyclopedic knowledge of distance running and runners. Our collaboration has linked David's experience and knowledge of cardiopulmonary physiology and aerobic athletes with my background and experience in nutrition and anaerobic athletes. The result has been a laboratory that brings a broad spectrum of experience and innovation to every athlete, regardless of the athletic discipline. Besides the positive nature of working closely with someone who is an extraordinary academician and scientist, working with David has been pure fun.

Dr. Walter Thompson, the author of the forward for this book, has the wonderful ability to bring scientists from different disciplines together, and, in his capacity as Director of the Center for Sports Medicine, Science & Technology, he does just that. His multidisciplinary capabilities are illustrated by his professorial status in two departments (Kinesiology and Health *and* Nutrition), and his inclusion on numerous national committees. I have never heard him say no to a good idea, regardless of the barriers to getting it accomplished. If it needed manpower, equipment, space, or someone to sell the idea to a higher power, he has always found a way to get it done.

Dr. Mildred (Missy) Cody is a food scientist without rival, and she's managed to couple this expertise with an understanding of electronic communications that is simply astounding. These skills are useful to all of us working on information dissemination, but Missy is also a scientist's scientist. When we need a solid, balanced view of the best procedures to learn more about a problem our athletes have been experiencing, Missy has always been there with a treasure of ideas. If I need to brainstorm with someone, she's the one and she's the best.

Dr. Satya Jonnalagadda, although relatively new to the faculty, has established herself as a powerful asset in determining the nutritional needs of the athletes we work with. If there's a limitation in assessment time or an assessment setting that may not be ideal, she knows the technique to use to get the information we need. What makes her even better is that *everyone* likes to work with her. Having a pleasant work environment is a key to getting work done, and her presence makes getting more work done easy.

I have other colleagues, including Ms. Meryl Sheard, Dr. Jeffrey Rupp, Dr. Andrew Doyle, Dr. Jerry Brandon, and Ms. Deborah Rupp who, on the occasions we've had to work together, have always contributed more than they were asked to. They have been wonderful, and their collegiality has made my work that much easier to do. The physician/scientists I work with on the F.I.G. Medical Commission, Dr. Kostas Markou, Dr. Neoklis Georgopoulos, and Dr. Michel Leglise have been extraordinary in their commitment to young athletes and the energy they put into making things better for them. Of course, I also have had numerous graduate students (too many to name here) who have assisted in every aspect of the lab and who make doing what I do possible. They've always been a great group.

The athletes I have had the pleasure of working with are not only first-class athletes (literally!), but they're also first-class people. Bright, energetic, enthusiastic, and inquisitive, these athletes are the motivation behind what I do. There are no better people on the planet, and I am thankful so many of them have let me get a glimpse of their unique world.

The staff at Human Kinetics has been wonderful to work with. Particularly, Martin Barnard, who originally proposed that I write this book, and Cassandra Mitchell, who has done so much to guide me along the way.

There is no question that many of the ideas in this book originated from these people. The ideas may have come while having a discussion over a cup of coffee, from a question at a dissertation defense, or when listening to one of them discuss an issue with an athlete. One way or another I know for certain these people were with me every step of the way whenever my fingers touched a keyboard to work on this book, and I am profoundly thankful.

Credits

Figures

Figure 2.1 is reprinted by permission from M. Hargreaves, 1996, "Physiological benefits of fluid and energy replacement during exercise," *Australian journal of nutrition and dietetics* 53 (4 Suppl): S3-S7.

Figure 2.2 is reprinted by permission from M. Hargreaves, 1996, "Physiological benefits of fluid and energy replacement during exercise," *Australian journal of nutrition and dietetics* 53 (4 Suppl): S3-S7.

Tables

Table 1.5 is adapted from B.W. Tobin and J.L. Beard, 1997, Iron. In *Sports Nutrition,* edited by I. Wolinsky and J.A. Driskell, (Boca Raton, FL: CRC Press), 148. Copyright Lewis Publishers, an imprint of CRC Press.

Table 2.3 is adapted by permission from H. O'Connor, 1996, "Practical aspects of fluid replacement," *Australian journal of nutrition and dietetics* 53 (4 Suppl): S27-S34.

Table 3.1 is adapted by permission from J.H. Wilmore and D.L. Costill, 1988, *Training for sport and activity: the physiological basis of the conditioning process,* 3rd ed. (Champaign, IL: Human Kinetics), appendix.

Table 4.1 is adapted from L. Bucci, 1993, *Nutrients as ergogenic aids for sports and exercise* (Boca Raton, FL: CRC Press), 11. Copyright Lewis Publishers, an imprint of CRC Press.

Table 5.1 is adapted by permission from B. Saltin, J. Henriksson, E. Nygaard, P. Anderson, and E. Jansson, 1977, "Fiber types and metabolic potentials of skeletal muscles in sedentary men and endurance runners," *Ann. NY Acad. Sci,* 301: 3-29.

Table 5.3 is adapted by permission from M.H. Williams, 1993, "Nutritional supplements for strength trained athletes," *Sports Science Exchange* 47 (6): 6.

Table 5.4 is adapted by permission from M.H. Williams, 1993, "Nutritional supplements for strength trained athletes," *Sports Science Exchange* 47 (6): 6.

Table 6.2 is adapted from R. Murray and C.A. Horswill, 1998, Nutrient requirements for competitive sports. In *Nutrition in exercise and sport,* 3rd ed., edited by I. Wolinsky (Boca Raton, FL: CRC Press). Copyright Lewis Publishers, an imprint of CRC Press.

Table 6.4 is adapted by permission from K. Foster-Powell and J.B. Miller, 1995, "International table of glycemic index," *American journal of clinical nutrition* 62: 871S-893S.

Table 6.5 is adapted from R. Murray and C.A. Horswill, 1998, Nutrient requirements for competitive sports. In *Nutrition in exercise and sport*, 3rd ed., edited by I. Wolinsky (Boca Raton, FL: CRC Press). Copyright Lewis Publishers, an imprint of CRC Press.

Table 8.1 is adapted by permission from J. Mielcarek and S. Kleiner, 1993, Time zone changes. In *Sports nutrition: a guide for the professional working with active people*, D. Benardot, ed., (Chicago: The American Dietetic Association), 195-196.

Table 8.2 is adapted by permission from E.R. Burke and J.R. Berning, 1996, *Training nutrition: the diet and nutrition guide for peak performance* (Carmel, IN: Cooper), 134.

Table 9.1 is adapted by permission from D.R. Lamb, 1995, "Basic principles for improving sport performance," *Sports Science Exchange* 55(8): 2.

Table 10.1 is adapted by permission from F.I. Katch, V.L. Katch, and W.D. McArdle, 1993, *Introduction to nutrition, exercise, and health*, 4th ed. (Philadephia: Lea & Febiger), 179.

Table 11.2 is adapted by permission from C. Williams and C.W. Nicholas, 1998, "Nutrition needs for team sport," *Sports Science Exchange* 11(3): 70.

Photos

© Claus Andersen 240, 281

© Eric Berndt/New England Stock 198

© Gus Bower 67

© Brian Drake/Sports Chrome 34, 224, 284

© Jay Foreman/Unicorn Stock Photos 21

© Richard B. Levine 171, 244

© Dennis Light/Light Photographic 220

© Craig Melivin/Sports Chrome 234

© John Mora 203

© Victah Sailer 105, 207, 229

© Robert Skeoch/The Picture Desk 147

© Rob Tringali/Sports Chrome 215

© Trozzo Photography 117

© Ron Vesely 151

© Aneal S. Vohra/Unicorn Stock Photos 259

© Terry Wild 129

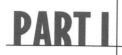

The Nutrition Toolbox

1 | Balancing Essential Nutrients

She Took So Many Supplements That She Forgot to Eat

She was young. She was smart. She was strong. She was fast. She was good-looking. She had big company support. She was the envy of the track world. In spite of all of this, she was miserable that she was getting older and bigger, that her breasts and hips were larger, and that she didn't smash any records at her last meet. So, in spite of her history of successes, she did what all too many athletes do to gain control over the biological clock that never stops ticking. She started "dieting." By the time she came through my lab, her times had slipped away with her weight, and she found herself in a downward funnel of eating that kept sucking her lower and lower. The first thing she said when she walked into the lab was, "The day I graduated from high school my metabolism stopped!" She had decided that the best way to gain control over her age-related biological changes was to eat less (big mistake), and to take supplements to obtain the nutrients she needed to stay healthy and strong (another big mistake).

The results were disastrous on many levels, mainly because she had changed much of what had made her successful. She had been an eater. She ate all the time. She ate before her morning run, after her morning run, at midmorning, at noon, at midafternoon, before her late-afternoon run, after her late-afternoon run, in the early evening, and in the late evening. She learned from the very beginning that this was the very best way to get the *energy* and *nutrients* she needed to meet the needs of her explosive power and magnificent endurance. But she had forgotten what worked for her and decided that eating less was better, and, besides, her health wouldn't suffer because she was taking "supplements."

When I asked her what supplements she was taking, she brought in a gym bag full of everything from B-complex to amino acid powders. When I explained that most of these supplements were useless without sufficient energy intake, she asked what *supplement* she should take to get the energy she needed for the supplements to work on! And then a stunned look appeared on her face, as if she had just awakened to what she had been doing to herself. It was like the sudden realization that smokers sometimes get when they're puffing on a cigarette and complaining of making it up the stairs. It's just one of those moments when the reality of the situation hits you. From that moment on, it was easy to get this world-class runner to do the right thing and start eating again, and she's happier and more successful as a result.

Food is the carrier of nutrients, and to get the nutrients we need, we require the right food *exposure*. It is this basic fact that is the basis of the most elementary nutritional principle: eat a wide variety of foods. While this may appear to be a simple and easy-to-accomplish principle, most people tend to consume the same few foods over and over again. This occurs because of habit, time limitations, work conditions, and basic food desires and dislikes. However, it is clear that monotonous intakes of this type will eventually lead to some degree of malnutrition and, for the athlete, some loss of performance potential. Perhaps it is due to this general understanding that eating a wide variety of foods is critical to optimal nutrition, along with the realization that doing this is difficult, that so many athletes resort to nutrient supplements and other nutritional products: they are trying to diminish their underlying fear that they simply don't eat right to perform well. Athletes, thus, commonly go from being undernourished from foods to being overnourished from supplements. Neither condition will help them accomplish their goals. However, it is clear that many coaches and athletes don't know how nutrients work and how the human body deals with nutritional mistakes. This chapter will review the essential elements of nutrients, what they do, and how they work.

The goal here is to demonstrate the importance of nutritional balance, because it is all too clear that nutritional imbalance (either too much or too little), is a major culprit in poor athletic performance. The best way to think about optimal nutritional status is by analogy with supply-and-demand microeconomics theory. Every cell has a nutritional requirement. If you provide too much, it must expend energy and effort to get rid of the excess. If you provide too little, the cell malfunctions. Every cell has a nutrient demand, and it's your job to supply what it needs at the time it needs it.

Six Classes of Nutrients

Everyone has heard of vitamins and minerals and knows that these are nutrients. But these are not all the nutrients. There are six classes of nutrients that include water, vitamins, minerals, proteins, fats, and carbohydrates. We are able to derive energy (fuel) from foods that contain three different compounds—carbohydrates, proteins, and fats. We can also derive energy from alcohol, but regular consumption of alcohol creates havoc with normal energy metabolic processes and increases the potential for dehydration. While many people attribute energy-providing properties to vitamins and minerals, they are not a source of energy. They are, however, needed to derive energy from carbohydrates, proteins, and fats that are consumed. Athletes who dramatically reduce food intake but think there won't be a problem because they're taking their vitamins are wrong. With no energy source, vitamins don't have much to work on. Water, discussed in chapter 2, is a nutrient that literally ties everything together. Water circulates the other nutrients to the tissues where they are used and removes the by-products of this tissue utilization. Water is also a key ingredient for maintaining body temperature during hard physical activity.

Nutrient Balance

Each nutrient is equally essential, and we can't eliminate any class of nutrient from the foods we eat and hope to do well athletically (much less survive in good health!). Critical to understanding nutrients is the concept that nutrients work together, both within nutrient classes and between nutrient classes. For instance, it's impossible to imagine burning fat for energy without having some carbohydrate present because 'fat burns in a carbohydrate flame.' It's also impossible to imagine having healthy red blood cells with sufficient iron intake but inadequate vitamin B-12 and folic acid intake. Having enough total energy intake (from carbohydrate, protein, and fat) is an excellent strategy for optimizing athletic performance. However, doing this with an inadequate fluid intake will impede your ability to burn these energy compounds by limiting their delivery to cells, limiting the removal of metabolic by-products from cells, and limiting your ability to cool yourself from the heat created when energy compounds are burned.

On the other hand, having too much of any one nutrient may damage the opportunity for the normal nutrient absorption and metabolism of other nutrients being consumed at an adequate level. For instance, calcium supplements are commonly taken to help ensure strong and healthy bones that are resistant to stress fractures (a common injury in sport) and to reduce the risk of osteoporosis. However, taking too much calcium at the same time as taking iron, magnesium, and zinc may inhibit the absorption of these other nutrients, which are equally important in maintaining health and athletic performance. Again, these are issues of nutrient balance. Having one nutrient without the other simply doesn't work, and having too much of one nutrient may cause difficulties with other nutrients.

Therefore, when you review table 1.1 and see a summary of nutrients and their various functions, it is dangerous thinking to believe that taking a single nutrient will, by itself, encourage that function. Think *balance.*

Table 1.1   Nutrient Functions

Nutrient	Major functions
Carbohydrate	Energy/muscular fuel (from starch, sugars, and glycogen) Cholesterol/fat control (from dietary fiber) Digestion assistance (from dietary fiber) Nutrient/water absorption (from sugars)
Protein	Energy source (if carbohydrates are depleted) Delivery of essential amino acids (amino acids the body needs but can't make) Essential for developing new tissue (important during growth and injury repair) Essential for maintaining existing tissue (helps control normal wear and tear) Basic substance in the manufacture of enzymes, antibodies, and hormones Fluid balance (helps control water level inside and outside cells) Carrier of substances in the blood (transports vitamins, minerals, and fats to and from cells)
Fat	Delivery of fat-soluble vitamins (vitamins A, D, E, and K) Delivery of essential fatty acids (fatty acids the body needs but can't make) Energy/muscular fuel (for low-intensity activity) Satiety control (helps make you feel satisfied from eating) Substance in many hormones
Vitamins	Tissue function and health (vitamin A helps the eye work correctly) Immune function (vitamins A and C are well known for this function) Energy metabolism control (B vitamins, in particular, are involved in helping cells burn energy) Nutrient absorption (vitamin D helps calcium and phosphorus go from the food you eat to your bloodstream) Nervous system maintenance (folic acid and thiamin are important in nerve system development and function) Antioxidants (help protect cells from oxidative damage)

Nutrient	Major functions
Minerals	Skeletal strength (calcium, phosphorus, and magnesium are keys to strong bones; fluoride keeps teeth strong by protecting them from bacterial acids) Nerve function (magnesium and calcium are both involved in nerve communication) Control of the body's pH (acidity level) Oxygen transport (iron is essential for getting oxygen to cells and removing carbon dioxide from cells) Control of the body's water balance (sodium and potassium play important roles in blood volume maintenance) Energy metabolism (zinc is in many enzymes involved in deriving energy from fuel, and iodine helps to control the rate at which energy is used)
Water	The body's coolant (helps maintain body temperature through sweat production) Carrier of nutrients to cells Remover of waste products from cells Important constituent of muscle Involved in many body reactions (both in digestion of food and in processes inside cells

Nutrient Intake Guidelines

In 1995, dietary guidelines were established by the U.S. Department of Agriculture and the U.S. Department of Health and Human Services to provide people with a simple set of rules for assuring good nutritional health and lowering the risk of high blood pressure, diabetes, and heart disease. These rules are also excellent rules for athletes to follow:

- Eat a variety of foods.
- Balance the food you eat with physical activity to maintain or improve your weight.
- Consume plenty of grain products, vegetables, and fruits.
- Keep fat, saturated fat, and cholesterol in your diet low.
- Choose a diet moderate in sugars.
- Have a diet that is moderate in salt (sodium).
- If you drink alcohol, do so only in moderation.

The Food Guide Pyramid

The most recent of the dietary guidelines, the Food Guide Pyramid, follows in the footsteps of past guides that are based on patterns of food intake. One of the early guides (established in the 1960s) that used food patterns was called the Basic Four Food Groups, which recommended that people consume a certain number of servings of foods from the dairy group, meat group, fruit and vegetable group, and bread and cereal group. This basic concept has evolved into the Food Guide Pyramid, which uses the shape of the pyramid (larger at the base smaller at the top) to communicate the amount of food that should be consumed from each of six food categories. The number of servings a person should eat depends on the amount of energy or calories* needed, which is dependent on a person's physical activity, age, gender, and size. The minimum number of suggested servings in each food group yields about 1,600 calories per day, and the maximum number of suggested servings in each food group provides about 2,800 calories per day.

- Bread, cereal, rice, and pasta (6 to 11 servings/day)
  (A serving is equivalent to 1 slice of bread; 1/2 cup of cooked cereal, rice, or pasta; 1 ounce of ready-to-eat cereal; 1/2 bun, bagel, or English muffin; 1 small roll, biscuit, or muffin; 3 to 4 small or 2 large crackers.)
- Vegetables (3 to 5 servings/day)
  (A serving is equivalent to 1/2 cup of cooked or raw vegetables; 1 cup of leafy raw vegetables; 1/2 cup of cooked dried beans, lentils, and peas; and 3/4 cup of vegetable juice.)
- Fruits (2 to 4 servings/day)
  (A serving is equivalent to 1 medium apple, banana, or orange; 1/2 grapefruit; 1 melon wedge; 3/4 cup juice; 1/2 cup berries; 1/2 cup diced, cooked, or canned fruit; 1/2 cup of dried fruit.)
- Milk, yogurt, and cheese (2 to 3 servings/day)
  (A serving is equivalent to 1 cup of milk or yogurt; 2 ounces of processed cheese food; or 1 1/2 ounces of cheese.)
- Meat, poultry, fish, dry beans, eggs, and nuts (2 to 3 servings/day)
  (A serving is equivalent to 2 to 3 ounces of lean, cooked meat, poultry, or fish for a total of 5 to 7 ounces per day; 1 egg, 1/2 cup

* In nutrition, the term "calorie" is actually a kilocalorie (kcal) or 1000 times the energy of the physics calorie. In this book, the term "calorie" is the standard term and is synonymous with kilocalorie and kcal.

of cooked legumes, or 2 tablespoons of peanut butter may be counted as 1 ounce of meat.)

- Fats, oils, and sweets (use sparingly)
  (High fat foods include butter, margarine, oils, mayonnaise, salad dressings, sour cream, cream cheese, gravy, and sauces. High sugar foods include candy, candy fruit rolls, soft drinks, fruit drinks, jelly, syrup, desserts, sugar, and honey.)

The Food Guide Pyramid makes no distinction between the kinds of fats but encourages a low level of total fat consumption. Other recommendations suggest a low fat intake but, within the context of a lower fat intake, a relatively higher level of olive oil.[1] This recommendation is based on the "Mediterranean diet," where people consume more olive oil (a monounsaturated fat) than other fats and have lower levels of chronic disorders than are present in North America.

The base of the pyramid (see figure 1.1), bread, cereals, and pasta, indicates that the majority of consumed foods should come from this group of high-carbohydrate products. As you go higher on the pyramid, the next categories are fruits and vegetables, followed by dairy and meats or legumes, and ending with fats, oils, and sweets,

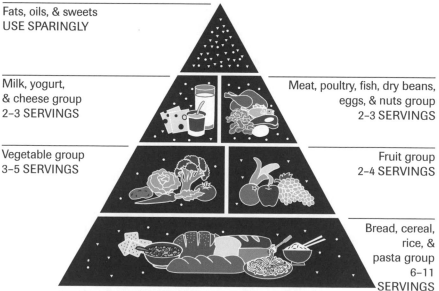

Fats, oils, & sweets
USE SPARINGLY

Milk, yogurt,
& cheese group
2–3 SERVINGS

Meat, poultry, fish, dry beans,
eggs, & nuts group
2–3 SERVINGS

Vegetable group
3–5 SERVINGS

Fruit group
2–4 SERVINGS

Bread, cereal,
rice, &
pasta group
6–11
SERVINGS

United States Departments of Agriculture and Health and Human Services

Figure 1.1 Food Guide Pyramid.

which should constitute the smallest part of a person's food intake. Within the context of the distribution of food categories, people are encouraged to vary the intake of foods from each category and to select foods with a high nutrient density. That is, for every calorie consumed, there should be a high concentration of nutrients. Sugar, for instance, provides energy but is associated with no other nutrients. Therefore, sugar has a low nutrient density. Whole grain and enriched breads, on the other hand, provide the same amount of energy (4 calories/gram) as sugar, but also provide B-vitamins, minerals, and fiber.

This is a clear departure from the early food guides, which gave almost equal importance to the consumption of dairy products, meats, and fruits and vegetables. The Food Guide Pyramid appropriately places a great deal of emphasis on carbohydrates, with 3 to 5 servings of vegetables, 2 to 4 servings of fruits, and 6 to 11 servings of bread, cereal, rice, and pasta. Taken together, the food guide pyramid recommends between 11 and 20 servings of high-carbohydrate foods per day! The message with the pyramid is clear: eat more complex carbohydrates. The word complex is important here, because sugars (also carbohydrates) are not complex and are relegated to the distant top of the pyramid. Athletes (regardless of whether they are involved in power sports or endurance events) would be hard pressed to find better eating guidelines. Add sufficient fluids to this mix, and you have a virtually perfect food intake pattern for athletes.

RDA: Appropriate for Athletes?

The Food and Nutrition Board of the American Academy of Sciences evaluates clinical, epidemiological, and case study data to establish levels of energy and nutrients that meet the requirements for most healthy people. These recommended levels of intake are referred to as the "Recommended Dietary Allowances" (RDA). Where there are inadequate data to make a good decision on recommended nutrient intakes, the Food and Nutrition Board periodically publishes "Estimated Safe and Adequate Intakes" (ESADI) and "Estimated Minimum Requirements" (EMR) for specific nutrients. Currently, there are published RDAs for energy; protein; and, vitamins A, D, E, K, B-1, B-2, niacin, B-6, B-12, and folate. There are published ESADIs for biotin, pantothenic acid, copper, manganese, fluoride, chromium, and molybdenum. There are EMRs for sodium, potassium, and chloride.

The energy RDA is based on the average requirement for healthy people of average height, weight, and activity. The level of nutrient requirement established for the RDA is based on the average requirement for healthy people in different age categories, plus two standard deviations. The purpose of establishing the nutrient RDA at a level that is above the average requirement is to have a level of intake that meets the requirement for 98 percent of all healthy people. The energy requirement is set at the average requirement (not two standard deviations above the average as with the nutrient RDA) because excessive intake of energy is associated with obesity. The way the nutrient RDA is established is an important point to consider, since the Food and Nutrition Board recognizes that there are inherent differences among people, and that these differences express themselves in the requirement for nutrients. Therefore, most healthy people have nutrient requirements that are considerably less than the RDA (i.e., close to the average requirement and not two standard deviations above the requirement), and a small proportion of people have nutrient requirements above the RDA. In spite of the way the RDAs are established, many (if not most) people consider the RDA to be a *minimum* requirement for good health and having more than the RDA (which is already higher than most people need to maintain good health) is even better. This mind-set is, of course, the reason so many people take nutrient supplements: they believe that more than enough is better than enough. However, it is important to consider that nutrient balance and energy adequacy are the keys to good health. Having too much may be just as bad as having too little.

For the athlete, the RDA is an excellent starting point to determine nutrient adequacy. Because athletes tend to burn more energy than the average person, energy requirements are likely to be higher than those established in the energy RDA. Since burning more energy requires more nutrients (particularly B-vitamins), and performance is closely tied to several minerals (iron and zinc in particular), consuming the nutrient RDA of these nutrients is a good idea. Serious athletes should periodically have a blood test to determine whether nutrient intake is adequate and to see if consuming the RDA level is right for them. In particular, checking adequate iron intake status by evaluating hemoglobin, hematocrit, and ferritin is important and may also be an indicator of the intake adequacy of other nutrients.

Carbohydrates

It is important to note that carbohydrates are expressed in the plural form because there are different types, and these different types are treated differently by our bodies. For instance, sugar and bran are both carbohydrates, but they're on different ends of the energy spectrum. Sugar enters the bloodstream quickly and initiates a fast and high insulin response, while the energy in bran doesn't make it into the bloodstream at all and tends to mediate the insulin response by slowing the rate at which other energy sources enter the bloodstream. Because these differences within substances exist, it is important to think about what *specific* type of carbohydrates might be best under different circumstances. Therefore, while athletes rely heavily on carbohydrates for fuel, not all carbohydrate foods are good for all occasions.

Taken together, athletes should obtain about 65 percent of total calories from carbohydrate foods. The minimum carbohydrate requirement for athletes is 30 calories of carbohydrate per kilogram of body weight. The key to remember is that glucose is the main source of fuel for muscular activity, and the higher the exercise intensity, the greater the reliance on glucose as a fuel. When glucose runs out, the athlete stops. Carbohydrates, if digestible, provide 4 calories of energy per gram and are categorized as either simple or complex.

Simple Carbohydrates

Simple carbohydrates, commonly referred to as sugars, include the monosaccharides (literally, single—mono—sugar sugars), and disaccharides (two-sugar sugars). The major monosaccharides are glucose (also called dextrose, or blood sugar), fructose (also called levulose), and galactose. The major disaccharides are sucrose (table sugar), lactose (milk sugar), and maltose (grain sugar). Assuming all the digestive enzymes are available and working, we break down the disaccharides into their component monosaccharides in the digestive process:

- sucrose = glucose and fructose
- lactose = glucose and galactose
- maltose = glucose and glucose

If you wish to have a quick boost to your blood glucose level, consumption of maltose might be a better option than lactose, because the digestion of maltose gives you two ready-to-use molecules of glucose, while lactose digestion results in one molecule of glucose and one molecule of galactose. The galactose must go through a secondary conversion (which takes time) to glucose before it can be used. Determining what carbohydrate source to consume is not easy, since there are additional issues related to solubility, sweetness (palatability), and availability. For instance, maltose provides more immediate glucose than the other disaccharides, but has less than half the sweetness of sucrose, limiting its palatability. Therefore, rather than being removed from some foods for use as a sweetener as sucrose is (sucrose is removed from sugar beets and sugar cane and sold as table sugar), maltose is typically fermented for the production of malt beverages, such as beer.

The type of food consumed influences the type of carbohydrate available to the system. Simple carbohydrates are derived naturally from many foods, including fruits (fresh, dried, and fruit juices) and vegetables. We also obtain simple carbohydrates from processed foods, including candies and sport beverages.

Complex Carbohydrates

Complex carbohydrates (also called polysaccharides) are subcategorized as digestible or indigestible and consist of long-chained branches of monosaccharides held together by two major bond types. The digestible complex carbohydrates have monosaccharides held together by bonds that can be disrupted by the digestive enzymes our bodies produce, while the indigestible complex carbohydrates are held together by bonds that are impervious to our digestive enzymes. Both the digestible and indigestible complex carbohydrates are important for maintaining health but should clearly be perceived as different by the athlete. Digestible complex carbohydrates are found in starchy foods, including potatoes, pasta, bread, cereal, and beans, while indigestible complex carbohydrates are found in the bran portion of cereals, in fruits, and in vegetables. Some sports beverages use glucose polymers, a type of artificially formed polysaccharide. These are chains of glucose molecules that are easily separated in the gut, making a lot of glucose quickly available to the athlete. Indigestible complex carbohydrate is commonly referred to as fiber. Even fiber is subcategorized as soluble fiber (pectin, mucilage, and gum) and insoluble fiber (cellulose and hemicellulose). Soluble fiber is found mainly in fruits, vegetables, and in some grains (particularly oats), while insoluble fiber is found mainly in the bran portion of cereal grains.

One of the most important fuels for athletes is a complex carbohydrate called glycogen. Glycogen is composed of many glucose molecules (often more than 3,000) and is the main storage form of glucose. It is found in the liver, where it helps to maintain normal blood glucose, and in muscle, where it is used as a source of fuel for muscular activity. An athlete's ability to store glycogen is mediated by conditioning, hydration state, and the availability of glucose and glycogen synthetase, an enzyme required to form glycogen from glucose.

There are other complex carbohydrates, including raffinose and stachyose (found in legumes), which are called oligosaccharides. Oligosaccharides are larger than disaccharides and smaller than polysaccharides, containing between 3 and 10 molecules of monosaccharides. The oligosaccharides found in legumes are either indigestible or only partially digestible, and are partially responsible for the gas production associated with eating beans. Gut bacteria that feed on these undigested carbohydrates produce this gas. This is an important consideration in the type of carbohydrate consumed, since intestinal gas and bloating may make an athlete uncomfortable and prevent the athlete from performing at the optimal level. See appendix B for the carbohydrate content of commonly consumed foods.

Proteins

Proteins are considered by many athletes to be the key to athletic success. It's hard to find power athletes who don't take some form of protein powders or protein supplements, and most who do swear that the successes they have are, at least partially, attributable to the protein they take. In fact, most athletes consume too much protein and, in doing so, are reducing their athletic potential. Interestingly, the athletes who need more protein (as a percent of total energy consumption) are those who typically have lower protein intakes. It has been demonstrated that endurance athletes actually have a higher requirement (per pound of body weight) than power athletes.[2,3] The endurance athletes actually burn a small amount of protein as part of their normal endurance activities, while power athletes do not. However, it is the power athletes who are typically the ones consuming more protein than they need.[4-6] To make matters worse, many of these athletes consume protein powders or amino acid supplements to increase their protein intake. When you consider that 1 ounce of meat provides about 7,000 milligrams of amino acids and that the typical amino acid supplement provides between 500 and 1,000 milligrams, none of this makes any sense.

Amino Acids

Proteins are unique substances that contain nitrogen, which is part of the bonding structure of protein building blocks called *amino acids.* These amino acids are the units the body uses to create protein-based substances, which include muscle, hormones, and enzymes. Protein is also the basic fibrous structure of the skeleton, onto which minerals are deposited to develop strength and rigidity. We can get amino acids from the foods we eat and from the breakdown of our own body tissues (mainly muscle and organ tissue). Some amino acids can be manufactured from carbohydrates, fats, and ammonia (a nitrogen-containing by-product of protein metabolism). These are called nonessential amino acids because it is not essential that we consume them from food (since we can make them from other substances.) The other amino acids, however, cannot be manufactured, so they are called essential amino acids. In other words, it is essential that we consume them from the foods we eat. The best food sources for protein include meats (beef, pork, lamb, poultry, fish, etc.), but dried beans and peas (legumes) are also good sources of protein. (Refer to appendix B for the protein content of commonly consumed foods.)

While protein derived from meats yields proteins that have a desirable balance of amino acids, plant proteins and soybeans must be properly combined to provide a desirable amino acid balance. For instance, combining beans and rice or combining beans and corn (a legume with a cereal) provides a combination of amino acids that is superior to eating a legume or a cereal by itself. Combining foods to provide a good amino acid balance is referred to as combining complementary proteins. That is, the amino acid weakness in one food is the amino acid strength of another food. When you put them together at one meal, you get a complete or balanced protein.

When we eat foods containing proteins, the proteins are digested into amino acids. These amino acids join other amino acids produced by the body to constitute the amino acid pool. The body takes the amino acids from this pool to synthesize the specific proteins it needs (muscle, hair, nails, hormones, enzymes, etc.). However, this amino acid pool is also available for use as energy to be burned if a sufficient amount of other fuels (carbohydrates and fat) are unavailable.

Determining Protein Needs

Protein yields approximately 4 calories per gram, which is the same energy concentration as carbohydrates. The recommended level of protein intake for the general population is 12 to 15 percent of total calories provided as protein. Therefore, someone consuming 2,000 calories per day would have a protein energy equivalent of 240 to 300 calories (60–76 grams) of protein per day. The requirement for protein is also expressed per unit of body weight. Looking at protein requirement this way, most people do well with 0.8 grams of protein per kilogram of body weight. Therefore, a 75 kilogram person (165 pounds) would have a protein requirement of 60 grams per day. It is generally considered that athletes have a slightly higher protein requirement because of a greater lean mass (which requires more protein to build and maintain), and because a small amount of protein is inevitably burned during physical activity. So, while the average person's protein requirement is 0.8 grams per kilogram of body weight, the athlete requirement is thought to be 1.5 to 2.0 grams per kilogram of body weight (approximately double that of healthy nonathletes).[3-5] Therefore, a 75 kilogram athlete might have a protein requirement of 120 grams per day. This 120 grams of daily protein may seem high, but still represents a relatively small proportion of total daily calories and is easily obtained by following the Food Guide Pyramid recommendations. For instance, 120 grams × 4 = 480 calories from protein. By comparison, the minimum recommended intake for carbohydrates is 30 calories per kilogram of body weight, so for this 75 kilogram person, the carbohydrate requirement represents 2,250 calories. See table 1.2 for an example of the protein content of a typical 2,000 calorie meal plan. There are a number of reasons for the increased protein requirement in athletes, including the following:

- Amino acids (from protein) contribute 5 to 15 percent of the fuel burned during exercise. The amount of protein used for energy rises as muscle glycogen decreases. It is generally thought that endurance exercise is more glycogen depleting than power exercise, so endurance activities are likely to cause a higher proportionate usage of protein.
- Exercise may cause muscle damage, which increases the protein requirement for tissue repair.
- Endurance exercise may cause a small amount of protein to be lost in the urine (where there is typically none or very little).

Table 1.2   Protein Content of a 2,000-Calorie Meal Plan

Food	Calories	Protein (gm)
Cracked wheat bread, toasted (2 slices)	132	4.37
Orange juice (1 cup)	112	1.74
Strawberry jam (1 tablespoon)	55	0.12
Hard-boiled egg (1 egg)	88	6.29
Roast beef sandwich (1 sandwich, plain)	346	21.5
1 cup low-fat (1%) milk	102	8.03
1 raw apple	87	0.26
Small tossed salad (3/4 cup)	27	1.3
Salad dressing (1 tbsp)	67	0.09
Chocolate chip cookies (5 small)	125	1.43
Gatorade (16 ounces)	100	0.00
Chicken breast (1/2 broiled)	152	26.67
Baked potato	145	3.06
Broccoli (1/2 stalk)	22	2.32
French bread (2 slices)	203	6.37
Vanilla ice cream (1/2 cup)	135	2.4
Totals	2000	93.98

Note: A 120-pound athlete would require approximately 1.5 grams of protein per kilogram of body weight. To convert pounds to kilograms, divide pounds by 2.2 (120 ÷ 2.2 = 55 kg). Then multiply kilograms by 1.5 (55 × 1.5 = 82.5). The protein requirement for this 120-pound athlete is 82.5 grams. The protein provided by this 2,000 calories is more than 10 grams greater than the requirement.

In spite of the increased protein requirement for athletes, most athletes consume much more protein (from food alone) than they require. A look at the protein content of some commonly consumed foods demonstrates this point (see appendix B).

While most athletes have no difficulty consuming sufficient protein, some groups of athletes should monitor protein intake carefully because it may be difficult for them to get enough. These groups include

- young athletes who have the combined demands of muscular work and growth;
- athletes who are restricting food intake in an attempt to achieve a desirable weight or body profile;
- vegetarian athletes who do not eat meat, fish, eggs, or dairy foods;
- athletes who restrict food intake for religious or cultural reasons.

As mentioned earlier, we can derive energy (calories) from proteins. However, burning protein as a fuel is a bit like sprinkling your family jewels on your breakfast cereal because you think it improves the texture. It's a complete waste of resources. Protein is so important for building and maintaining tissues and for making hormones and enzymes that burning it up as a fuel is wasteful. Besides, when you burn protein as a fuel, the nitrogen must be removed (a process called *deamination)* from the amino acid chains and excreted. When you increase the excretion of nitrogenous wastes, you also must increase the amount of water lost in the urine. Thus, two undesirable things occur: you waste valuable protein by burning it up, and you increase the risk of dehydration because of the volume of water that is lost when nitrogenous wastes are excreted. In addition, high-protein diets are shown to cause high losses of calcium in the urine (a clear problem for females who are at risk for later bone disease). In addition, high-protein diets tend also to be high-fat diets, which may increase the risk of cardiovascular disease. Therefore, the best way to make certain your protein needs are met is to consume a sufficient amount of food that focuses on carbohydrates but also contains small amounts of dairy and meat foods (or plenty of legumes if you're a vegetarian).

Protein and Total Energy Intake

To a large degree, the utilization of protein is a function of the adequacy of the amount of total energy a person consumes. A failure to consume sufficient amounts of energy (typical for most athletes) means that a good deal of the protein consumed will be burned as an energy source. We basically have an energy-first system, which means that there must be an adequate supply of energy (calories) before other parts of the system will work properly. Therefore, providing protein in an environment of inadequate total energy means that the protein will be burned as a fuel rather than used for other body-building and body-maintaining purposes (refer to table 1.1 for functions of protein).

A standard tenant in nutrition is that carbohydrates have a protein-sparing effect. What this really means is that if you can supply sufficient carbohydrates to the system for fuel, then protein will be spared from being burned and used for more important functions.

Let's think about what happens when an athlete overconsumes protein. Most studies indicate that the maximal rate of protein utilization for nonenergy uses is approximately 1.5 grams of protein per kilogram of body weight.[3-5] When you exceed this amount, your body has to make some decisions about what to do with the excess. You can store some of the excess as fat, or you can burn some of the excess as energy. In either case, nitrogen must be removed from the amino acids, and this nitrogenous waste must be removed from the body. Virtually all studies that have looked at the total energy consumption of athletes indicate that athletes consume less total energy than they should to support the combined needs of activity, growth, and maintenance. Since burning protein causes a lot of metabolic waste, it would be better to meet the energy requirement by providing a cleaner burning fuel—carbohydrates.

Fats

Despite some recent literature espousing (wrongly) the benefits of high-fat intakes (i.e., intakes of 30 percent or more of total calories from fat), fat is a highly concentrated fuel that tends to be overconsumed. In addition, there is little scientific information that suggests that more fat is better than less. For athletes in particular, consuming less fat (i.e., less than 30 percent of total calories) is generally associated with better performance, regardless of the sport. Consumption of less fat is not easy and, unless steps are taken to provide the energy from other substrates (mainly from more carbohydrates) that the eliminated fat represents, athletes may place themselves in an energy-deficit state that is, in itself, a detriment to performance. Therefore, while a reduction in fat intake is generally useful, a conscious effort should be made to provide enough total energy when a reduced-fat intake is consumed. Since fat is more than twice as concentrated in calories than either protein or carbohydrate (9 calories per gram versus 4 calories per gram), more than twice as much food needs to be consumed to make up the difference in reduced fat. This fits precisely with the general recommendations of the Food Guide Pyramid, which encourages a consumption of up to 20 servings of carbohydrate foods per day.

Fats include cholesterol, oils, butter, and margarine. All of these are fats but they have slightly different characteristics. In general, fats (or more specifically *lipids*) have one common attribute that makes them soluble in organic solvents but not soluble in water. Anyone who has tried to mix Italian dressing knows this to be true. The oil in the dressing eventually rises to the top, no matter how hard the bottle is shaken. The term fat is usually applied to lipids that are solid at room temperature, and the term oils is applied to lipids that are liquid at room temperature. An example of a lipid is cholesterol. The most commonly consumed form of lipid is triglyceride, which is made from three fatty acids and one glycerol molecule (thus the name *triglyceride*).

Despite these different forms of lipids, we consume them all from the food supply, and we are also capable of making nearly all of them by combining carbon units from other substances. Nearly every cell in the body has the capability of making cholesterol, which is why a person can have a high-cholesterol level even when they consume a low-cholesterol diet. We can also make phospholipids, triglycerides, and oils. In fact, it is this ability to effectively manufacture different types of lipids that limits our requirement to consume large amounts of lipids.

Essential Fats

This is not to suggest that we need no fats. A certain amount of fat, between 20 and 25 percent of total consumed calories, is necessary to assure a sufficient energy and nutrient intake. Fat-soluble vitamins (vitamins A, D, E, and K) must be delivered in a fat package. Also, we must consume essential fatty acids that are needed for specific body functions but that we are unable to manufacture. We need a certain amount of dietary fat to give us a feeling of satiety during the meal, which creates the important physiological signal that it is time to stop eating. Also, dietary fats stay in the stomach longer than carbohydrates, possibly giving us a feeling that we have satisfied our eating needs for a time after the meal. Not to mention the obvious fact that fat helps to make foods taste good (is there anyone out there who doesn't honestly like fried chicken or French fried potatoes?)

Fatty Acids

Linoleic (omega-6 fatty acid) and linolenic (omega-3 fatty acid) fatty acids are considered essential fatty acids because the body is incapable of manufacturing them. They are, however, easily obtained from vegetable oils (corn, safflower, canola, etc.) and the oils of cold-water fish. The omega-6 classification means that these fatty acids, which are polyunsaturated, have the last double bond 6 carbons from the end of the carbon chain.

Triglycerides

Most of the lipids we consume are in the form of triglycerides, which contain three fatty acids and a glycerol molecule. This also happens to be the main storage form of fat, so when you over-consume food, the body stores this excess energy in the form of triglycerides. When we burn fat as a source of energy, the stored triglycerides are taken out of storage and the molecule is cleaved into its component fatty acids and glycerol molecules. Each fatty acid can then be broken

Balancing Essential Nutrients   **21**

apart (two carbon units at a time) and thrown into the cellular furnaces that create heat and muscular work. This process is referred to as the beta oxidative metabolic pathway because burning fats, besides requiring some carbohydrate, also requires a lot of oxygen.

Glycerol is a unique fatty acid in that it is burned more like a carbohydrate than a fat. (We will discuss this in greater detail when we look at energy metabolism in chapters 5 and 6.) Glycerol is also an effective humectant (it holds water with it), and many endurance athletes (particularly marathoners and iron men and women) find that adding some glycerol to water helps them retain more water (i.e., to superhydrate) than if they consumed water alone. Refer to chapter 2 on hydration for more detailed information. If they drink glycerol-containing water before an event, they can store more water, so their water status is better at the end of a race when most athletes are suffering from some degree of underhydration.

Lipid Structure

You've probably heard that some fats are saturated, others are unsaturated, and still others are monounsaturated. These labels refer to the degree to which the carbon atoms, which make up the skeleton

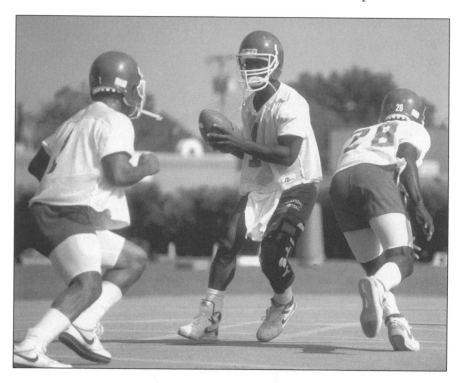

of the fatty acids, are held together by double or single chemical bonds. Single bonds are stronger and less chemically reactive than double bonds (just the opposite of what the terminology would lead you to believe), so the greater the number of double bonds, the greater the opportunity for the chemical environment to react with the fatty acid. It is this ability to react with the fatty acid that makes the difference when it is consumed.

Saturated fatty acids have no double bonds: that is, they are saturated with single bonds and the hydrogen atoms associated with them. Monounsaturated fatty acids (*mono* = one) have one double bond holding together two of its carbon atoms, and polyunsaturated fatty acids (*poly* = many) have two or more double bonds holding together four or more of its carbon atoms. In general, saturated fatty acids are commonly found in highest concentration in fats of animal origin, palm kernel oil, and coconut oil. Monounsaturated fats are highest in olive oil and canola oil, but are also present in fats of animal origin. Polyunsaturated fats are highest in vegetable oils (with the exception of olive oil, which is more than 75 percent monounsaturated.) In the context of a low-fat intake, monounsaturated fatty acids and polyunsaturated fatty acids should make up the majority of the fats consumed. To achieve this requires a reduction in the consumption of foods that are high in saturated fatty acids, including red meats, chocolate candies (which often contain saturated tropical oils), fried foods, and high-fat dairy products.

Medium-chain triglycerides, or triglycerides with fatty acid chains that range from 6 to 12 carbon atoms, are not the most abundant form of triglycerides in the diet (long-chain triglycerides are more common), but there is some early evidence that medium-chain triglycerides (MCTs) are beneficial for athletes. MCTs are easily and quickly oxidized for energy and appear to mimic the effects of carbohydrate metabolism rather than fat metabolism. There is also some evidence that they enhance the movement of fats from storage to be burned as energy, and they also increase the rate at which energy is burned (i.e., a higher energy metabolism).[7-10] While MCT oil does not exist in concentrated amounts in any food(s), MCT oil is available in many stores and, because it is saturated, is stable and has a long shelf life. For athletes who may find it difficult to consume sufficient total energy, consumption of two to three tablespoons of MCT oil may prove to be beneficial. Since MCT oil is burned differently than other fats, taking this small amount of MCT oil (two to three tablespoons) will not negatively impact on the recommendation for low-fat intakes, and may be a good way to assure that athletes who have difficulty taking in enough calories get in what they need.

Fish Oils

Fish liver oils that are high in omega-3 acids (called omega-3 because the last double bond is 3 carbons from the last carbon in the chain) have received much attention recently. They have been shown to reduce the ability of red blood cells to congregate, and therefore they reduce the chance for an unwanted blood clot to form. This reduces the risk of a heart attack, which is most commonly caused by a clot formation in one of the major heart arteries. The oils from cold-water fish that appear to have the biggest impact in reducing the heart disease death rate are called *eicosapentanoic acid* (EPA) and *docosohexanoic acid* (DHA). Even a once-weekly consumption of cold-water fish (salmon, albacore tuna, Atlantic herring, etc.) is sufficient to make a significant reduction in the risk of heart attack and stroke.[11] Despite these findings, excessive intake (more than 1 supplement daily or cold-water fish consumed daily) of these fish oils may cause problems, including an increase in oxidative damage of cells. The best rule of thumb is to make fish consumption a regular part of your weekly intake (meals with fish once to twice weekly), so that supplement intake of omega-3 fatty acids is unnecessary.

Some attention has been given to the potential benefits of omega-3 fatty acids in athletic performance. According to Bucci,[12] these potential benefits include:

- Improved delivery of oxygen and nutrients to muscles and other tissues because of reduced blood viscosity.
- Improved aerobic metabolism because of enhanced delivery of oxygen to cells.
- Improved release of somatotropin (growth hormone) in response to normal stimuli, such as exercise, sleep, and hunger, which may have an anabolic effect and/or improve post-exercise recovery time.
- Reduction of inflammation caused by muscular fatigue and over-exertion, which may improve post-exercise recovery time.
- Possible prevention of tissues from becoming inflamed.

In general, studies that have evaluated the effectiveness of omega-3 fatty acids tend to show improvements in both strength and endurance.[13-15] The major impact of omega-3 fatty acid consumption appears to be an enhancement of aerobic metabolic processes, which is an important factor in both athletic performance and in an individual's ability to effectively burn fat as an energy substrate. This should not suggest that an increase in *total* fat intake is desirable to obtain these benefits. On the contrary, higher fat intakes are typically associated with reduced athletic performance. However, athletes should consider altering the *types* of fats consumed by including periodic but regular 4 to 5 ounce servings (once or twice weekly) of salmon, albacore tuna, Atlantic herring, and other cold-water fish.

Determining Fat Needs

From an exercise standpoint, there is little reason to believe that increasing fat consumption results in improving athletic performance, unless the increase in fat intake is the only reasonable means for the athlete to obtain the energy needed to meet needs. For the athlete who needs more than 4,000 calories each day to meet the combined demands of growth, exercise, and maintenance, moderate increases in dietary fats may be needed. Since fat is a more concentrated form of energy than either carbohydrate or protein, more energy can be consumed in a smaller food package if the foods contain more fat. So much volume of food needs to be consumed if an athlete tries to restrict fat completely, that it may be impossible to schedule enough meals or enough time during meals to consume the needed energy, leading to an inadequate energy intake. Table 1.3 includes a simple guide to the amount of fat that is reasonable to consume.

Vitamins

Vitamins are substances needed by cells to encourage specific chemical reactions that take place in the cell. Some vitamins (particularly B-vitamins), are involved in energy reactions that enable cells to derive energy from carbohydrate, protein, and fat. Since athletes burn more energy than nonathletes, these vitamins are of particular interest here. Other vitamins are involved in maintaining mineral balance. For instance, vitamin D (which we can derive from both sunlight and food) encourages the cells in a specific part of the small intestine to allow more calcium and phosphorus to be absorbed from food into the blood.

Table 1.3   Desirable Distribution of Energy Substrates for Athletes With Different Energy Needs

Total energy requirement	Carbohydrate distribution	Protein distribution	Fat distribution	Explanation
1,600-2,200 cal	65%	15%	20%	This level of energy intake is typically seen in young athletes or small female athletes involved in anaerobic activities (gymnastics, skating, etc.). They have a relatively high demand for carbohydrates and a low demand for fats.
2,200-3,000 cal	60%	15%	25%	This level of energy intake is commonly seen in males and females involved in intermediate-intensity sports, with both an anaerobic and aerobic component (basketball, soccer, etc.). They still have a relatively high need for carbohydrate, but are better able to use fats for energy because of their aerobic training.
3,000-4,000 cal	55-60%	15%	25-30%	This level of energy intake is commonly seen in males and females involved in long-distance, predominantly aerobic sports (long-distance running, biking, iron man, triathlon, etc.). They have a high need for carbohydrate but are better able to meet their high energy demands with a slight increase in fat intake. Their aerobic training improves their ability to use fats for energy.
4,000+ cal	55%	15%	30%	This level of energy intake is commonly seen in male football players (especially linemen) and some power lifters. It is extremely difficult for them to consume sufficient energy without some fat in their diet. Because of the predominantly anaerobic nature of their activities, however, fat intake should still not represent more than 30% of the total energy consumed. Additional energy from fat could be provided in the form of MCT oil.

Alcohol

Alcohol provides approximately 7 calories per gram, but to consider alcohol an energy substrate of equal importance to proteins, carbohydrates, and fats is dangerous thinking. Most importantly, regular alcohol consumption alters the normal metabolic processing of vitamins, minerals, proteins, carbohydrates, and fats to a degree that it must be considered a toxic substance. A common serving of 12 ounces of beer, a 4-ounce glass of wine, or one ounce of liquor yields approximately half an ounce of alcohol, and this is equivalent to approximately 14 grams (1 gram = .035 ounce). At 7 calories per gram, this one drink has the potential of providing approximately 98 calories but may reduce the ability to effectively use the energy from this and other foods.

While there is recent evidence of a reduction in cardiovascular disease risk with a low to moderate (1–2 drinks per day) consumption of alcohol, there is no evidence that alcohol consumption is useful in enhancing athletic performance. On the contrary, the negative metabolic effects of alcohol consumption are long lasting and may impair reaction time, endurance, coordination, and strength.[16] Serious athletes should try to avoid regular consumption of alcoholic beverages, particularly during seasonal periods of training and competition.

Water-Soluble Vitamins

Vitamins are typically organized into fat-soluble and water-soluble categories. The fat-soluble vitamins literally require a fat-based environment in which to function, and the water-soluble vitamins require a water-based environment. To one degree or another, we have the capacity to store all vitamins. That is to say, if we ate a meal two days ago that had a large amount of vitamin C, and had no vitamin C in the foods we consumed yesterday, we wouldn't expect to suffer from symptoms of vitamin C deficiency today. The reason for this is that cells that require vitamin C have a capacity to store slightly more than they need. However, in the case of water-soluble vitamins such as vitamin C, there are no clear storage depots where large amounts of the vitamin can be stored. Fat-soluble vitamins, however, do have a large storage capacity.

It is this difference in storage capacity that is responsible for the commonly repeated recommendation that water-soluble vitamins should be consumed every day because they are not stored. Interestingly, it is also this difference in storage capacity that has led to the myth that any excess in water-soluble vitamin intake is without problems, since we just excrete the excess in the urine. While it is true that excess intake of fat-soluble vitamins, especially vitamins D and A, can produce severe toxicity, it is not true that taking excess water-soluble vitamins creates no difficulties. A prime example of this is the neurological problem (peripheral neuropathy—loss of feeling in the fingers) created with excess intake of vitamin B-6 (500 milligrams per day over time is enough to create permanent damage). Another problem is that humans are adaptable to intake. Therefore, *the more you have, the more you may need* to get the same biological effect. A discussion of individual water-soluble vitamins follows. The table on pages 38 and 39 summarizes the functions, sources, and possible problems associated with each vitamin.[16a]

Vitamin B-1 (Thiamin)

Vitamin B-1 is commonly referred to as thiamin and is present in a variety of food sources, including whole grains, nuts, legumes (beans and dried peas), and pork. It works in unison with other B vitamins in energy metabolic processes that involve converting the energy in the foods we consume to muscular energy. Thiamin does this through its involvement in the removal of carbon dioxide in energy reactions with its active coenzyme called *thiamin pyrophosphate* (TPP); it is particularly important in deriving energy from carbohydrate foods.

A deficiency of thiamin for athletes has not been reported in the literature, but in populations consuming a low-quality diet of unenriched polished rice or other processed and unenriched grains, thiamin deficiency occurs. A thiamin-deficiency disease called beriberi involves nervous system malfunction (especially in the hands and legs, as well as in balance) and heart failure. One form of beriberi also causes water retention (edema). As would be expected for a vitamin involved in energy reactions, early deficiency is characterized by muscular fatigue, and this progresses to muscular weakness as the deficiency becomes more severe. Other common symptoms of deficiency include loss of appetite, nausea, constipation, irritability, depression, loss of coordination, and confusion. A deficiency of thiamin is not likely to occur in U.S. athletes. However, since alcohol inhibits normal thiamin metabolism, it is possible that thiamin-deficiency symptoms may occur in those who frequently consume alcoholic beverages.

Maximizing Vitamin Intake

To maximize vitamin intake from your diet, try the following:

- Eat a wide variety of colorful fruits and vegetables.
- When possible eat *fresh* fruits and vegetables, especially those in season.
- Don't overcook vegetables—long cooking times reduce nutrient content
- Steam or microwave your vegetables rather than boiling them—nutrients seep out in boiling water only to be poured down the drain.

It is conceivable that some athletes may require more than the RDA for thiamin, since the requirement is based on 0.5 milligrams/1,000 calories consumed. Athletes often consume more than 3,000 calories (often 5,000–6,000 calories), making the actual thiamin requirement greater than 1.5 milligrams/day for these athletes. However, even in an athlete consuming 6,000 calories per day, the thiamin requirement would not exceed 3 milligrams/day. Therefore, it appears reasonable to suggest an intake of two times the RDA (3 milligrams/day) for athletes consuming high levels of energy. Since athletes commonly consume high-carbohydrate foods that are high in thiamin, high energy intakes are typically also high thiamin intakes, making it likely that many athletes already consume 3 milligrams/day.

Vitamin B-2 (Riboflavin)

Riboflavin is involved in energy production and normal cellular function through its coenzymes *flavin adenine dinucleotide* (FAD) and *flavin mononucleotide* (FMN). These coenzymes are mainly involved in obtaining energy from consumed carbohydrates, proteins, and fats. Food sources of riboflavin include dairy products (e.g., milk, yogurt, cottage cheese), dark leafy green vegetables (e.g., spinach, chard, mustard greens, broccoli, green peppers), whole-grain foods, and enriched grain foods.

There are no studies suggesting that athletes commonly suffer from riboflavin-deficiency symptoms. Also, no apparent toxicity symptoms occur from taking more than the RDA. Several studies that suggest that athletes and those involved in regular activity may have higher requirements than the RDA, which is based on 0.6 milligrams per 1,000 calories. In a series of studies performed on exercising women and women seeking to lose weight, the riboflavin requirement appeared to range between 0.63 and 1.40 milligrams per 1,000 calories. [17-19]

It is never easy to make a determination about what level of intake is right for athletes because there are so many considerations. In the case of riboflavin, understanding the requirement is made more complex because riboflavin is easily destroyed by ultraviolet light (the reason behind all those new opaque milk bottles in the grocery store). Therefore, the amount of riboflavin in fresh dairy products is not the same as older products that have had multiple light exposures. This makes it difficult to understand the actual amount of riboflavin that is commonly delivered by food. Nevertheless, there is some beginning evidence that physical activity increases the requirement to a level slightly higher than 0.5 milligrams per 1,000 calories, but not more than 1.5 milligrams per 1,000 calories.[11-13,20] However, even with this apparently higher requirement for athletes, there are no studies that clearly demonstrate an improvement in athletic performance with intakes greater than the RDA.

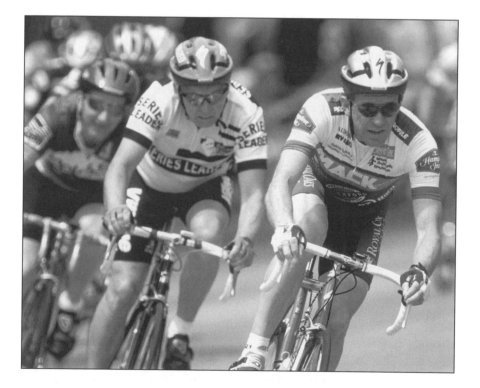

Niacin (Niacinamide, Nicotinic Acid, Nicotinamide, or Vitamin B-3)

Niacin is involved in energy production from carbohydrate, protein, and fat, glycogen synthesis, and normal cellular metabolism through its active coenzymes. These enzymes, *nicotinamide adenine dinucleotide* (NAD) and *nicotinamide adenine dinucleotide phosphate* (NADP), are essential for normal muscle function. While niacin deficiency is well documented in human populations suffering from famine or monotonous intakes of unenriched grain products, there is no evidence of niacin deficiency in athletes.

Niacin is found in meat, whole or enriched grains, seeds, nuts, and legumes. It can be produced by the body from the amino acid tryptophan (60 milligrams of tryptophan yields 1 milligram niacin), which is found in all high-quality protein foods (e.g., meat, fish, poultry). Given the broad spectrum of foods that provide niacin, it is relatively easy for people to consume the RDA requirement of 6.6 niacin equivalents (NE) per 1,000 calories (between 13 and 19 milligrams/day for the average adult) niacin equivalents are equal to 1 milligram of niacin or 60 milligrams of dietary tryptophan; you can obtain niacin directly or indirectly by consuming the amino acid tryptophan. NE takes both sources into account. When a deficiency does occur, it results in muscular weakness, loss of appetite, indigestion, and skin rash. If a deficiency becomes more severe, it results in the disease pellagra, which is characterized by a sore tongue, diarrhea, loss of mental acuity, and dermatitis. It is possible to produce toxicity symptoms from excessive intake of niacin. These symptoms include becoming red faced, flushed, and feeling hot. It may also result in a tingling feeling around the neck, face, and fingers. These symptoms appear to be common in patients taking large doses of niacin to lower blood lipids.

In studies evaluating the performance effects of niacin supplementation, it was found that endurance was reduced because excess niacin caused a reduction in fat metabolism.[21-23] Therefore, there was a greater reliance on carbohydrate fuels (glucose and glycogen) to support activity. Since the storage of carbohydrate fuels is limited, athletes taking niacin supplements became fatigued earlier. To date, there is no evidence that the requirement for niacin is increased in physical activity.

Vitamin B-6

Vitamin B-6 refers to several compounds (pyridoxine, pyridoxal, pyridoxamine, pyridoxine 5-phosphate, pyridoxal 5-phosphate, and pyridoxamine 5-phosphatepyridoxine) that display the same metabolic activity. Vitamin B-6 is found in highest quantity in meats (especially liver) and is also available in wheat germ, fish, poultry, legumes, bananas, brown rice, whole-grain cereals, and vegetables. Because the function of this vitamin is closely linked to protein and amino acid metabolism, the requirements are also linked to protein intake (the higher the protein intake, the higher the vitamin B-6 requirement). The adult requirement is based on 0.016 milligrams of B-6 per gram of protein consumed each day,[24] and is adequate for those consuming typical protein intakes. When you consider that high-protein foods are also typically high in vitamin B-6, those consuming protein from food (regardless of the amount) are most likely to have adequate B-6 levels as well. However, since many athletes consume additional protein in purified, supplemental forms (protein powders, amino acid powders, etc.), it is conceivable that some athletes with high supplemental protein intakes will have an inadequate B-6 intake.

Vitamin B-6 functions in reactions related to protein synthesis by aiding in the creation of amino acids and proteins, and is also involved in protein catabolism through involvement in reactions that break down amino acids and proteins. It is involved, therefore, in manufacturing muscle, hemoglobin, and other proteins critical to athletic performance. The major enzyme of vitamin B-6, pyridoxal phosphate (PP), is also involved in the breakdown of muscle glycogen for energy through the enzyme glycogen phosphorylase.

A deficiency of vitamin B-6 will lead to symptoms of peripheral neuritis (loss of nerve function in the hands, feet, arms, and legs), ataxia (loss of balance), irritability, depression, and convulsions. An excess intake of vitamin B-6 does lead to toxic symptoms that have been documented in humans. These symptoms are similar to those seen in B-6 deficiency and include ataxia and severe sensory neuropathy (loss of sensation in the fingers). Toxicity symptoms have been documented in women taking doses (that, on average, equal 119 milligrams/day) to treat premenstrual syndrome and several types of mental disorders.[25,26]

There is a theoretical basis for investigating vitamin B-6 and athletic performance. B-6 is involved in the breakdown of amino acids in muscle as a means of obtaining needed energy and in converting lactic acid to glucose in the liver.[27] Vitamin B-6 is also involved in the breakdown of muscle glycogen to derive energy. Other functions of vitamin B-6 that may be related to athletic performance include the formation of serotonin and the synthesis of carnitine from lysine. There is evidence that some athletes may be at risk for inadequate vitamin B-6 status.[28-30] Poor B-6 status also reduces athletic performance.[31]

Because many athletes are always looking for that extra edge, there is an understandable attractiveness to natural substances that are legal. Vitamin B-6 is sometimes marketed as one of those natural (and legal) substances because, besides its importance in energy metabolism, it is linked with the production of growth hormone, which can help to increase muscle mass.[32] It appears as if the combined effect of exercise and vitamin B-6 on growth hormone production is greater than either of these factors individually.[33,34]

Given the importance of this vitamin to athletic performance, it is easy to see why athletes may rush to obtain more. However, these factors should be considered:[35]

- Most athletes have adequate vitamin B-6 intakes and adequate vitamin B-6 status.
- Those athletes with poor vitamin B-6 status are generally those with inadequate energy intakes.
- A greater proportion of female athletes and athletes participating in sports that emphasize low weights (gymnastics, wrestling, skating, etc.) are likely to have inadequate energy intakes and, therefore, inadequate vitamin B-6 intakes.
- High doses of vitamin B-6 have been shown to have toxic effects.
- There is no good evidence that having more than the recommended intake has a beneficial effect on athletic performance.[36]
- Vitamin B-6 supplementation does not appear necessary to enhance athletic performance if a balanced diet, with adequate energy, is consumed.[37]

Taken together, these factors should encourage athletes to consume an adequate intake of energy *before* they consider taking supplements of vitamin B-6.

Vitamin B-12 (Cobalamin)

Vitamin B-12 is perhaps the most chemically complex of all the vitamins. It contains the mineral cobalt (thus the name "cobalamin") and has a major involvement in red blood cell formation, folic acid metabolism, DNA synthesis, and nerve development, but it is essential for the function of all cells.

Dietary sources of this vitamin are mainly foods of animal origin (meats, eggs, dairy products), and it is essentially absent from plant foods. There may also be some very small amount of absorbable vitamin B-12 that is produced by gut bacteria.[38] It should be clear from this that vegetarian athletes who avoid *all* foods of animal origin (i.e., they do not eat meat, nor do they consume eggs or dairy products) would be at risk for vitamin B-12 deficiency.

The disease associated with vitamin B-12 deficiency is pernicious anemia. This form of anemia most commonly occurs in the elderly who have experienced a reduction in normal stomach function. The stomach produces a substance called *intrinsic factor* that is required for vitamin B-12 to get absorbed. Without intrinsic factor, a person can have a diet high in B-12 but still develop a deficiency because none of it is absorbed. Symptoms of deficiency include fatigue, poor muscular coordination (possibly leading to paralysis), and dementia.

There is a long history of vitamin B-12 abuse by athletes. It was (and continues to be) common for many athletes to be injected with large amounts of vitamin B-12 (often 1,000 milligrams) before competitions.[39,40] However, the athletic performance benefits of vitamin B-12 injections and supplementation have not been established.[41-43]

It certainly makes sense that athletes consume foods that will avoid deficiencies of any kind, including the avoidance of B-12 deficiency. The resulting anemia would clearly impact on performance by producing a reduction in endurance and, potentially, a lowering of muscular coordination. However, consumption or injections of such large doses as have been reported in the literature for vitamin B-12 is without logic and without proven beneficial outcomes. Unless someone has a genetic predisposition to B-12 malabsorption (typically because of an inadequate production of intrinsic factor), there is no basis for taking supplements if a balanced mixed-food diet is consumed. Pure vegetarian athletes, on the other hand, have a good reason to be concerned about vitamin B-12 status. A supplement that provides, on average, the daily RDA (2 micrograms) for this group makes good sense, as does the consumption of foods that are fortified with vitamin B-12 (such as some soy milk products).

Folic Acid (Folate)

Folic acid is widespread in the food supply, but is present in the highest concentrations in liver, yeast, leafy vegetables, fruits, and legumes. It is easily destroyed through common household food preparation techniques and long storage times, so it is most commonly associated with fresh foods. Folate functions in amino acid metabolism and nucleic acid synthesis (RNA and DNA), so a deficiency leads to alterations in protein synthesis.[44] Tissues that have a rapid turnover are particularly sensitive to folic acid. This includes red and white blood cells, as well as tissues of the gastrointestinal tract and the uterus. More recently, adequate folate intake during pregnancy has been associated with the elimination of fetal neural tube defects (most notably spina bifida).[45,46] The average U.S. folate intake exceeds the requirement (of between 180 and 200 micrograms/day) by between 25 and 50 percent, but its importance in red cell formation and in eliminating neural tube defects has led to the common (and appropriate) supplementation with folic acid during pregnancy. The recommended intake of folate during pregnancy (400 micrograms) is double that of the adult requirement.

A deficiency of folic acid leads to anemia (it functions with vitamin B-12 in forming healthy new red blood cells); gastrointestinal problems (diarrhea, malabsorption, pain); and a swollen, red tongue. Toxicity of folate from excess intake has not been reported in the literature.

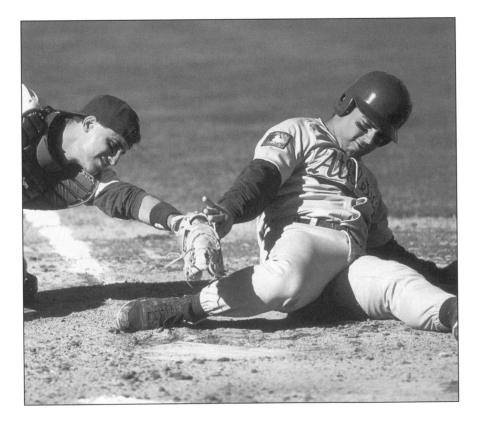

There are no studies that have reported on the relationship between folic acid and athletic performance. However, given that athletes may have a higher than normal tissue turnover because of the pounding the body takes in various sports, and the evidence that red blood cell turnover is faster in athletes than nonathletes,[47,48] there is good reason for athletes to be certain that their folic acid status is adequate. The best way to do this is through the regular consumption of fresh fruits and vegetables. If this is not possible, a daily supplement at the level of the recommended intake (200 milligrams/day) is an effective means of maintaining folate status.

Biotin (Vitamin H)

Biotin works with magnesium and *adenosine triphosphate* (ATP) to play a role in carbon dioxide metabolism, new glucose production (gluconeogenesis), carbohydrate metabolism, and fatty acid synthesis.[49] Food sources of biotin include egg yolk, soy flour, liver, sardines, walnuts, pecans, peanuts, and yeast. Fruits and meats are, however, poor dietary sources of the vitamin. Biotin is also synthesized by bacteria in the intestines. A deficiency of this vitamin is rare but can be induced through the intake of large amounts of raw egg whites, which contain the protein avidin. This protein binds to biotin and makes it unavailable for absorption. When a deficiency occurs, symptoms include loss of appetite, vomiting, depression, and dermatitis. However, since there aren't many people who consume large quantities of raw egg white, deficiencies of this vitamin are rare.

There is no evidence that athletes are at risk for biotin deficiency, and no information on the relationship between biotin and athletic performance. Therefore, no recommendation on biotin intake for athletes can be made.

Pantothenic Acid (Vitamin B-5)

Pantothenic acid is a structural part of *coenzyme A* (CoA), a compound of central importance in energy metabolic processes. Pantothenic acid is involved, through CoA, in carbohydrate, protein, and fat metabolism. Since pantothenic acid is widely distributed in the food supply, it is unlikely that an athlete would suffer from a deficiency, particularly if sufficient total energy is consumed. The highest concentrations of pantothenic acid are found in meat, whole-grain foods, beans, and peas. If a rare deficiency does occur, symptoms include easy fatigue, weakness, and insomnia. Supplemental doses of the vitamin are typically 10 milligrams/day (150–200 percent of the RDA) and, at this level, have not been shown to produce toxic effects.

Studies on animals suggest that pantothenic acid supplementation is effective in improving time to exhaustion.[50,51] Human studies do not agree on the potential benefits of pantothenic acid supplementation. In one study using a double-blind protocol, there was no difference in time to exhaustion in conditioned runners given either a pantothenic acid supplement or a placebo.[52] However, in another study that used a double-blind protocol, there was a difference in lactate (a 16.7 percent reduction) and oxygen consumption (an 8.4 percent increase) in subjects given pantothenate (2,000 milligrams) versus those given a placebo prior to riding a cycle ergometer to exhaustion.[53]

While there is a possible relationship between pantothenic acid supplementation and exercise performance, more information is needed before a sound recommendation can be made on pantothenate intake for athletes. In studies that have experimented with pantothenic acid supplements to determine a requirement level, the typical dosage has been 10 milligrams/day. When this level is provided, 5 to 7 milligrams/day is excreted in the urine.[54] Therefore, it appears that taking supplements at or above this level is excessive.

Vitamin C (Ascorbic acid, Ascorbate, Dehydroascorbate, L-Ascorbate)

Vitamin C functions as an antioxidant and is also involved in reactions that help to form the connective tissue protein collagen. Fresh fruits and vegetables are the best sources of vitamin C. Cereal grains contain no vitamin C (unless fortified with vitamin C), and meats and dairy products are low in vitamin C. Vitamin C is easily destroyed by cooking (heat) and exposure to air (oxygen). It is also highly water-soluble, which means it is easily removed from foods by water. The vitamin C deficiency disease, scurvy, is caused by a long-term dietary deficiency of the vitamin. For a variety of reasons (fresh food availability, supplement intake, use of vitamin C as an antioxidant in packaged foods), scurvy is almost nonexistent now. Toxicity from high, regular supplemental intakes of the vitamin is rare, but may include a predisposition to developing kidney stones and a reduced tissue sensitivity to the vitamin. Doses of 100 to 200 milligrams/day will saturate the body with vitamin C,[55] yet many people take supplemental doses of 1,000 to 2,000 milligrams/day. This level of supplemental vitamin C intake represents doses that are 16 to 33 times higher than the RDA of 60 milligrams/day.

There are a number of studies that have evaluated the relationship between vitamin C intake and athletic performance, and the results from these studies are inconsistent. Part of the problem with many of the studies performed on vitamin C is a lack of standardization between subjects and a general lack of comparative controls. Given these research design flaws, it's easy to understand why the study results are so inconsistent. Nevertheless, according to a review of studies that used controls and provided vitamin C supplements at or below 500 milligrams/day (remember that the RDA is 60 milligrams), there was no measurable benefit on athletic performance.[56] One study noted that when a 500-milligram dose of vitamin C was provided shortly (4 hours) before testing, there was a significant improvement in strength and a significant reduction in maximal oxygen consumption ($\dot{V}O_2$max)—which is a good thing—but there was no impact on muscular endurance.[57] ($\dot{V}O_2$max is the maximum volume of oxygen that the lungs can bring into the system. Working at a lower level of $\dot{V}O_2$max means the person is not working as hard as maximal aerobic capacity.) However, when participants were provided with the same amount for seven days, there was an improvement in strength but a decrease in endurance. When these same subjects were provided with 2,000 milligrams each day for seven days, there was only a lowering of $\dot{V}O_2$max, but no change in endurance performance.

There may be a benefit in consuming a slightly higher level of vitamin C for athletes involved in concussive sports where muscle soreness occurs or there is an injury. Studies on animals generally indicate that having more vitamin C improves the healing process and that inadequate vitamin C inhibits healing.[58] Also, a few recent studies indicate that muscle soreness may be more rapidly relieved when consuming moderate supplemental doses of vitamin C and other antioxidants.[59]

Given these inconsistent results, it is difficult to make a rational recommendation on vitamin C and performance. However, slightly increasing vitamin C intake may reduce muscle soreness faster and may also improve healing. The question is: How much is just right? Unfortunately, it's impossible to know the answer for everyone. Since studies demonstrate that high doses may cause endurance problems, it is important to keep the level of intake below one that may cause performance deficits. In 1993, Victor Herbert reported on three deaths that were due to iron overload. Vitamin C is known to enhance iron absorption, and the people who died were taking large daily doses of vitamin C.[60] Also consider that many athletes already consume more than 250 milligrams of vitamin C each day from food alone because of the high intake of fresh fruits and vegetables. A reasonable recommendation is to consume an abundant amount of fresh fruits and vegetables (wonderful sources of carbohydrates and many other nutrients besides vitamin C). If that's not possible, a reasonable strategy is to try taking a moderate daily supplement containing the RDA level (60 milligrams). Even someone consuming a low but regular intake of fruits and vegetables is likely to obtain sufficient vitamin C, but this kind of low-level supplement may act as an appropriate safety buffer.

Water-Soluble Vitamins

Vitamin	Functions	Sources	Possible problems
Vitamin B-1 (Thiamin)	Energy metabolism, nerve system function, appetite.	Pork and pork products, enriched grains, whole grains, legumes (dried beans/peas), and nuts.	Inadequate levels may lead to a disease called beriberi, with enlarged heart, arrhythmias, confusion, weakness, and depression.
Vitamin B-2 (Riboflavin)	Energy metabolism, vision (especially in bright light), health of skin.	Dairy products, meats, green leafy vegetables, and enriched and whole-grain products.	Inadequate levels may lead to bright light sensitivity, skin rash (especially around the corners of the mouth), and sore tongue.
Niacin (Vitamin B-3)	Energy metabolism, nerve system function, digestive system function, and health of skin.	Dairy products, meats, enriched and whole-grain products, meat, poultry, and fish.	Inadequate levels may lead to diarrhea, mental confusion, weakness, and dermatitis (dry flaky skin). Excessive levels may lead to flushed skin, rash, and hepatitis.
Vitamin B-6 (Pyridoxine, pyridoxal, pyridoxamine)	Protein manufacture, fat metabolism, and manufacture of niacin from tryptophan.	Meats, fish, poultry, green leafy vegetables, and whole-grain products.	Inadequate level may lead to poor tissue repair, irritability, convulsions, and dermatitis. Excessive levels may lead to neurological disorders, fatigue, and depression.

Vitamin	Functions	Sources	Possible problems
Vitamin B-12 (Cobalamin)	New tissue manufacture, especially involved in making red blood cells. Also involved in nerve cell maintenance.	Meat, fish, poultry, eggs, and dairy products. Small amounts also found in soy products.	Inadequate level may lead to red cell anemia, sore tongue, fatigue, and confusion.
Folic acid (Folate)	New tissue manufacture, especially involved in making red blood cells. Needed for proper nerve cell formation of fetuses (in utero). Also needed to maintain a healthy gastrointestinal tract.	Green leafy vegetables, legumes (dried beans/peas), seeds.	Inadequate level may lead to red cell anemia, gut stress (diarrhea, constipation, etc.), fatigue, depression, and confusion.
Biotin (Vitamin H)	Energy metabolism and glycogen synthesis.	Available in most foods.	Inadequate level may lead to irregular heart beat, dermatitis, fatigue, nausea, and depression.
Pantothenic acid (Vitamin B-5)	Energy metabolism (through substance of central importance called "coenzyme A".	Available in most foods.	Inadequate level may lead to fatigue and GI distress.
Vitamin C (Ascorbic acid)	Formation of connective tissue protein called "collagen", improved resistance to infection, improved absorption of vegetable-based iron, and powerful antioxidant.	Fresh fruits and vegetables (particularly citrus fruits, strawberries, and green peppers).	Inadequate level may lead to anemia, frequent illness, muscle pain, bleeding gums, and poor wound healing. Excessive intake may lead to nausea, headache, and skin rashes, and dependence on high doses.

Fat-Soluble Vitamins

Fat-soluble vitamins are delivered in a fat solute and represent one of the important reasons why athletes should not attempt placing themselves on a diet that is excessively low in fat. (Going below 10 percent of total calories from fat is dangerous, while athletes do very well when fat intake is between 20 and 25 percent of total calories.) There are only 4 fat-soluble vitamins—vitamins A, D, E, and K—and these vitamins can be effectively stored for later use. The table on page 44 summarizes the functions, sources, and possible problems associated with each vitamin.[16a] Therefore, unlike water-soluble vitamins that should be consumed daily or almost daily, the intake of fat-soluble vitamins does not have to be as frequent. However, the storage capacity for these vitamins does have limitations, and providing a level of these vitamins that exceeds our ability to store them may quickly lead to symptoms of toxicity and, in extreme cases, death. In fact, the two most potentially toxic substances in human nutrition are vitamins A and D. Achieving toxic-level doses of these vitamins is difficult if consuming the usual foods, but toxic doses may be easily achieved if supplemental intakes exceed recommended doses. In general, the storage capabilities we have for these vitamins eliminates the need for supplemental intake in most circumstances.

Vitamin A (Retinol or Beta-carotene)

The active form of this vitamin is called retinol. We obtain the active form from foods of animal origin, including liver, egg yolks, dairy products that have been fortified with vitamin A (e.g., vitamin A and D milk), margarine, and fish oil. The recommended level of intake ranges between 800 retinol equivalents (RE) for women and 1,000 RE for men. (One RE equals one microgram of retinol or six micrograms of beta-carotene.) Expressed as international units (IU), the recommended level of intake for women is 2,667 IU and for men is 3,333 IU. Vitamin A has a well-established relationship to normal vision; helps keep bones, skin, and red blood cells healthy; and is also needed for the immune system to function normally.

There is no evidence that taking extra vitamin A aids athletic performance. In a study performed in the 1940s, supplementation of vitamin A produced no improvement in endurance.[61] In the same study, subjects provided with a diet deficient in vitamin A noted no decrease in performance, probably because a deficit state of the vitamin was not reached.

Since the vitamin has clearly toxic side effects when taken in excess (i.e., at levels consistently higher than the RDA), athletes should be cautioned against taking supplemental doses of this vitamin. Toxicity of vitamin A manifests itself in several ways, including dry skin, headache, irritability, vomiting, bone pain, and vision problems. Excess vitamin A intake during pregnancy is also associated with an increase in birth defects.

A precursor to vitamin A is beta-carotene. A *precursor* is a substance that, under the proper conditions, is converted to the active form of the vitamin. Therefore, consuming foods with beta-carotene is an indirect way of obtaining vitamin A. Beta-carotene is found in all red, orange, yellow, and dark green colored fruits and vegetables (carrots, sweet potatoes, spinach, apricots, cantaloupes, tomatoes, etc.). It is a powerful antioxidant, protecting cells from oxidative damage that could lead to cancer and, of course, can be converted to vitamin A as we need it.

Unlike preformed vitamin A (retinol), beta-carotene does not exhibit the same clear toxic effects if excess doses are consumed. However, a consistently high intake of carrots, sweet potatoes, and other foods high in beta-carotene may cause a person to develop a yellowish skin tone. Although no other effects of this excess beta-carotene storage have been found, this effect may make you wonder if someone will eventually find that excess consumption is, in fact, dangerous because it breaches the all-important balance rule in nutrition.

It is conceivable that beta-carotene may, as an antioxidant, prove to be effective in reducing postexercise muscle soreness and improve postexercise recovery. However, this is a theoretical connection only, since there is no study making a direct link between beta-carotene intake and reduced soreness and improved recovery. Despite this, the U.S. Olympic Committee has recognized beta-carotene's potential as an antioxidant.[61a]

Vitamin D (Cholecalciferol)

Vitamin D is the most potentially toxic vitamin in human nutrition. We can obtain the vitamin in an inactive form from food and sunlight exposure. Ultraviolet radiation (sunlight) exposure of the skin alters a cholesterol derivative (7-dehydrocholesterol) to an inactive form of vitamin D called cholecalciferol. To be functional, this inactive form of vitamin D must be activated by the kidneys. Therefore, kidney disease may be the cause of vitamin D–related disorders. Dietary sources of vitamin D include eggs, vitamin D fortified milk, liver, butter, and margarine. Cod liver oil, which was once given commonly as a supplement, is a concentrated source of the vitamin. The adult RDA for vitamin D is 5 micrograms/day of cholecalciferol, or 200 international units (IU) of vitamin D.

Vitamin D functions to promote growth and mineralize bone and teeth by increasing the absorption of calcium and phosphorus. A diet with an adequate intake of calcium and phosphorus, but without adequate vitamin D, will thus lead to calcium and phosphorus deficiency. The childhood deficiency disease rickets and the adult deficiency disease osteomalacia are diseases of calcium deficiency that are due to either inadequate levels of vitamin D or the inability to convert vitamin D to the active (functional) form. However, because vitamin D is so potentially toxic, caution must be taken not to consume too much. Excess vitamin D intake may lead to vomiting, diarrhea, weight loss, kidney damage, high blood calcium levels, and death.

There are no studies indicating that vitamin D supplementation aids athletic performance, and there is no theoretical basis for performance enhancement to occur. As vitamin D is potentially the most dangerous (possibly deadly) in excess, don't mess with supplements. However, vitamin D may play an indirect role in injury resistance. Athletes in some sports may have dramatically lower sunlight exposure because all training takes place inside. This lower sunlight (i.e., UV) exposure may reduce vitamin D availability to a point where both growth and bone density are affected. Lower bone densities are known to place athletes at higher risk for developing stress fractures, [62-64] an injury that can end an athletic career. In a recent survey of U.S. national team gymnasts, it was found that the factor most closely related to bone density was sunlight exposure. Those with higher densities had the greatest exposure.[65] Also, sunlight exposure was more important as a predictor of bone density in this group than vitamin D or calcium intake from food.

Vitamin E (Tocopherol)

Vitamin E is a generic term for several substances (tocopherols) that have similar activity, and the unit of measure is based on the level of tocopherol with an activity equivalent to that of alpha-tocopherol. For instance, beta-tocopherol has a lower level of activity than alpha-tocopherol, so more of it would be necessary to get the same effect. The adult RDA for vitamin E is 8 to 10 milligrams. Vitamin E is found in green leafy vegetables, vegetable oils, seeds, nuts, liver, and corn. It is difficult to induce a vitamin E deficiency in humans, and it also appears to be a relatively nontoxic vitamin.

Vitamin E is a potent antioxidant that serves to protect membranes from destruction by peroxides. Peroxides are formed when fats (especially polyunsaturated fats) become oxidized (rancid). These peroxides are called free radicals because they bounce around unpredictably inside cells, altering or destroying them. Since vitamin E is an antioxidant, it helps to capture oxygen, thereby limiting the oxidation of fats to protect cells.

Several studies on vitamin E and physical performance have been conducted, but none has found an improvement in either strength or endurance with vitamin E supplementation.[66-69] Several studies evaluating whether vitamin E supplementation reduced exercise-induced peroxide damage had mixed findings. Some suggest that a clear reduction in peroxidative damage occurs,[70,71] but others suggest that vitamin E has no benefit.[72] It seems clear that more information on vitamin E is needed before a definitive exercise-related benefit can be claimed. However, the theoretical basis related to a reduction in peroxidative damage through a slight increase in additional vitamin E consumption is sound.

Vitamin K (Phylloquinone)

Vitamin K is found in green leafy vegetables and also, in small amounts, in cereals, fruits, and meats. Bacteria in the intestines also produce vitamin K, so the absolute dietary requirement is not known. This vitamin is needed for the formation of prothrombin, which is required for blood to clot. It is possible for people who regularly take antibiotics that destroy the bacteria in the intestines to be at increased risk for vitamin K deficiency. A deficiency would cause an increase in bleeding and hemorrhages. Vitamin K appears to be relatively nontoxic, but high intakes of synthetic forms may cause jaundice. The adult RDA for vitamin K is 65 to 70 micrograms.

There are no studies on the relationship between vitamin K and athletic performance. Further, it is difficult to think of a theoretical framework where such a relationship might exist. It seems clear that, especially for athletes involved in contact sports, adequate vitamin K status is necessary to avoid excessive bruising and bleeding. However, there is no documented evidence that athletes are at risk for a deficiency.

Fat-Soluble Vitamins

Vitamin	Functions	Sources	Possible problems
Vitamin A (Retinol; beta-carotene can be made into vitamin A)	Eyesight, health of skin and soft-tissue membranes, bone development, reproduction, immune system, Beta-carotene is a powerful anti-oxidant.	Vitamin A and D milk, fortified cheese, cream and butter, eggs. Beta-carotene is found in dark green leafy vegetables and orange and yellow pigmented fruits and vegetables.	Inadequate level leads to eye problems, frequent infections, poor growth, and red blood cell deficiency. Excess may lead to nausea, cramping, poor bone develop-ment, and dry skin.
Vitamin D (Cholecalciferol)	Absorption of calcium and phosphorus; mineralization of bones.	All dairy products, dark green vege-tables, eggs, and canned fish.	Inadequate level leads to muscle cramping, poor skeletal and tooth development, and pain in the joints. Excess may lead to nausea, weakness, headaches, and irritability. *This is the most potentially toxic of the vitamins, and excessive intake may lead to death.*
Vitamin E (Tocopherol)	Powerful antioxi-dant that protects cells from oxidative damage. Also protects vitamin A from oxidative damage.	Oils of vegetable origin, green vegetables, nuts, seeds, and whole-grain foods.	Inadequate level leads to shortened red cell life and may be related to premature problems of the eyes related to aging.
Vitamin K (Phylloquinone)	Involved in blood clotting.	Made from bacteria resident in the gut, but small amounts also present in green vegetables and milk.	Inadequate level may prevent blood from clotting properly, leading to excessive bleeding.

Minerals

Minerals are unique in that, unlike other nutrients, they are inorganic. However, like the organic nutrients, they work together. For example, vitamin D works with the mineral calcium. In general, minerals have several major functions. These include:

- Adding to the strength and structure of the skeleton, keeping it strong and resistant to fracture.

- Maintaining the relative acidity or alkalinity of the blood and tissue. For athletes, hard physical activity has the tendency to lower the pH level (i.e., increase the relative acidity), so having a healthy system to control acid-base balance is critical for endurance performance.

- Serving as bridges for electrical impules that stimulate muscular movement. Since all athletic endeavors rely on efficient and effective muscular movement and coordination, this function is critically important.

- Metabolizing cells —Physical activity increases the rate at which fuel is burned. Therefore, the effective control of this fuel burn at the cellular level is necessary to athletic endeavors.

All of these functions are important for athletes. Athletes with weak bones are at increased risk of stress fractures; poor fluid buffering (acid-base *im*balance) leads to poor endurance; poor nerve and muscle function leads to poor coordination; and altered cell metabolism limits a cell's ability to obtain and store energy.

The established roles of minerals in the development of optimal physical performance include involvement in glycolysis (obtaining energy from stored glucose), lipolysis (obtaining energy from fats), proteolysis (obtaining energy from proteins), and in the phosphagen system (obtaining energy from phosphocreatine).[73] Inorganic mineral nutrients are required in the structural composition of hard and soft body tissues. They also participate in such processes as the action of enzyme systems, the contraction of muscles, nerve reactions, and the clotting of blood. These mineral nutrients, all of which must be supplied in the diet, are of two classes: the major elements (macrominerals) such as calcium, phosphorus, magnesium, iron, iodine, and potassium; and trace elements (microminerals) such as copper, cobalt, manganese, fluorine, and zinc.[16a]

Macrominerals

The total mineral content of the body is approximately 4 percent of body weight. Macrominerals are those minerals that are present in the body in relatively large amounts (compared to microminerals). These are minerals that are required at a level of 100 mg per day or more, or the body content of the mineral is greater than 5 grams. Macrominerals include calcium, phosphorus, magnesium, um, sodium, chloride, and sulfur. Calcium makes up approximately 1.75 percent of total body weight, phosphorus makes up approximately 1.10 percent of total body weight, and magnesium makes up approximately 0.04 percent of total body weight.

Calcium (Chemical symbol = Ca)

Calcium is an important mineral for bone and tooth structure, blood clotting, and nerve transmission, and has an adult RDA of 800 to 1,200 milligrams. Deficiencies are associated with skeletal malformations (as in rickets), increased skeletal fragility (as in osteoporotic fracture and stress fractures), and blood pressure abnormalities. There are few reports of toxicity from taking high doses of calcium, but it is conceivable that a high and frequent intake of calcium supplements may alter the acidity of the stomach (making it more alkaline), thereby interfering with protein digestion. Since there is competitive absorption between many minerals in the small intestine (calcium, zinc, iron, and magnesium), it is also possible that having a high amount of calcium may interfere with the absorption of other minerals if they are present in the gut at the same time. Therefore, taking high-dose calcium supplements at the same time you eat a food that contains iron, for example, may result in the malabsorption of iron and eventually lead to iron deficiency anemia.

Food sources of calcium include dairy products (milk, cheese, yogurt), dark green vegetables (collards, spinach, chard, mustard greens, broccoli, green peppers), and dried beans and peas (lentils, navy beans, soy beans, and split peas). It's important to note that calcium and several other minerals (especially iron, magnesium, and zinc) are easily bound to a compound found in dark green vegetables called oxalic acid or oxalate. If these minerals are bound to oxalate, they become unavailable for absorption. Therefore, while dark green vegetables are potentially good sources of calcium and several other minerals, these foods don't make the minerals easily available to us. However, it is possible to improve the bioavailability of these oxalate-bound minerals through an easy food preparation technique called blanching. Oxalate is highly water soluble so by dipping the vegetables for a few seconds into boiling water, a good deal of the oxalate is removed but the minerals remain. You can then prepare the vegetables as you like. This technique dramatically improves the delivery of calcium from vegetables, and has been used by cultures that traditionally have not consumed dairy products (especially in Asia) for thousands of years. As a side benefit, vegetables that are blanched may also be more acceptable for children to eat. Children are more sensitive to bitter tastes than adults (we lose some of our taste sensitivities as we age!), and oxalic acid has a bitter taste. Therefore, by removing the oxalate you also remove some of the bitter taste that children find unacceptable.

There have been numerous studies looking at the relationships among calcium intake, physical activity, and bone density. However, the relationship between calcium supplementation and physical performance has not been well studied. In fact, when athletes take calcium supplements it is typically for the purpose of reducing the risk of fracture (i.e., improving bone density) and not for the purpose of improving physical performance. Physical activity is known to enhance bone density, just as physical inactivity is known to lower bone density. However, the development and mineralization of bone are complex and involve several factors including growth phase (childhood and adolescence are associated with faster bone development), hormonal status (especially estrogen for women), energy adequacy, vitamin D availability, and calcium intake.

Since 1993, there has been an increased availability of an accurate bone-density measuring device called DEXA (Dual Energy X-ray Absorptiometry) that has dramatically improved the ability to measure bone density and determine risk of fracture. Studies that have used DEXA appear to indicate that children and adolescents who have a calcium intake at or slightly above the RDA (up to 1,500 milligrams) may improve bone density. However, the relationship between calcium supplementation and bone density in adults is less clear (i.e., taking calcium supplements by themselves does not necessarily lead to a greater bone density). Despite this, it seems prudent to make certain that calcium intake is maintained at the RDA level, that adequate physical activity is maintained (not a problem for most athletes), and that there is an adequate intake of vitamin D. A recent survey on the United States Gymnastics team indicated that sunlight exposure was more highly correlated (and significantly so) to bone mineral density than calcium intake. Even in gymnasts with an inadequate calcium intake (i.e., below the RDA), having more sunlight exposure was associated with higher bone densities.[74]

Another concern with many female athletes is amenorrhea (cessation of menses), because this is strongly associated with either poor bone development (in young athletes) or bone demineralization (in older athletes). The causes of amenorrhea are complex and include inadequate energy intake, eating disorders, low body fat levels, poor iron status, psychological stress, high cortisol levels, and overtraining. In other words, hard-working elite female athletes are *at risk*.

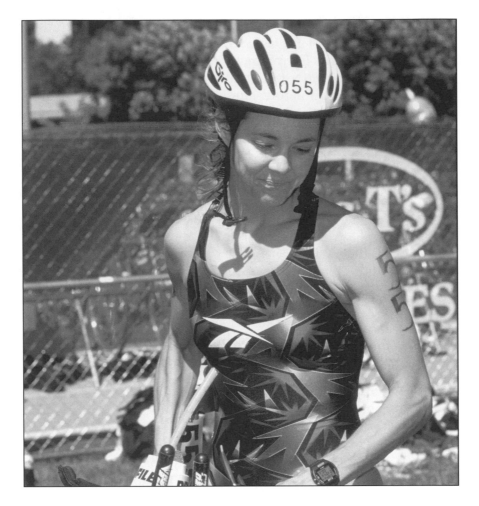

Anything that might lower risk, such as maintaining a good iron status and consuming enough energy, is useful for lowering the risk of developing amenorrhea. Even if an amenorrheic athlete has sufficient calcium intake, that alone would not suffice to maintain or develop healthy bones because the lower level of circulating estrogen associated with amenorrhea would inhibit normal bone development or maintenance.

Phosphorus (Chemical symbol = P)

Phosphorus is present in most foods and is especially high in protein-rich foods (meat, poultry, fish, and dairy products) and cereal grains. It combines with calcium (about two parts calcium for every part phosphorus) to produce healthy bones and teeth. It also plays an important role in energy metabolism, affecting carbohydrates, lipids, and proteins. The energy derived for muscular work comes largely from phosphorus-containing compounds called *adenosine triphosphate* (ATP) and *creatine phosphate* (CP). As with calcium, the absorption of phosphorus is largely dependent on vitamin D, and the adult RDA is 800 to 1,200 milligrams/day.

Because phosphorus is so omnipresent in the food supply, a deficiency is rare. However, it has been seen in people taking antacids that contain aluminum hydroxide for long periods of time.[75] This type of antacid binds with phosphorus, making it unavailable for absorption.[76]

There is a long history of supplementing with phosphorus-containing substances to improve physical performance. In World War I, Germany provided its soldiers with foods and supplements high in phosphorus with the aim of improving strength and endurance.[77] This experience with phosphorus suggests that relatively large amounts are well tolerated over time, but there is no evidence that strength and endurance are actually improved. The results of more recent studies on the effect of phosphorus supplementation are mixed. A study on runners, rowers, and swimmers who took 2 grams of sodium dihydrogen phosphate one hour prior to exercise *all* showed performance improvements, while only half the unsupplemented athletes showed improvements.[78] In another study, VO_2max was improved on a treadmill test following short-term phosphorus supplementation.[79] However, in another study evaluating the effect of phosphate supplementation on muscular power, there was no apparent benefit from taking the phosphate.[80] Taken together, the mixed results of these studies make it difficult to say whether a small preexercise supplement of phosphorus will improve performance. Clearly, more studies are needed before an answer to this question can be attempted.

Magnesium (Chemical symbol = Mg)
Magnesium, which is present in most foods, is essential for human metabolism and is important for maintaining the electrical potential in nerve and muscle cells. A deficiency in magnesium among malnourished people, especially alcoholics, leads to tremors and convulsions. It is involved in more than 300 reactions in which food is synthesized to new products, and it is a critical component in the processes that create muscular energy from carbohydrate, protein, and fat.[81] The adult RDA for magnesium is 280 to 350 milligrams per day.

It is possible that athletes training in hot and humid environments could lose a large amount of magnesium in sweat. Were this to occur, a magnesium deficiency could, given the importance of magnesium in muscle function processes, cause athletes to underachieve athletically. In one study where magnesium supplements were given to athletes, there was an improvement in physical performance.[82] There is some limited evidence that taking magnesium supplements at the level of the RDA (about 350 milligrams/day) may have a beneficial effect on endurance and strength performance in athletes who have blood magnesium levels at the low end of the normal range.[83,84] However, with the exception of these studies, there is little other research evidence that magnesium deficiency is common among athletes or that supplementation improves performance. In fact, with the exception of athletes who are known to reduce total energy intake in an attempt to maintain or lower weight (wrestlers, gymnasts, skaters, etc.), it appears as if most male athletes consume the RDA or more, and most female athletes consume at least 60 percent of the magnesium RDA.[85,86]

Sodium (Chemical symbol = Na)

Sodium is an essential mineral commonly referred to as salt, which is actually sodium chloride. It is involved in body water balance and acid-base balance and is the major extracellular (outside the cell, including blood and fluid) mineral. Sodium is present in small quantities in most natural foods and is found in high amounts in processed, canned, cooked, and fast foods. While most people are capable of excreting excess sodium, some are sensitive to sodium, because they do not have this capability. This excess retention of sodium causes edema, which is an overaccumulation of extracellular fluid and may contribute to high blood pressure. If you are salt sensitive, you can limit your sodium intake by concentrating food

Table 1.4   Understanding Food Labels: Sodium

Term	Definition
Sodium-free	Less than 5 mg sodium per standard serving.
Low sodium	140 mg sodium or less per standard serving. If the serving weighs 30 grams or less, 140 mg sodium or less per 50 grams of food. If the serving is 2 tablespoons or less, 140 mg sodium or less per 50 g of the food.
Very low sodium	35 mg sodium or less per standard serving. If the serving weighs 30 grams or less, 35 mg sodium or less per 50 grams of food. If the serving is 2 tablespoons or less, 35 mg sodium or less per 50 g of the food.
Reduced or less sodium	A minimum of a 25 percent lower sodium content than the food it is compared to.

choices on natural, whole foods and avoiding high-sodium comercially prepared foods. Food labels provide information about sodium content (see table 1.4). The Food and Drug Administration's (FDA's) daily reference values for the sodium content of 2,500-calorie diets is less than 2,400 milligrams. The RDA estimated daily sodium requirement is 500 milligrams.

One of the key ingredients of sports beverages is sodium, because it helps to drive the desire to drink, and because it helps to maintain blood volume. Maintenance of blood volume is an important factor in athletic performance, because it is related to the ability to deliver nutrients to cells, remove metabolic by-products from cells, and maintain the sweat rate so the body doesn't overheat. Additional information on sodium is included in chapter 2.

Chloride (Chemical symbol = Cl)

Chloride, another extracellular mineral, is essential for the maintenance of fluid balance, and is also an important component of gastric juices. Virtually all the chloride we consume is associated with table salt (sodium *chloride*), so there is a parallel between sodium and chloride intakes. In addition, chloride losses are closely linked to sodium losses, so a deficiency of one is related to a deficiency of the other. Deficiencies typically occur with heavy sweating, frequent diarrhea, or frequent vomiting.[87] In fact, sweat losses are likely to deplete chloride and sodium to a greater degree than other minerals (electrolytes including potassium and magnesium) that are lost in sweat.[88] Since most people consume excessive amounts of sodium because of a heavy table salt intake, chloride intake is typically 6,000 milligrams (6 grams), a level that is well above normal requirements.[89] The RDA estimated chloride requirement is 750 milligrams per day. Additional information on chloride is included in chapter 2.

Potassium (Chemical symbol = K)

Potassium is the main mineral found inside cells (an intracellular electrolyte) at a concentration that is 30 times greater than the concentration of potassium found outside cells. It is involved in water balance, nerve impulse transmission, and muscular contractions. Dietary deficiency is rare and typically only occurs with chronic diarrhea and vomiting or laxative abuse. Individuals taking medications for high blood pressure force the loss of sodium, and in this process potassium is also lost. These individuals are encouraged to replace this lost potassium through the intake of potassium supplements or foods high in potassium (fruits, vegetables, and meats). The typical intake of potassium ranges from 1,000 to 11,000 milligrams per day (1–11 grams/day), with people consuming large amounts of fresh fruits and vegetables having the highest intakes. There is good evidence that high levels of potassium (around 3,500 milligrams/day) are beneficial in controlling high blood pressure.[90] Toxicity, which occurs with intakes of potassium that are around 18,000 milligrams (18 grams) may lead to cardiac arrest.[91] The RDA estimated daily potassium requirement is 2,000 milligrams.

Although it is well established that potassium is critical to heart and skeletal muscle function, the amount of potassium lost in sweat during exercise is relatively small and does not seriously affect the body's potassium stores. Therefore, sweat-related losses of potassium should not seriously affect athletic performance in the well-nourished athlete.[92] Additional information on potassium is included in chapter 2.

Macrominerals

Mineral	Functions	Sources	Cautions
Macrominerals (major)			
Calcium	Skeletal structure, muscle contraction and relaxation, blood pressure, nerve function, and immune system.	All dairy products, tofu, dark green leafy vegetables, legumes (dried beans and peas), and canned fish (with edible bones).	Poorly developed and deformed skeleton, increased skeletal fragility, and growth stunting in children.
Phosphorus	Present in the cell wall as "phospholipids," involved in high energy bonds of energy metabolic processes, and helps to maintain body pH (acidity-alkalinity).	Present in all foods of animal origin, and also present in legumes.	Deficiency is only seen in conjunction with the intake of certain drugs. Calcium deficiency may occur with excess intake of phosphorus.
Potassium	Involved in protein synthesis, water balance, pH balance, nerve impulse transmission, and muscle contraction. The most prevalent intercellular electrolyte.	Present in meats, poultry, dairy products, fruits, vegetables, grains, and legumes. Bananas and oranges are good nonmeat sources.	Deficiency is associated with weakness, paralysis, and confusion, and is commonly seen in conjunction with dehydration. Severe deficiency may cause death.

Mineral	Functions	Sources	Cautions
Sulfur	Part of some amino acids, biotin, thiamin, and insulin. Involved in the shape of some proteins (through sulfer bonding structures). Detoxifies certain substances.	Present in all foods that contain protein (as most foods do).	Deficiency would only occur in the presence of severe protein deprivation (a rare occurrence), and toxicity would only occur in the presence of a protein excess (a documented condition in animals but not humans).
Sodium	The major extracellular (blood) electrolyte, involved in fluid balance, pH balance, and nerve impulse transmission.	Present in salt, most fast foods, and in many preserved foods.	Those individuals with sodium sensitivity develop hypertension with excessive intake. A deficiency of sodium leads to muscle cramping, lethargy, and anorexia.
Chloride	Involved in digestive enzymes (hydrochloric acid in the stomach).	Present in table salt (sodium chloride), processed and preserved foods, and fast foods.	Inadequate intake may lead to growth retardation in children, cramps, lethargy, and anorexia.
Magnesium	Involved in bone strength, protein synthesis, muscle contraction, and nerve impulse transmission. The second most prevalent intercellular electrolyte.	Present in nuts, legumes, whole grains, dark green leafy vegetables, seafood, and cocoa.	Inadequate intake may lead to muscle weakness, convulsions, hallucinations, and growth failure. Excess intake (typically through frequent intake of magnesium-containing antacids and laxatives) may lead to kidney problems, confusion, and poor muscular coordination.

Microminerals

The microminerals (trace elements) are present in extremely small amounts but have important roles to play in human nutrition. These microminerals are needed inamounts less than 100 mg per day, and have body contents of less than 5 grams. They include iron, iodine, zinc, copper, fluorine, manganese, molybdenum, selenium, and chromium.

Iron (Chemical symbol = Fe)

Iron is needed to form the oxygen-transporting compounds hemoglobin (in blood) and myoglobin (in muscle), and is also found in a number of other compounds involved in normal tissue function. Iron absorption is limited because we have no effective mechanism for excreting any excess; it is also driven by the amount of iron we have stored (in ferritin and hemosiderin). The lower the storage level, the higher the absorption; however, overall absorption rates rarely go above 10 to 15 percent of the iron content of consumed food. This variable absorption mechanism is aimed at maintaining a relatively constant level of iron and avoiding an excess uptake. In spite of this variable absorption rate, people with marginal intakes of iron are at risk for developing iron deficiency and eventual anemia. Iron deficiency anemia is characterized by poor oxygen-carrying capacity, a condition that is known to cause performance deficits in athletes. Iron deficiency is also associated with poor immune function, short attention span, irritability, and poor learning ability. In the United States, children experiencing fast growth, women of menstrual age, vegetarians, and pregnant women are at increased risk for developing iron deficiency anemia. Periods of growth and pregnancy are associated with a higher requirement of iron because of a fast expansion of the blood volume, and iron is an essential component of red blood cells. Women of menstrual age have higher requirements because of the regular blood (and iron) losses associated with the menstrual period. For this reason, women of childbearing age have a higher requirement for iron (18 milligrams) than men of the same age (10 milligrams). Some people are at risk for developing iron toxicity because they are missing the mechanisms for limiting absorption. Young children, in particular, may be at risk for iron toxicity if they ingest supplements intended for adults. While the iron RDA for children is similar to that for adults (10 milligrams per day for children and 10 to 15 milligrams per day for adults), many iron supplements intended for adults have levels of iron that are more than 300 percent of the RDA. Where iron overload disease occurs, it may be fatal.

Iron is available in a wide variety of foods, including meats, eggs, vegetables, and iron-fortified cereals. Milk and other dairy products are poor sources of iron. The most easily absorbed form of iron is "heme" iron, which comes from meats and other foods of animal origin. Non-heme iron, which is not as easily absorbed as heme iron, is found in fruits, vegetables, and cereals. However, non-heme iron absorption may be enhanced by consuming foods high in vitamin C. On the other hand, non-heme iron absorption may be inhibited by phytic acid (a substance associated with bran in cereal grains), antacids, and calcium phosphate. In general, red meats are considered to provide the most abundant and easily absorbable source of iron. It is for this reason that vegetarians are considered to be at increased risk for iron deficiency anemia. Nevertheless, with proper planning, the consumption of vegetables and fruits high in iron, and sound cooking techniques that aid iron absorption, vegetarians can obtain sufficient iron.

Maximizing Iron Intake in a Vegetarian Diet

For vegetarians who want to improve iron absorption from foods, consider the following:

- Dark green vegetables have iron, but they also have oxalic acid, which reduces iron availability. To remove the oxalic acid from the vegetables, blanche them by putting them in a pot of boiling water for 5 to 10 seconds. Much of the oxalate is removed but the iron remains.

- High-fiber cereals (those with a high bran content) have large amounts of phytic acid, which binds with iron and reduces iron availability. Switch to whole-grain cereals rather than consuming bran-added cereals.

- Iron in vegetables is in a form that has a lower rate of absorption than iron in meats. To improve the rate of absorption, add vitamin C to the vegetables by squeezing lemon or orange juice on them before eating.

Athletes have good reason to be concerned about iron status, since oxygen-carrying capacity (via hemoglobin in blood and myoglobin in muscles) is a critical factor in physical endurance. Iron deficiency is one of the most common nutrient deficiencies, and it appears as if athletes have about the same rate of iron deficiency anemia as the general public.[93] There may be several reasons why some athletes suffer from low iron levels. These include:

• *Low dietary intake of iron.* It is possible that some athletes may consume foods with an inadequate total intake of iron. This may be especially true with athletes who are limiting total energy intake as a means (albeit ineffective) of maintaining or reducing weight.

• *Consumption of foods with low iron absorption rates.* Many athletes consume large amounts of carbohydrates and are limiting the intake of red meat. While iron exists in nonmeat sources, the absorption rate of iron in these foods is typically less, as well as the total iron content.

• *Increased iron losses (hematuria).* Some forms of exercise, particularly long-distance running and concussive sports, cause small amounts of hemoglobin and/or myoglobin to be lost in the urine due to a rupturing of red blood cells.

• *Loss of iron in sweat.* While iron losses in sweat are low (about 0.3 to 0.4 milligrams per liter of sweat), a typical absorption rate of iron from food (about 10 percent) would require that 3 to 4 milligrams of dietary iron be consumed for each liter of sweat produced.[94] Runners commonly lose, particularly in hot and humid environments, up to 2 liters of sweat per hour.

• *"Sports anemia".* It is common for many athletes to appear as if they are anemic at the beginning of training season because there is a large increase in blood volume at the initiation of training. This increase in blood volume has the effect of diluting the constituents of the blood, including red blood cells, making it appear as though there is an anemia. However, after a short time, the body increases the production of red blood cells to remove the appearance of anemia.

There are differences in how an athlete might respond in the presence of frank anemia (reduction in the number and size of red blood cells) versus iron deficiency (low serum iron and low stored iron, but normal red blood cells) anemia. These differences have been summarized by Wolinsky and Driskell in the table that follows (see table 1.5).[95]

While iron-deficient athletes are known to experience a performance deficit, there appears to be no benefit in providing iron supplements to athletes who have a normal iron status.[96] Further, iron supplementation is often associated with nausea, constipation, and stomach irritation. However, in athletes who have had blood tests that demonstrate either an anemia or a marginal level of stored iron, iron supplementation is warranted. The best means of providing iron supplements to reduce the chance of potential negative side effects is to provide 25 to 50 milligrams every third or fourth day rather than daily doses.[97]

Table 1.5   The Impact of Anemia and Iron Deficiency on Exercise Performance

Anemia	Iron deficiency
Lower oxygen delivery to cells	Higher rate of glucose oxidation
Decreased oxygen uptake (lower $\dot{V}O_2$max)	Higher lactic acid production
Lower endurance performance	Higher respiratory quotient (higher proportion of carbohydrate consumed to meet energy needs)
Lower oxidative metabolism	Decreased endurance performance possible
Higher glucose oxidation	
Higher lactic acid production	
Increased respiratory quotient (higher proportion of carbohydrate consumed to meet energy needs)	

Adapted from Tobin and Beard 1997.

Zinc (Chemical symbol = Zn)

Zinc is also important in forming enzymes. Zinc is a mineral that helps to form certain enzymes, a type of protein. Enzymes help chemical reactions—such as the healing of wounds—occur at a proper rate. Zinc-containing enzymes are involved in the metabolism of carbohydrates, fats, and proteins. Insufficient dietary intake of zinc causes a variety of health problems, including stunted growth, slow wound healing, and failure of the immune system. Zinc also plays an important role in the removal of carbon dioxide from cells, and is part of an important antioxidant enzyme called superoxide dismutase. Excessive intake can cause anemia, vomiting, and immune-system failure. Meat, liver, eggs, and seafood are good sources of zinc. The adult RDA for zinc is 12 to 15 milligrams per day.

Zinc levels at the lower end of the normal range, or lower, have been observed in male and female endurance runners. Athletes with lower serum zinc values had lower training mileage (i.e., could probably not train as hard) than those who had higher values.[98-100] Therefore, there appears to be a performance deficit in the small number of athletes who have poor zinc status. The effect of zinc supplementation on performance has not been extensively studied, and the level of supplementation in these studies has been extremely high (around 135 milligrams/day). Also, the athletes tested were never assessed for zinc status prior to the initiation of the research protocol. Nevertheless, this level of intake did lead to an improvement in both muscular strength and endurance.[101] Athletes should be cautioned that this level of zinc intake has never been tested over time, so it may well have negative side effects. Toxicity and malabsorption of other nutrients are both likely and possible with this level of intake.[102-104]

Iodine (Chemical symbol = I)

Iodine is needed to synthesize a key hormone of the thyroid gland, thyroxin, which is involved in regulating metabolic rate, growth, and development. A deficiency of iodine leads to goiter, a swelling of the thyroid gland in the front of the neck. Goiter was once common in the United States because certain areas have foods grown in soils with a low iodine content. It remains a prevalent nutritional deficiency disease in certain parts of Asia, Africa, and South America. Pregnant women with low iodine intakes give birth to cretinous or mentally retarded infants. In the United States, an early public health measure to assure that everyone had an adequate intake of iodine was to add iodine to salt. This *iodized salt* eliminated goiter in this country. An excessive intake of iodine has the effect of depressing thyroid activity, so taking additional supplemental doses of iodine is not recommended.

Selenium (Chemical symbol = Se)

Selenium is an important mineral antioxidant in human nutrition. Since exercise (particularly endurance exercise) is associated with an increased production of potentially damaging oxidative by-products (peroxides and free radicals) in muscle fibers, it is possible that selenium may play a role in reducing muscular oxidative stress.[105] A selenium deficiency may result in muscle weakness and increase recovery time from exhaustive exercise.[106] There is little evidence, however, that increasing the intake of supplemental selenium increases exercise performance.[107] The adult RDA for selenium is 55 to 70 micrograms. It is difficult to determine dietary adequacy, since the selenium content of food is determined by soil and water where the food was grown. Nutritional supplements, including sodium selenite and high-selenium yeast, are effective sources of selenium, but excessive intake may be toxic, so proper care in taking appropriate levels of supplements is important.

Copper (Chemical symbol = Cu)

Among the more important trace elements is copper, which is present in many enzymes and in copper-containing proteins found in the blood, brain, and liver. Copper deficiency is associated with the failure to use iron in the formation of hemoglobin and myoglobin. It is also important in preventing oxidative damage to cells through the enzyme superoxide dismutase. The adult RDA for copper is 1.5 to 3.0 milligrams per day. Good sources of copper include shellfish, soybean products, legumes, nuts, seeds, liver, and potatoes. As another good example of why nutritional balance is important, excessive consumption of calcium, phosphate, iron, zinc, and vitamin C all reduce copper absorption.

Very few studies have been performed on the relationship between copper and athletic performance. Studies of blood copper concentrations in athletes and nonathletes have not revealed any significant differences, but the athletes have a slightly higher (3–4 percent) concentration of serum copper than nonathletes.[108] In a study evaluating the copper status of swimmers during a competitive season there was no difference in pre- and post-season copper status. In this study, the majority of swimmers were consuming adequate levels of copper (more than 1 milligram per day) from food.[109]

Manganese (Chemical symbol = Mn)

Manganese is a trace mineral that is involved in bone formation, immune function, antioxidant activity, and carbohydrate metabolism.[110] While manganese deficiency is rare, deficiencies are associated with skeletal problems (undermineralized bone and increased risk of fracture) and poor wound healing. It appears that those at greatest risk for deficiency are those on diets (inadequate intake) or where malabsorption occurs. Manganese is in competition with calcium, iron, and zinc for absorption, so an excess intake of these other minerals may decrease manganese absorption and lead to deficiency symptoms. Much like iron, manganese absorption is enhanced with vitamin C and meat intake. Food sources of manganese include coffee, tea, chocolate, whole wheat, nuts, seeds, soybeans, dried beans (navy beans, lentils, split peas, etc.), liver, and fruits. As with several other minerals, the intake of foods high in oxalic acid (present in dark green leafy vegetables) may inhibit manganese absorption. (See calcium section for ways of reducing the oxalic acid content of foods.) The adult RDI for manganese is 2 milligrams. (RDI = recommended dietary intake—used by the NRC (National Research Council) when there is insufficient data to develop an RDA. For many microminerals there is only an RDI because there has been limited research on human requirements.) Food sources include tea, coffee, chocolate, soybean products, legumes, whole grains, liver, and fruits. As with copper, excessive intakes of calcium, phosphorus, iron, zinc, fiber, and oxalic acid all decrease manganese absorption.

Chromium (Chemical symbol = Cr)

Chromium is also known as *glucose tolerance factor* (GTF) because of its involvement in helping cells use glucose. A deficiency of chromium is known to be associated with poor blood glucose maintenance (either hypo- or hyperglycemia), an excessive production of insulin (hyperinsulinemia), excessive fatigue, and a craving for sweet foods. (*Hypo*glycemia is low blood sugar; *hyper*glycemia is high blood sugar). It is also associated with irritability (a common condition with poor blood glucose control), weight gain, adult-onset diabetes, and increased risk of cardiovascular disease.[111] There is some evidence that frequent intense exercise, which is common for serious athletes, may place a person at risk of chromium deficiency. High consumption of simple sugars (sweets) may also place people at risk for deficiency. It appears, from a number of surveys, that a large proportion of the U.S. population consumes inadequate levels of chromium, a factor that may be associated with the excess weight commonly found in greater numbers of the population. The best food sources of chromium include whole grains and meats. Nutritional supplements, commonly in the form of chromium picolinate, are taken as a means of reducing weight or body fat, but the results of studies on this supplement have produced mixed results. Initial studies of chromium picolinate supplementation suggested that this supplement was effective at increasing muscle mass and decreasing body fat in bodybuilders and football players.[112] However, subsequent controlled studies have failed to reach the same conclusions.[113, 114] Other supplements for chromium include chromium polynicotinate, chromium chloride, and high chromium yeast. The adult RDI for chromium is 120 micrograms per day. Dietary sources include whole-grain breads and cereals, meats, and high chromium yeast.

Because chromium is not well absorbed, there is little evidence to suggest that an excessive intake of chromium will result in toxicity.

However, the toxicity of chromium has not been directly tested, so athletes should be cautious about taking supplements. One study suggests that chromium picolinate has the potential of altering DNA, and thus producing mutated, cancerous cells.[115] Taken together, these studies suggest that to maintain optimal chromium nutriture, athletes should consume foods low in sugar and a diet that contains whole grains and, if not a vegetarian, some meat. Supplementation has not been shown to aid athletic performance.

Microminerals

Mineral	Functions	Sources	Cautions
Iron	Part of hemoglobin, involved in oxygen and carbon dioxide transfer in the blood. Makes oxygen available to muscles for aerobic activity.	Found in red meats, dark poultry, fish, eggs, legumes, and dried fruits. (Absorption of plant-based iron is enhanced with vitamin C.)	Inadequate intake leads to iron deficiency anemia, which results in easy fatigue, increased infection risk, poor concentration, and lower learning ability.
Copper	Involved in transferring iron from storage to its functional form (hemoglobin). Also part of several enzymes.	Found in meat and most drinking water.	Inadequate intake contributes to iron deficiency anemia.
Iodine	An important component of thyroid hormone (thyroxine), which is the major controlling hormone of energy metabolism.	The most certain dietary source is iodized salt, but it is also available in seafood. Soil levels of iodine vary, so foods grown in different areas have a different iodine content.	Deficiency symptoms include fatigue, low body temperature (hypothermia), and weakness. Serious deficiency results in goiter (gland enlargement), mental retardation (cretinism), and cardiovascular disease. Toxicity is not documented, but regular supplemental intakes exeeding the RDI of 150 micrograms/day should be avoided.

(continued)

Microminerals   *(continued)*

Mineral	Functions	Sources	Cautions
Zinc	Part of many enzymes involved in energy metabolism. Also involved in taste, wound healing, and immune function.	Found in most high-protein foods, especially red meat, fish, and poultry. Found in smaller concentrations in grains and vegetables.	Inadequate intake leads to growth failure in children and a delay in development of secondary sexual characteristics. Deficiency also leads to altered taste and poor healing of injuries. Excess may lead to nausea, diarrhea, poor muscular coordination, and kidney failure.
Flouride	Involved in developing strong bones and teeth. Teeth formed when fluoride is available in the system creates decay-resistant enamel.	Fluoridated water, fluoridated dentifrices (if swallowed), and seafood.	Deficiency may increase risk of developing dental cavities. Excess may cause fluorosis (discolored teeth) and nausea.
Chromium	Also called glucose tolerance factor because of its involvement in controlling blood glucose (it helps insulin work effectively).	Found in whole-grain foods and meats, and is available in supplement form as chromium picolinate, chromium chloride, and high chromium yeast.	Deficiency is most commonly seen with frequent intense exercise and high consumption of simple sugars and is associated with poor blood glucose control (hyperglycemia and hypoglycemia). Typical intakes in the U.S. range from < 50 to 100 micrograms, so a deficiency is possible. Toxicity is possible but not documented. Supplemental intake should not regularly exceed the RDI of 120 micrograms.

Mineral	Functions	Sources	Cautions
Manganese	Involved in bone and cartilage growth and maintenance, carbohydrate metabolism, antioxidant activity, fat metabolism, and the production of glucose from protein (gluconeogenesis).	Found in whole grain wheat, nuts, seeds, legumes (including soy products), and fruits. Also found in tea and coffee. Available in supplements, but RDI of 2.0 mg/day should not be exceeded on regular basis.	Deficiency associated with skeletal problems (osteoarthritis, osteoporosis, increased fracture risk) and poor healing.
Molybdenum	Involved in the enzyme that oxidizes xanthine to uric acid. Also important for nitrogen-fixing bacteria, which are the basis of our protein foods.	Molybdenum concentrations vary widely in foods, depending on the soil where the foods are grown. Concentrations are highest in legumes, whole-grain cereals, and liver.	Deficiency of molybdenum only documented with long-term intravenous feeding, and is unlikely in people who regularly consume a wide variety of foods. Toxicity symptoms from excess molybdenum intake are not well documented in humans, but regular supplemental intakes exceeding the RDI of 75 micrograms per day should be avoided.
Selenium	An important cellular antioxidant that works as part of a compound called "glutathione peroxidase." Aids the antioxidant functions of vitamin E and vitamin C.	Food content based on selenium content of soil and water where food was grown, so is highly variable. May be obtained from supplements (commonly sodium selenite, selenomethionine, and high selenium yeast).	Deficiency disorders *may* be related to cardiac dysfunction (Keshan disease) and osteoarthritis. May also be associated with increased cancer risk, muscle weakness, and impaired immune function. Potential toxicity risk with excess supplementation (regular daily intakes exceeding 0.2 mg/day) exists.

Digestion and Absorption

Digestion is the process where the body breaks down the physical and chemical constituents of consumed foods to bring them to a sufficiently small size and molecular structure that they can pass through the lining of the small intestine to be absorbed into the blood. We have tremendously complex systems for doing this, with the result that over 90 percent of the energy consumed is actually absorbed (see table 1.6).

The absorption rates for vitamins and minerals vary, in large part due to physiological need. Our ability to control the absorption of certain minerals is a built-in safety mechanism to make certain we don't exceed a safe level of the mineral in our tissues. Iron, for instance, is absorbed at relatively low rates (5 to 20 percent of the iron consumed) because we have no effective means of excreting the excess. Absorbing too much iron into the system would cause too much iron to accumulate and would cause serious (even deadly) problems as discussed earlier. On the other hand, there are minerals that we absorb freely, such as sodium, because we have an effective means of excreting the excess.

Some vitamins, such as vitamin B-12, require the assistance of another substance to be absorbed. For instance, vitamin B-12 attaches itself to a substance called intrinsic factor, which is produced by a specific set of cells in the stomach (parietal cells). The intrinsic factor takes vitamin B-12 to the right place in the small intestine for absorption. Without sufficient intrinsic factor production, a person would suffer from pernicious anemia (a vitamin B-12 deficiency disorder) even with a sufficient intake of vitamin B-12.

The cooperative nature of intrinsic factor and vitamin B-12 points to another critical point: a failure of one part of the digestive or absorptive system is likely to lead to problems elsewhere in the system. To carry the vitamin B-12 example further, someone with a stomach problem (irritation, ulcer, cancer, etc.) may not produce sufficient intrinsic factor to aid in the absorption of vitamin B-12. Since the parietal cells that produce intrinsic factor are also responsible for producing hydrochloric acid, a key element in achieving the proper digestive acidity, other nutrients (particularly protein) would also not get properly digested or absorbed.

For athletes, the issues surrounding digestion and absorption are also of practical importance, particularly as they relate to the pre-game or precompetition meal. The selection of appropriate foods during this time is critical for assuring that athletes receive the

Table 1.6   Digestion and Absorption Sites for Nutrients

Gastrointestinal tract	Digestion and absorption
Mouth	Involved in mechanically breaking apart foods to allow digestive enzymes to mix and chemically "digest" the foods. The enzyme produced in the mouth by the saliva glands (salivary amylase) can chemically digest carbohydrates. No absorption of nutrients takes place in the mouth.
Stomach	Food travels from the mouth to the stomach via the esophagus. Stomach cells produce an enzyme (gastric protease) that digests proteins into smaller units called peptones. The stomach also can digest small-sized fats (called short- and medium-chain triglycerides) into individual fatty acids and a small, 3-carbon unit called glycerol. A very small amount of the digested protein and fat can enter (i.e., can be "absorbed") into the veins in the stomach. However, the level of nutrient absorption in the stomach is considered to be extremely small.
Small intestine	In the small intestine, the pancreas introduces enzymes for the continued digestion of carbohydrate, protein, and fat. These enzymes (called pancreatic amylase, protease, and lipase), plus bile from the gall bladder and other enzymes produced in the small intestine, complete the digestion of consumed foods. It is the small intestine where the majority of all nutrient (carbohydrates, proteins, fats, vitamins, and minerals) absorption takes place. The absorption site for some minerals (iron, calcium, zinc, magnesium) is extremely small, which causes these minerals to compete for the same absorption site.
Large intestine	In the large intestine, there is a major exchange of fluid and electrolytes (minerals). The large intestine (colon) also has a significant population of friendly bacteria that aids in the disposal of food remnants. These bacteria are also involved in producing certain vitamins, such as vitamin K.

nutrients that they need, but it's also an important time to know that they shouldn't consume anything that might stay in the stomach too long. Different foods require different amounts of time to digest and absorb. The key is to make certain that the stomach is empty at the time the practice or competition begins. Otherwise, the athlete may develop an upset stomach, a factor that could easily impede optimal performance. The reason for this is straightforward: when exercise begins, blood is shunted to the working muscles and away from the

GI (gastrointestinal) tract. This shift of blood away from the GI tract may impede or slow normal digestive and absorptive processes, leaving food where it doesn't belong.

The preparation of the foods consumed and the combination of the foods eaten at one time may influence how well energy and nutrients are digested and absorbed, and this in turn may influence how you feel while you practice or compete. For example, there is a move in many endurance sports to reduce (or eliminate) red meat consumption and rely solely on grains, fruits, vegetables, and some dairy products for providing needed nutrients. In the hands of a knowledgeable person, a nourishing eating plan that contains these restrictions can be developed. However, many people don't know what it takes and *mal*nutrition is the result. An example of this is the problem associated with the oxalic acid found in dark green vegetables discussed earlier. If not removed, oxalic acid can interfere with the absorption of bivalent minerals (iron, zinc, magnesium, and calcium).

The fiber portion of grains contains a substance called phytic acid. In many ways, phytic acid and oxalic acid are similar, because both have a high binding affinity for iron, zinc, magnesium, and calcium. Imagine, for example, eating a high-fiber cereal with milk. The phytic acid in the bran binds with some of the calcium in the milk and makes it unavailable for absorption. Therefore, except for the occasions that constipation occurs or on the advice of your physician, it makes more nutritional sense to consume whole-grain products rather than bran-added products. The added bran, while useful from a regularity standpoint, may be associated with a substance that inhibits the absorption of some key minerals.

Another key point to make here is that the substances moving through the GI tract are constantly moving. They don't wait around in one particular place to get absorbed. Therefore, the reduction in mineral bioavailability imparted by oxalate and phytate is only temporary. For the oxalate or phytate to bind with minerals, either of these substances *and* minerals must be in the gut at the same time. Eating a high-bran cereal in the morning won't have an effect on the soup you eat for lunch.

Common Nutritional Myths

The most common thing I hear athletes say is, "I eat this because I know it's good for me." The second most common thing I hear athletes say is, "I don't eat that because it's bad for me." While these statements may be true, they are also bad mind-sets to have, because they fail to consider context. What's good or bad has to do with the *context* of other foods that are consumed, both in the short term and in the long term. If an athlete believes that cottage cheese is a perfect food and eats it every day for lunch and most days for dinner then that athlete is a prime target for malnutrition. It may just be possible that the best nutritional thing a "meat-avoider" (not a vegetarian) could do is to have a hamburger for lunch every once in a while. It has rightly been said that human breast milk is the perfect food for a newborn infant. But after six months, even infants need to try some other foods or they'll become anemic (breast milk is a poor source of iron). The truth is, there is no perfect food *in and of itself*, and athletes who eat a monotonous diet because they are convinced that a limited set of foods is the ticket to crossing the finish line first are badly fooling themselves.

Another common mind-set that athletes have is that you can't get enough of a nutrient (or related substance) that is good for performance. So, if a little is good for me then give me a lot. This also breaches a key rule of nutrition that "more than enough is not better

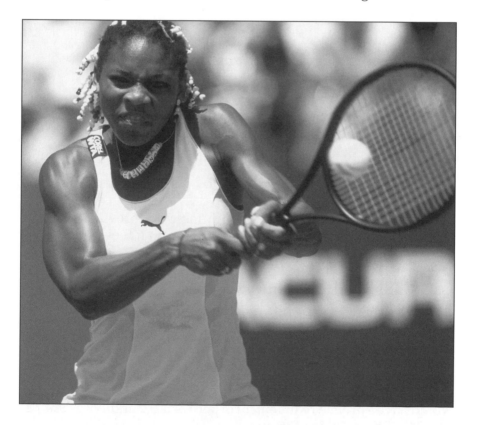

than enough." There is an ancient Latin saying that is true and relevant here: *Sola docis facit venenum* (the dose makes the poison). Just as having too little is bad, so is having too much. The way athletes think about the RDA is a prime example of how easy it is to get too much. It is (wrongly) believed that the RDA is a minimum requirement, even though it represents more than most healthy people need. Therefore, athletes are drawn to products that provide multiples of the RDA. This is even true for the way they feel about some breakfast cereals, which advertise that they provide 100 percent of the RDA for most nutrients in a single serving. Athletes jump at the chance of eating 200, 300, or 400 percent of the RDA by eating bowl after bowl. Unless this is some form of new math (which I don't understand), 100 percent usually means that you've met the requirement. Supplement intake behavior is also often consistent with this (wrong) philosophy that "more than enough is better than enough." The level of nutrient intake is often excessive, and even more often mistargeted, when taking high doses of substances that are not the most needed.

The best way to think about nutrients and energy is to remember these simple rules:

- Eat a wide variety of foods.
- More than enough is *not* better than enough.
- Eat foods that provide a lot of complex carbohydrates, some proteins, and little fat. A good way to reduce fat intake is to avoid fried foods, prepared meats (bologna, salami, sausage, etc.), and visible fats, and to consume low-fat dairy products.
- Eat enough to meet energy needs.

Let's put all of this into perspective by looking at a sample daily intake.

The sample daily intake shown in table 1.7 provides approximately 2,800 calories, is high in carbohydrates (65 percent of total calories), moderately high in protein (18 percent of total calories), and relatively low in fat (17 percent of total calories). This level of intake is appropriate for an athlete weighing about 150 pounds. Carbohydrate needs can be calculated as 3 grams per pound of body weight or approximately 450 grams. This diet meets that requirement by providing 466 grams of carbohydrates. This diet also meets protein needs of a 150-pound athlete. Protein requirement is estimated to be between 1.5 grams/kilogram and 1.8 grams/kilogram (or 0.68 grams/pound and 0.82 grams/pound). A 150-pound athlete would have a protein requirement of between 102 and 123 grams per day. This diet provides 126 grams.

Table 1.7   Sample Daily Intake

	Food	Cal.	Carb	Prot	Fat
Breakfast	2 slices cracked-wheat toast	132	26.0	4.0	1.0
	1 cup 1% milk	102	11.7	8.0	2.6
	1 tbsp strawberry jam	54	14.0	0.1	0.0
	1 cup orange juice	110	25.0	2.0	0.7
	Breakfast totals	**398**	**77**	**15**	**4**
Mid-AM snack	16 ounces Gatorade	100	28.1	0.0	0.0
	1 plain bagel	200	38.0	7.0	2.0
	Midmorning snack totals	**300**	**66**	**7**	**2**
Lunch	1/2 chicken breast (skinless, broiled)	142	0.0	26.7	3.01
	1 cup white rice	200	43.3	4.0	0.5
	1 cup green beans (steamed)	43	9.8	2.3	0.4
	1 roll (2.5-inch diameter)	119	19.6	2.9	3.0
	1% milk	102	11.7	8.0	2.6
	1 pear	98	25.1	0.7	0.7
	Lunch totals	**704**	**109**	**45**	**10**
Mid-PM snack	4 medium pretzels	250	48.6	6.3	2.9
	1 cup apple juice	117	29.0	0.2	0.3
	1 medium carrot	31	7.3	0.7	0.1
	Midafternoon snack totals	**397**	**85**	**7**	**3**
Dinner	2 cups chef salad (with ham, cheese)	400	7.1	39.0	24.1
	1 tbsp Italian dressing	70	1.5	0.1	7.1
	3 slices French bread	300	58.2	10.0	3.2
	Dinner totals	**774**	**67**	**49**	**34**
Evening snack	16 ounces Gatorade	100	28.1	0.0	0.0
	1 orange (raw)	62	1.2	0.2	0.0
	4 cups popcorn (plain)	93	18.4	3.0	1.2
	Evening snack totals	**254**	**62**	**4.3**	**1**
	Overall Totals	**2,827**	**466**	**126**	**56**
	% Calories from		**65**	**18**	**17**

As you can see, the foods in this daily intake consist of common foods that can be obtained anywhere. That's key, since dependence on special foods that may only be available at the local health food market will be inclined to make your life miserable, especially if you do any traveling. There are a few other important features of this sample meal plan that are important to note:

1. *Frequent eating.* You'll notice that, in this sample day, the athlete would eat six separate times. Eating three meals a day, although typical for so many people, is not the way humans should eat. If you evaluate the way free-living peoples (noninstitutionalized; people who can make decisions for themselves) eat, they eat frequently and some aborigines eat constantly. One of the features of this kind of eating pattern is that meal sizes are small but frequent. Industrialized cultures typically eat large meals, and they eat infrequently to fit into an "industrial" work schedule. For athletes, the more ideal food intake pattern is small meals consumed frequently. Ideally, athletes should strive to eat something every three hours (see chapter 7, "Timing of Meals and Snacks."). The goal is to *never get hungry* and *never get thirsty.*

2. *Energy distribution.* Athletes should derive the majority of energy from carbohydrates. In this meal plan (see "% Calories from" at the end of table 1.7), carbohydrates provide 65 percent of the total energy (ideal for athletes), proteins provide 18 percent, and fat provides 17 percent. Fat intake is even a little lower than it needs to be with these foods, so an athlete could actually put some margarine or butter on the popcorn or the toast and still stay within the 20 to 25 percent fat level you're trying to achieve.

3. *Small meals.* No meal is more than 800 calories. This is important, because large meals provide so much energy that a proportion of that energy inevitably contributes to stored fat. With many athletes, especially those doing power- rather than endurance-type work, getting fat out of storage once it's in there is difficult and detracts

Table 1.8 **Selected Nutrients in Sample Meal Plan Compared to the Recommended Dietary Allowances**

Nutrient	Intake	RDA	% of RDA
Energy (cal)	2,827	2,982	95
Protein (gm)	126	58	218
Calcium (mg)	1,344	1,200	112
Phosphorus (mg)	1,890	1,200	158
Iron (mg)	19	10	189
Potassium (mg)	4,002	2,000	200
Vitamin A (IU)	24,385	5,000	488
Thiamin (mg)	2.94	1.5	196
Riboflavin (mg)	2.66	1.7	156
Vitamin C (mg)	337	60	561

from both appearance and the strength:weight ratio. By having small but frequent meals, you help to limit the amount of fat that is stored.

4. *Carbohydrate throughout the day*. If you look at normal fluctuations in blood glucose (blood sugar), it rises after a meal and then starts to drop below the normal level about three hours after eating. By having some source of carbohydrate throughout the day, it helps to maintain a normal blood glucose level. Besides making you feel better and more alert, maintaining blood sugar may be an important strategy for maintaining metabolic rate. It's important to remember that the same fuel that fuels the brain (glucose) also fuels muscles. Muscle and mental fatigue go together. It's no accident that most athletic injuries occur at the end of the event or at the end of practice when muscles are fatigued and the mind can't focus on the task at hand. These foods in this eating pattern help to assure that carbohydrate (glucose) is available throughout the day.

If these foods were consumed by a 21-year-old male athlete who weighs 150 pounds and is 70 inches (5'10") tall, he would meet or exceed the RDA for most vitamins and minerals (see table 1.8). The point here is that, with a little planning (and no clinical condition that would prohibit you from doing so), it's relatively easy to meet or exceed your nutrient requirements simply by eating food.

Even though energy intake is 95 percent of the predicted requirement for this (hypothetical) person, nutrient intakes are far greater than the Recommended Dietary Allowances. Why would anyone feel as if they need to consume vitamin C supplements when, from food alone, vitamin C intake is 561 percent of the RDA! Protein supplements, which are so commonly taken by athletes, can be thrown in the trash bin when the foods consumed provide over 200 percent of the requirement.

Summary

Eating well most of the time is critical to maintaining optimal nutritional status. Without a generally good level of nutrient intake, it is impossible for the pretraining/precompetition meal to make a difference in an athlete's performance. Further, eating well most of the time helps to guarantee that the athlete will get the most benefit from training by enabling the athlete to train harder and longer. Importantly, eating well reduces the chance for muscle soreness and injury.

As a general rule, athletes should strive to eat foods that are high in carbohydrate, low in fat, and moderate in protein. Ideally, this distribution (expressed as a percent of total consumed energy) should be 25 percent or less from fat, 12 to 15 percent from protein, and 60 percent or more from carbohydrate. All athletes, including those who wish to increase muscle mass, will benefit from this type of energy distribution. In particular, a high-carbohydrate intake helps to guarantee that the athlete maintains a high stored energy level (glycogen) to delay fatigue.

It is important for athletes to rely on foods rather than vitamin and mineral supplements for obtaining needed nutrients. Eating a varied, nutrient-dense diet that contains lots of complex carbohydrates (whole-grain breads and cereals, pasta, fruits, vegetables, and beans) helps to guarantee that you obtain all the vitamins and minerals you need in the right proportions. Calcium and iron have been found to be low in some athletes, so a regular consumption of low-fat foods that are high in calcium (low-fat dairy products, dark green vegetables, canned salmon, etc.) and iron (lean meats, dark green vegetables, dried fruit, etc.) is desirable.

2 | Staying Hydrated

Making the Water Bottle a Part of the Uniform

A number of years ago, I was asked to work with the football team at a major university. The coach for this team was as much of an institution as the university itself, and he had experienced enough success to keep the university alumni and administrators happy. However, he was beginning to feel the pressure of winning fewer and fewer games in recent years, and he started looking for ways to regain a competitive edge. The tradition in college football had been, for some time, to avoid drinking fluids during practice, a training regimen this well-seasoned coach followed. He believed it would make the players "tougher" and help players cope with games played on hot days. Football practices often last for more than three hours, and when the season is approaching, two-a-day practices are common. When I agreed to work with the team, much of my time was spent observing practices to determine where the best opportunities for nutritional intervention might occur. It became immediately and glaringly obvious to me that one of the major nutritional problems the football players were experiencing was inadequate fluid consumption, and I was sure this was negatively impacting any conditioning gains the players might get from practice. I was also concerned that *not* drinking fluids was a dangerous practice (every year there were publicized deaths among high school and college football players that were due to severe dehydration), particularly when I saw some salt tablets being passed around to the athletes. (Salt tablets are commonly given to people in hot environments, but should only be given with water. Salt is the major electrolyte in the blood and draws water from inside cells to normalize the blood electrolyte concentration. Salt without water leaves cells dehydrated and dangerously dysfunctional.)

At my first opportunity to share my concerns with the team coaches and athletes, I put the fluid issue at the top of my agenda. I started by saying, "I'm amazed to see the football players arriving at practice without being fully dressed." Of course, everyone looked at me with surprised expressions wondering what I had seen that they, who *were* the sport, had missed. I explained that, without their water bottles in hand, I considered the athletes *not* to be fully dressed and ready to practice. There was, of course, vigorous rebuttal, and it is absolutely critical to let everyone express their opinions about why they do the things they do. The basic argument in favor of *not* drinking boiled down to "tradition". "That's the way we did it when we were players," said the

73

coaches, "so that's what we do now." There was a belief that drinking fluids during practice would give the football players stomach cramps, which would make it more difficult for them to practice and run their drills. There was no evidence that this was the case, but it was a belief among the coaching staff. A less frequently expressed belief was that this dehydration strategy would help football players train their muscles to work effectively without fluids, so there was a benefit in having them practice without water. Supposedly, these trained muscles had the added benefit of allowing athletes to run faster and move more quickly because they were a bit lighter (because of less water weight). None of these arguments stand up to scientific scrutiny, but it was good to know that they weren't restricting fluids to be punitive!

After hearing their explanations, I explained that muscles were over 70 percent water and that they simply do not work efficiently when they are dehydrated. Further, trying to train muscles that have an inadequate water level simply meant that the potential benefits that can be derived from training are diminished. Muscle soreness, muscle pulls, and easy fatigue are also associated with insufficient water intake. After a lengthy discussion of this issue, we all left the meeting on friendly terms, but I still didn't know how they would utilize the information. At the next practice the following day, the crusty head coach approached me and told me to look closely because the players were now "fully dressed." And there they all were, walking onto the practice field with water bottles in hand.

All nutrients are important for performance, but water is often mentioned as critically important to performance because the performance deficits that a dehydrated athlete experiences occur quickly and are easily measured. The body's reliance on water for cooling, nutrient transport, joint lubrication, metabolic waste removal, digestion, and absorption are all clearly established, and dehydrated athletes simply don't perform as well as well-hydrated athletes, regardless of the sport. Studies have shown, however, that athletes tend to replace less fluid than that is lost in sweat, and this creates a gradual reduction in performance. There are several reasons for this, including drinking tradition in the sport, the lack of a timely thirst mechanism, fluid unavailability, or the availability of fluids that don't taste good to the exercising athlete. *All* of these factors can be overcome with training and planning and will go a long way toward sustaining the athlete's performance over the entire practice or competition.

No level of *low* body water is acceptable for achieving optimal athletic performance and endurance, so you should consider a strategy for *maintaining* optimal body water while you exercise. Imagine that you have a full glass of water that represents your body at a state of optimal hydration. When you're not exercising, it's like having a pinhole in the bottom of the glass. The water level will drop, but only at a very slow rate and at a pace that makes it easy for you to maintain an optimal hydration state. Because the water level drops so slowly, drinking an occasional glass of water or other fluid is an adequate means of maintaining your hydration state. Since 8 cups (8 × 8 ounces = 2 quarts, or about 1.5 liters) of water is a common recommendation for nonathletes, who have relatively low sweat rates, it makes sense to make a dramatic increase in the water requirement for athletes. An athlete working in a warm environment can lose 1.5 liters of water per hour! This is equivalent to putting a larger pencil hole in the bottom of the glass, so the rate of water loss is much faster. Within even a short period of time, there will be a significant amount of water loss that could be enough to affect exercise performance and endurance. Even minor reductions in hydration state can cause measurable reductions in performance, so the goal is to stay within 2 percent of your preexercise body weight. It doesn't matter if you're an aerobic athlete trying to go long distances, or an anaerobic athlete wanting to jump higher, go faster, or push better—losing more water than is replaced causes performance reductions and can be the difference between winning and losing.

Since water is being lost at a faster rate while exercising, an important strategy for avoiding a performance loss is, clearly, to replace water at a faster rate. If the frequency of drinking when not exercising is once every two hours, then imagine that the frequency of drinking during exercise should be once every 10 to 15 minutes. Water is lost so fast during exercise that it becomes difficult, if not impossible, to replace the amount of water being lost and virtually impossible to *increase* body water while exercising. Therefore, waiting too long between drinks is a bad strategy, since it allows body water to decrease in such a way that it cannot be adequately replaced. When you exercise, the water in the glass drops quickly, so all you can hope to do when you drink is keep the water level stable. If you wait to drink, you may be able to maintain the body's water level at its current state, but that state will be too low.

Where's the Water?

- Sixty-six percent of an athlete's total body weight is from water.[1]
- Thirty-seven percent of total body weight is from water inside cells.
- Twenty-four percent of total body weight is from water outside cells.
- Five percent of total body weight is from the water that makes up blood plasma.
- Well-hydrated muscles are about 75 percent water.
- Bones are about 32 percent water.
- Fat has very little water, about 10 percent.
- Blood is about 93 percent water.

Temperature Regulation and Water Balance

Physical activity creates heat, and this heat must be dissipated for the athlete to continue doing the activity. Failure to dissipate this heat will eventually lead to heatstroke and, potentially, death. One of the main mechanisms we have for dissipating heat is to produce sweat, which cools the body down as it evaporates off the skin. It should be obvious that the inability to produce sweat causes the body to overheat. The body has a finite storage capacity for water but continues to produce heat as physical work continues. Unless the water lost as sweat is replaced, the sweat rate will be reduced and body temperature will rise. Therefore, it is perfectly logical to suggest that athletes must drink enough fluids to sustain the sweat rate. It should be remembered that, even when not exercising, the body loses water through insensible (i.e., not noticed) perspiration. When you exercise, the rate of water loss increases and becomes sensible (i.e., noticed) perspiration.

Temperature regulation represents the balance between heat produced or received (heat-in), and heat removed (heat-out). When the body's temperature regulation system is working correctly, *heat-in* and *heat-out* are in perfect balance and body temperature is maintained. There are both internal and external factors that can contribute to body heat. Radiant heat from the sun contributes to body temperature, and the heat created from burning fuel also contributes to body temperature. Somehow, the body must find a way to dissipate the same amount of heat that has been added to maintain a constant body temperature.

We have two primary systems for dissipating or losing heat while at rest:

- Moving more blood to the skin to allow heat dissipation through radiation.
- Increasing the rate of sweat production.

These two systems account for about 85 percent of the heat lost when a person is at rest. Heat losses through *conduction* (the natural transmission of heat from a hotter body to the cooler air environment) and *convection* (heat transfer from tissue to the blood and through the skin) account for the remaining 15 percent of heat-out. During exercise, virtually *all* heat loss occurs via evaporation (sweat).

Both of these systems rely on maintenance of an adequate blood volume. When blood volume drops, the movement of blood to the skin is reduced and sweat production is also reduced, altering the balance between heat-in and heat-out. There is, however, competition for blood for metabolic and heat-releasing requirements. Working muscles demand more blood flow to deliver nutrients and to remove the by-products of burned fuel. However, at the very same time there is a need to shift blood away from the muscles and toward the skin to increase the sweat rate. With low blood volume, one or both of these systems fails, and there is a dramatic decrease in athletic performance. In fact, the maintenance of blood volume is so important for athletic performance that it is considered by many to be the primary indicator of whether an athlete is capable of continuing physical work at a high rate.

Energy metabolism is only about 20 to 25 percent efficient. This means that, of the energy consumed from food, only 20 to 25 percent can be converted to the mechanical energy of muscular work. The remaining 75 to 80 percent of the food energy that is burned is lost as heat. To a certain extent, that loss is a good thing, since humans are warm-blooded animals that require heat production to maintain body temperature at about 98.6° F. When the rate of energy burn goes up, however, the amount of heat added to the system is dramatically increased, so the heat-out systems must be turned up. In fact, heavy exercise can create heat production that is 20 times higher than the amount of heat produced at rest.[1] Without an efficient means to remove this excess heat, body temperature will rise quickly. The upper limit for human survival is about 110° F, only 11.5° F higher than normal body temperature. With the potential for body temperature to rise at the rate of about 1° F every 5 minutes, it is conceivable that a dehydrated exercising athlete could be at risk for heatstroke and death only 55 minutes after the initiation of exercise.

Let's put what can happen into real numbers. Imagine doing very mild exercise that burns 300 calories of energy during 30 minutes. If the muscles are 25 percent efficient, then 75 Calories are used for muscular work and 225 calories are lost as heat that must be dissipated to maintain body temperature. Now imagine working twice as hard over that same 30 minutes. That means 450 calories of heat would need to be dissipated over that same 30 minutes to maintain body temperature! In general, every milliliter of sweat can dissipate half a calorie. So over that 30 minutes, the body would lose 900 milliliters (almost 1 liter) of water. In one hour of high-intensity activity, approximately 1.8 liters of water would be lost. To complicate matters, now imagine working hard during a sunny, hot day when the heat of the sun is *added* to the heat produced from muscular work. On a humid day, water doesn't evaporate off the body as easily, so more sweat must be produced to get the same cooling effect. Now imagine how much water would be lost as sweat if you were working hard on a sunny, hot, and humid day. In these conditions, a person can easily lose one to two liters of fluid (via sweat) per hour. A well-trained athlete who is training in a hot and humid environment can lose over three liters of fluid per hour.[1]

Monitoring Fluid Balance During Training

Without water intake, the blood volume can quickly become reduced, sweat rates drop, and body heat rises quickly and dangerously—at the rate of approximately one degree Celsius every five to seven minutes. However, it's difficult to consume sufficient fluids during hard physical work, so athletes should have a plan of what to do. If an athlete loses one liter of water per hour, they should find a way to drink over four cups of water per hour. The athlete who loses two liters of water per hour needs to find a way to drink over eight cups of water per hour. Of course, it's difficult to know precisely how much water is being lost during activity, but there is a simple rule that will help an athlete estimate how much is lost and what to do. One liter of water weighs approximately two pounds, and one pint of water weighs approximately one pound. Knowing these weights allows athletes to estimate how much fluid should be consumed during activity. Do the following:

1. Write down what time it is just before the exercise session.
2. Write down body weight (preferably nude weight) in pounds.
3. Do the normal exercise and monitor how much fluid is consumed during the exercise period.
4. On the completion of exercise, calculate exercise time by subtracting ending time from beginning time.
5. Take off the sweaty clothing and towel dry.
6. Once completely dry, write down body weight (preferably nude weight) in pounds.
7. Calculate the amount of fluid you lost via sweat by subtracting your body weight at the end of exercise from your body weight at the beginning of exercise.
8. The amount of *extra* fluid that should be consumed is equivalent to one pint of fluid for each pound lost, provided in volumes that range from 2 to 5 ounces and in time intervals that range from 10 to 20 minutes. (Differences in the amount to drink and the frequency of drinking are related to the total amount of fluid that must be replaced. It's easiest to have the lowest amount with the least frequency [i.e., 2 ounces every 20 minutes], but you shouldn't go longer than 20 minutes without drinking something.)

For example, John weighs 160 pounds at the beginning of his two-hour football practice and drinks 1 pint (2 cups) of fluid during the practice. At the end of practice, John weighs 158 pounds, so he needs to figure out how to take in an additional 2 pints of water during the practice for a total of 3 pints (6 cups or 48 ounces) over two hours. There are 12 10-minute increments in two hours, so John has 12 opportunities to consume a total of 48 ounces of fluids if he chooses to drink some fluids once every 10 minutes. Forty-eight ounces divided by 12 equals 4 ounces of fluid (1/2 cup) every 10 minutes. If John can't tolerate drinking that much fluid during practice to begin with, then he should try "training" himself to drink that much by gradually increasing the fluid consumption over several weeks to achieve an equal pre- and postexercise weight. The main point is any fluid amount greater than the current amount consumed is beneficial if the athlete experiences weight loss during the activity.

In a 150-pound (about 70 kilograms) athlete, fluid loss can represent between 2 to 5 percent of body weight every hour. When you consider that a 3 percent loss of body weight (from water loss) is considered clinical dehydration, you can see how easily an athlete can become seriously dehydrated (see table 2.1).

All of this is made more complex by environmental conditions and the level of conditioning an athlete has. Better-conditioned athletes are better able to cool themselves because they have developed more efficient sweat systems. This allows better-conditioned athletes to perform longer, but it also requires that they consume more fluids. When the environment is hot and humid, water doesn't evaporate off the body easily, so it doesn't have a real cooling effect. (All that sweat-soaked clothing doesn't mean you're controlling body temperature, it just means you're sweating and losing water.) For sweat to have a cooling effect it must *evaporate* off the skin. On hot and humid days, the water on your skin doesn't evaporate easily into the air because the moisture content of the air is already high. There are several factors that affect the rate at which an athlete loses water through sweat. These include temperature, humidity, clothing, conditioning/training, and fluid balance.

- The higher the temperature, the more the athlete sweats.
- The higher the humidity, the more the athlete sweats, but with reduced cooling efficiency.
- Clothing that traps sweat against the skin (i.e., does not breathe) has a reduced cooling efficiency, so it forces the athlete to sweat more. Some new materials made for athletes actually wick sweat away from the skin to improve evaporative efficiency. Check with

Table 2.1 Rehydration Recommendations

Initial weight (lb)	Weight (lb) after 3% body weight loss	Amount of water (in pints) to replace to avoid the weight loss
75	72.75	2.25
100	97.00	3.00
125	121.25	3.75
150	145.50	4.50
175	169.75	5.25
200	197.00	6.00
225	219.25	6.75
250	242.50	7.50
275	264.75	8.25

your sports clothing outfitter for materials with these properties that are suitable for your sport or activity.

- Well-conditioned athletes can actually sweat more, so they have a better cooling potential. However, this higher sweat rate requires a greater during-exercise fluid consumption.
- The better the fluid balance, the more sweat potential there is. As the athlete becomes progressively dehydrated, the sweat rate is reduced and body temperature rises. This is a problem, since fluid consumption during activity is rarely greater than two cups per hour, or only 30 to 40 percent of the amount of fluid lost in sweat. This level of rehydration inevitably leads to the athlete becoming dehydrated.

There are also several factors that affect fluid intake, and the rate at which fluid leaves the stomach and goes into the intestine. The two main factors influencing fluid intake are thirst and taste. Interestingly, most athletes induce a voluntary dehydration in themselves because they do not drink enough, even though there are plenty of drinks around them. It is likely, however, that athletes don't drink enough to maintain their hydration state simply because they are not thirsty. The thirst sensation, therefore, should not be considered an appropriate indicator of the need for fluids in athletes.[2] In fact, the thirst sensation could be considered delayed in athletes because it doesn't appear until an athlete has already lost 1.5 to 2.0 liters of water. There is no hope that an athlete could return to an adequately hydrated state during exercise if fluid consumption began at the same time the thirst sensation occurred. This apparent delay in the thirst mechanism is a good reason for athletes to train themselves to consume fluids on a schedule, whether they feel thirsty or not.

The appeal of a beverage is another important factor in whether it will be consumed. Color, taste, odor, temperature, and mouth feel all play a role in determining if the beverage will be considered desirable and whether it will be consumed. In general, it appears that athletes prefer cool beverages with a slightly sweet flavor. Heavily sweetened beverages of around a 12 percent carbohydrate solution, like soda or fruit juice, are not as widely tolerated during exercise as beverages with a 6 or 7 percent carbohydrate solution like Gatorade.[3,4] Interestingly, when not exercising, the reverse may be true. This points to an interesting phenomenon of exercise: food and drink taste differently while exercising than when not exercising. Given the extensive research on the benefits of consuming a sports drink with a 6 to 7 percent carbohydrate solution, regardless of whether the activity lasts half an hour or longer than four hours, there is no question that athletes should get into the habit of drinking a sports beverage rather than water. Consumption of sports beverages results in better performance than water whether you do sprints or endurance work.

Factors Affecting Gastric Emptying

A number of factors influence the rate at which fluids leave the stomach, but before these are reviewed, it's important to understand what slow or fast gastric emptying really means. When a food or drink is described as having a slower gastric emptying, it doesn't mean that *all* of the food stays in the stomach longer. It means that the food or drink trickles out of the stomach and into the intestines more slowly, so *some* of the food or drink is in the stomach longer. *Gastric emptying,* therefore, describes the volume of food or drink that leaves the stomach per unit of time. Since athletes are more comfortable exercising without an extensive amount of food or fluid in the stomach, a beverage that leaves the stomach more quickly (i.e., has a fast gastric emptying property) is considered desirable. In addition, fast gastric emptying offers the possibility for a faster delivery of energy and water to working muscles by more quickly presenting substances to the intestines for absorption.

Carbohydrate Concentration of the Solution

When the concentration of carbohydrate in a fluid rises above 7 percent, the gastric emptying time is slower. At concentrations below 7 percent carbohydrate, gastric emptying time is hardly affected.[5] This is one of the reasons why the recommended carbohydrate concentration in sports beverages is below 8 percent.

Type of Carbohydrate in the Solution

Carbohydrates come in different molecular sizes and in different molecular combinations. For instance, glucose is a monosaccharide (a single-molecule carbohydrate), sucrose is a disaccharide (two monosaccharides held together with a bond), and starch is a polysaccharide (many molecules of monosaccharides held together with bonds). The smaller the length of a carbohydrate chain is, the slower the gastric emptying time. Therefore, pure glucose (a monosaccharide) takes longer to leave the stomach than table sugar (a disaccharide), and table sugar takes longer to leave the stomach than a simple starch (a polysaccharide). The size of the sugar particle is so important that even if two beverages have the same carbohydrate concentration, the beverage with smaller carbohydrate molecules will take longer to leave the stomach than the beverage with larger carbohydrate molecules.[6]

Amount of Solution That Has Been Consumed

The amount of fluid that is consumed at one time has a major influence on gastric emptying time. When a large volume of fluid is consumed, gastric emptying time is initially faster. When the volume of fluid in the stomach is reduced, gastric emptying time slows. This suggests that, to become more quickly hydrated prior to competition or practice, a relatively large volume of fluid should be consumed (approximately half a liter), followed by frequent sipping of fluid to maintain the fluid volume in the stomach and, therefore, a faster gastric emptying time.[7]

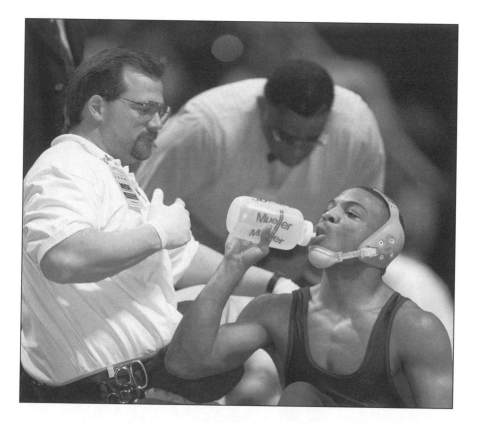

Temperature of the Solution

Most studies indicate that the solution temperature only slightly affects gastric emptying time. When people are at rest, fluids at body temperature leave the stomach more quickly than either very hot or very cold fluids.[8] There is evidence that, during exercise, cool fluids leave the stomach more quickly than room temperature or body temperature fluids.[9]

Carbonation of the Solution

While there are many athletes who believe that consuming a carbonated beverage will cause gastric distress and delayed gastric emptying (the first sports beverage was probably a "defizzed" cola), there is little scientific evidence that this occurs. However, the studies that have evaluated the impact of fluid carbonation on gastric emptying time have typically relied on few subjects. In general, the studies suggest that, all other things being equal (carbohydrate concentration, volume, temperature, etc.), carbonation has little impact on gastric emptying.[10,11]

State of Hydration or Dehydration of the Athlete

With the increasing dehydration and higher body temperatures associated with high-intensity activity, the rate of gastric emptying slows.[12] This is an excellent reason for athletes to try, as much as possible, to maintain their hydration state during activity. Allowing dehydration to occur makes it almost impossible for the athlete to return to an adequately hydrated state during exercise. If such hydration is attempted through consumption of a large volume of fluid, it will likely add to a sense of discomfort rather than faster rehydration.

Degree to Which the Athlete Is Mentally Stressed

The mental stress and anxiety associated with athletic competition are major factors in gastric emptying. Higher levels of mental stress and anxiety are associated with a reduced gastric emptying that can have a serious impact on the athlete's ability to adequately rehydrate during competition.[13,14] Obviously, the mental training techniques that may be learned from a sports psychologist to reduce stress are an important strategy for reducing the physiological effects of sports-related stress and anxiety.

Type of Activity the Athlete Is Doing

Studies have suggested that high-intensity activity is associated with a slower gastric emptying rate than lower-intensity activity, but the differences appear to be minor. In addition, the type of activity (running, swimming, cycling, etc.) does not appear to have a large influence on gastric emptying rate.[15]

Athlete Conditioning and Adaptation

The human body has wonderful adaptive mechanisms, and the ability to adapt to higher or lower glucose concentrations, and faster or slower rates of fluid ingestion, are no exception. To a certain extent, athletes can find a system for optimal rehydration that suits them best by consistently practicing that system. Practicing a reasonable system allows the body to adapt to it and reduce the chance of any difficulties that could arise from trying something new just before an important competition. Therefore, it is important for athletes to start with general recommendations for fluid intake to maintain their hydration state, but to make modifications that are best suited to their own individual circumstances.

Intestinal Absorption

Once the solution (fluid) leaves the stomach and goes into the small intestine, the water and carbohydrate that make up the solution must be absorbed into the blood. The main factor that influences the speed with which water and carbohydrate are absorbed is the concentration of carbohydrate in the solution that enters the intestines.[16] A solution that has a slightly lower concentration of carbohydrate and electrolytes, relative to the concentration of plasma, causes a faster absorption of water than a solution that has either a much higher or a much lower concentration.[17] Consumption of highly concentrated carbohydrate solutions during exercise may cause a temporary shift of fluids away from the muscles and into the intestines to dilute the solution prior to absorption. This would have a negative impact on both muscle function and sweat rates since it would cause, at least temporarily, a shift of water away from muscle to cause tissue dehydration.

Preexercise Fluid Considerations

The purpose of this section is to let the athlete and coach know how important it is for the athlete to be in a state of optimal hydration before the initiation of exercise or competition. If a single factor can be pointed to that, by itself, may make the difference between a good training session and a bad one, and a good competition and a bad one, it is this. All the evidence suggests that even a minor level of underhydration (as little as 2 percent of body weight) can cause a measurable difference in endurance and performance, and the greater the underhydration the greater the negative impact on endurance and performance.[18,19] Furthermore, it can take 24 hours or longer to bring a dehydrated athlete back to a well-hydrated state. Therefore, waiting until just before practice or competition to bring an athlete to a well-hydrated state, or simply failing to take any steps to make certain the athlete is in an optimally hydrated state, will doom that athlete to having a poor practice or competition performance.

Of course, there are sports where athletes are trying to have a particular "look" or trying to make a particular weight. The classic body profile in rhythmic gymnastics is to have long graceful lines with, essentially, no secondary sexual characteristics. It is common for rhythmic gymnasts to restrict water intake before a competition because they think it will help to give them the desired (but in my mind "cadaverous") look. Wrestlers have a well-established regimen for fluid restriction to try to achieve a particular weight class. Then they have about 24 hours to rehydrate themselves before the competition. Besides the inherent health dangers of doing this (there are well-documented deaths associated with this strategy), it is unlikely that dehydrated wrestlers would be able to adequately rehydrate themselves in just 24 hours. Therefore, performance is likely to be affected. Other than the desire to "make weight," there is no reason to want to quickly reduce body water, and there is certainly no safe way to do this. If excessive water retention is a concern (which it may well be for wrestlers and bodybuilders), then athletes should avoid consuming foods that are excessively salty for several days leading up to the event.

There are some athletes on the other side of the continuum who try to "superhydrate" with water before exercise. Long-distance runners, whose water loss during the competition is likely to be greater than their ability to replace it, typically do this. The runner with the best hydration state at the end of the competition will have a major advantage over less well-hydrated competitors. When athletes constantly superhydrate, they may develop a greater blood (plasma) volume with resultant lower core temperatures and heart rates during activity.[20,21] All of these values suggest the potential for improved endurance and performance. Consumption of large fluid volumes is also associated with frequent urination, but this may be mediated to a degree by consumption of sodium-containing fluids.[22]

Glycerol (a simple three-carbon lipid that is metabolized like a carbohydrate) has been used by some athletes to aid superhydration because it acts like a humectant (i.e., it attracts water). There is some limited evidence that adding glycerol to pre-exercise fluids at the rate of one gram per kilogram of body weight will improve endurance performance in hot and humid environments. This improvement occurs because glycerol enables the retention of more of the

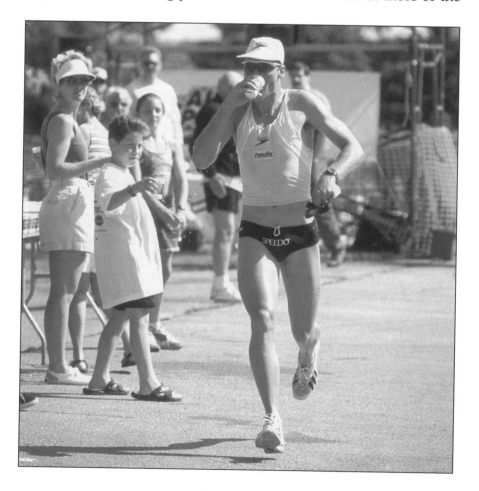

consumed fluids.[23,24] However, individual athletes respond to this protocol differently. Some athletes find that superhydrating with glycerol makes them feel stiff and uncomfortable, while others are more comfortable with this sensation.[25] See chapter 4 for more on glycerol.

In general, athletes should follow these hydration guidelines before exercise:

• The sensation of thirst should *not* be relied on as an indicator of fluid need. Thirst should be considered an "emergency" sensation that occurs when the body has already lost 1.5 to 2.0 liters of water. During exercise, the thirst sensation may be delayed, so the exercising athlete may require more water loss before the sensation of thirst occurs.

• Athletes should become accustomed to consuming fluids *without* the thirst sensation. As a practical matter, this is made easier if athletes carry water with them all the time, wherever they are and wherever they go. Fluid consumption is much more likely to occur if the water is there than if you have to go looking for it, especially if the athlete doesn't *feel* thirsty.

• Enough fluid should be consumed prior to exercise that the athlete produces urine that is clear. Clear urine is a good sign that the athlete is well hydrated and producing a dilute, large-volume urine. Dark urine is a sign that the athlete is producing a low-volume concentrated urine, which suggests that the body needs to retain as much fluid as possible because it is underhydrated.

• Approximately 1 to 1.5 hours prior to exercise the athlete should consume a large volume of fluid (up to half a liter) to assure adequate hydration and to improve gastric emptying. Following this, athletes should sip on fluids (approximately half a cup every 10 minutes) to maintain their hydration state before exercise or competition begins. Athletes should consume fluid as frequently and in as high a volume as can be tolerated to replace water losses.

• Athletes seeking to superhydrate should be very careful *not* to try this technique without careful monitoring, especially if they are superhydrating using glycerol. *Individuals who have cardiovascular systems that are not in perfect condition should never attempt this.* As a practical matter, the safest way to superhydrate is to consume fluids frequently.

• Avoid foods and drinks that may have a diuretic (water-losing) impact. For instance, caffeine and related substances commonly found in coffee, tea, chocolate, and sodas cause an increase in the rate at which water is lost. Therefore, these substances are counterproductive in terms of optimizing the hydration state before exercise.

Fluid Considerations During Exercise

When athletes consume fluids during exercise there are clear benefits that occur, including a better maintenance of exercise performance and a slowing of the exercise-induced rise in heart rate and body temperature (see figures 2.1 and 2.2). In addition, there is an improvement or maintenance of blood flow to the skin. The degree to which the cardiovascular and heat maintenance capacity is maintained is directly related to the degree to which dehydration can be avoided. It is clear that a failure to consume sufficient fluids during exercise is a major risk factor in the onset of heat exhaustion.[26] It is also clear that the best strategy for athletes to follow, to avoid heat exhaustion and maintain athletic performance, is to consume fluids during exercise.[27-29]

Most studies that have evaluated the interaction between hydration adequacy and athletic performance have used either plain water

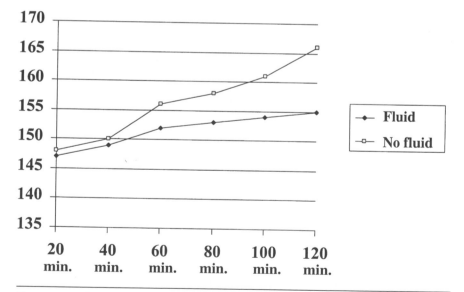

Figure 2.1 Comparison of heart rate in athletes consuming fluids and not consuming fluids during exercise.

Adapted from Hargreaves 1996.

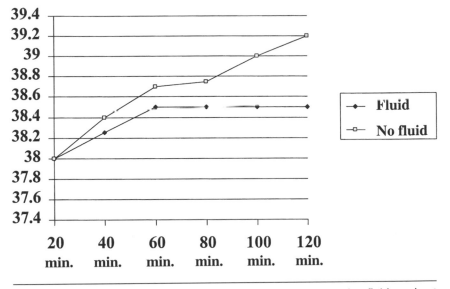

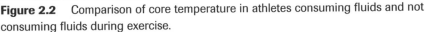

Figure 2.2   Comparison of core temperature in athletes consuming fluids and not consuming fluids during exercise.

Adapted from Hargreaves 1996.

or sports beverages that contain, in differing degrees, carbohydrates and electrolytes (see table 2.2). The results of these studies are similar in confirming the importance of fluid consumption during exercise. However, the inclusion of carbohydrates and electrolytes in the fluids affords the athlete certain advantages over plain water. Recent studies suggest that including carbohydrates in the rehydration solution improves both the athlete's ability to maintain or increase work output during exercise and increases the time to exhaustion.[30-33] This occurs because consumed carbohydrates help to avoid the depletion of muscle glycogen and provide a fuel to muscles when muscle glycogen is low.

Different activities result in different types of carbohydrate utilization, but in each case consuming a carbohydrate-containing fluid helps to maintain athletic performance. For instance, in strenuous cycling the rate of muscle glycogen use is not affected when a carbohydrate solution is used.[34] In long-distance running, there is a reduction in the rate of muscle glycogen usage when a carbohydrate-containing fluid is consumed.[35] And in stop-go intermittent exercise, there is a reduction in muscle glycogen usage when a carbohydrate-containing fluid is consumed.[36,37] In each of these scenarios, carbohydrate depletion is generally considered to be the

Table 2.2 Carbohydrate and Electrolyte Content of Common Sports Beverages

Beverage	Carbohydrate type	Carbohydrate concentration (%)	Sodium (mg) per 8oz serving	Potassium (mg) per 8 oz serving
10-K (Beverage Products, Inc.)	Sucrose, glucose, and fructose	6.3	52	26
AllSport (Pepsi-Cola Co.)	High fructose corn syrup	8-9	55	25
Body Fuel 450 (Vitex Foods, Inc.)	Maltodextrin and fructose	4.2	80	20
Cytomax	Fructose corn syrup and sucrose	7-11	10	150
Everlast	Sucrose and fructose	6	100	20
Exceed (Ross Laboratories)	Glucose polymer and fructose	7.2	50	45
Gatorade (Quaker Oats Co.)	Sucrose and glucose	6	110	25
Hydra Charge	Maltodextrin and fructose	8		Trace
Hydra Fuel	Glucose polymers, fructose, glucose	7	25	50
Powerade (Coca-Cola Co.)	High fructose corn syrup and maltodextrin	8	73	33
PowerBurst (PowerBurst Corp.)	Fructose	6.0	35	55
Quickick (Cramer Products, Inc.)	Glucose	2.5	80	25
SportaLyte	Maltodextrin, fructose, and glucose	7.5	100	60
Sqwincher (Universal Products, Inc.)	Glucose and fructose	6.8	60	36

Compared with soda and orange juice

Beverage	Carbohydrate type	Carbohydrate concentration (%)	Sodium (mg) per 8oz serving	Potassium (mg) per 8 oz serving
Coca-Cola	High fructose corn syrup	11	9.2	Trace
Orange juice	Fructose and sucrose	11-15	2.7	510

Performance Benefits of Water and Carbohydrate

- 6.7 percent improved performance with large volume of fluid compared to ingestion of small volume of fluid[38]
- 6.3 percent improved performance with ingestion of carbohydrate compared to no carbohydrate
- 12.4 percent improved performance with combination of large fluid volume with carbohydrate compared to small volume of fluid without carbohydrate

Based on 50 minutes of exercise at 80 percent $\dot{V}O_2$max

cause of performance degradation. However, there is good evidence that consuming a carbohydrate-containing beverage may also be important for improving athletic performance in high-intensity activities where carbohydrate is not expected to be depleted because of the relatively short duration of the activity.[39-41]

These data all suggest that athletes should become accustomed to consuming a carbohydrate-containing fluid during exercise. See table 2.3 for opportunities for replacing fluids in different sports. However, the concentration of carbohydrate and the type of carbohydrate are important considerations. There appear to be no major differences among glucose, sucrose, maltodextrins, and starch (all different types of carbohydrates) on exercise performance.[42-44] (See table 2.2.) Beverages that rely solely on fructose for carbohydrates, however, may cause intestinal distress and may not be quickly absorbed.[45,46] Maltodextrins are less sweet than sucrose and fructose, so they may be used to add carbohydrate energy to solutions without making them unpalatably sweet tasting.[47] In any case, carbohydrate energy, regardless of whether it is in liquid or solid form and almost regardless of the type of carbohydrate, will aid athletic performance.[48] However, since providing carbohydrates in liquid form allows the athlete to take care of two issues at once (energy and fluid), liquids that contain carbohydrates are preferred.

The amount of carbohydrate to be provided during exercise is important to consider, since providing too much too fast may induce gastrointestinal distress and, at least temporarily, take needed fluids away from muscle and skin to dilute this excessively concentrated solution. On the other hand, providing a fluid that has just a scant amount of carbohydrate in it may lend no performance benefit. In general, athletes should strive to consume about one gram of carbohydrate per minute of exercise. This level of intake can be achieved

Table 2.3 Opportunities for Fluid Replacement in Different Sports During Competitions

Event and duration	Opportunities for fluid breaks	Fluid and carbohydrate requirements
Events lasting less than 30 minutes • Sprints • Jumping • Throwing • Gymnastics	Consumption of fluids between events, but no fluids consumed within 15 minutes of event.	Not needed during the event, but required between events during the course of the entire competition.
Intermediate events lasting less than 1 hour • 10-kilometer run • Rowing • Aerobics class • Tennis lesson • Track cycling	Consumption of fluids between events. Runners should consume some fluid at least every 5 kilometers (more often if hot and humid). All athletes in this category should bring beverage container.	Fluid replacement is needed before, during, and after event, and carbohydrate is needed before and after event. However, carbohydrate will aid fluid uptake during event, so beverages should contain carbohydrate.
Endurance events • Marathon • 80-kilometer cycling • Olympic distance triathlon • 5 sets of tennis	Marathon runners should consume some fluid at least every 5 kilometers (more often if hot and humid). Triathletes should consume fluids every 10 kilometers during cycling and every 2 to 4 kilometers during running. Tennis players should take as much time as allowable during court changes and after 3rd set to take fluids.	Fluids, electrolytes (sodium), and carbohydrate replacement are all recommended during these events. The amounts needed will vary based on environmental conditions, initial glycogen stores, and exercise intensity (i.e., difficulty of the match).

(continued)

Table 2.3   *(continued)*

Event and duration	Opportunities for fluid breaks	Fluid and carbohydrate requirements
Ultraendurance events • Ironman • English channel swim • Road cycling • Stage races such as Tour de France	Consumption of fluids at every opportunity, with a plan to consume fluids once every 10 minutes. Where fluids are not made available by race organizers (as may occur with cycling races), a fluid consumption plan with carried fluids must be in place.	Fluids, electrolytes (sodium), and carbohydrate replacement are all recommended during these events. The amounts needed will vary based on environmental conditions, initial glycogen stores, and exercise intensity.
Team sports lasting around 90 minutes • Hockey • Basketball • Football • Volleyball • Baseball • Soccer	Plan to consume fluids at breaks that naturally occur, but no less frequently than once every 15 minutes. Ideally, fluids should be consumed every 10 minutes. Naturally occurring longer breaks (half-time, between innings, between quarters, etc.) should be considered an opportunity to replenish fluids.	Fluids, electrolytes (sodium), and carbohydrate replacement are all recommended during these events. The amounts needed will vary based on environmental conditions, initial glycogen stores, and exercise intensity.

Adapted from O'Connor 1996.

by consuming solutions that contain between 4 percent and 8 percent carbohydrate, at a volume of .6 to 1.2 liters per hour.[49,50] Some sports beverages have carbohydrates precisely within this range, while others have higher concentrations (see table 2.2). Higher concentrations, however, may cause a delay in gastric emptying and do not necessarily lead to a faster or better carbohydrate metabolism during exercise.[51] Another real advantage of consuming a 4 to 8 percent carbohydrate solution is that it has a faster rate of intestinal absorption than water alone. This means that fluid status can be more efficiently maintained and the delivery of carbohydrate to the blood and muscles is enhanced. If you know of anyone who's ever had a baby with diarrhea, you know that physicians commonly prescribe Pedialyte (sugar water) because it delivers water faster than water alone and can more quickly rehydrate the baby. This effect, apparently, does not change with age.

Above all, remember these important considerations:

• Have fluids closely available to consume during the exercise. These should preferably be cool and have a flavor that you enjoy drinking while you exercise.

• Avoid sharing your drinking container with others since this is a terrific way to make the entire team (or all your sports mates) sick.

• Drink on a fixed schedule, whether you're thirsty or not. The goal is to *avoid* thirst.

• Monitor your fluid intake adequacy by checking your pre- and postexercise weight, as covered earlier in this chapter.

Postexercise Fluid Considerations

It is very likely that athletes who have exercised intensely for half an hour or longer will experience some degree of underhydration. For those athletes who exercise every day or most days (i.e., most elite athletes), postexercise fluid consumption becomes a critically important part of the exercise regimen because it allows the athlete to begin each subsequent day of activity in a well-hydrated state. The important point to consider is that it takes time to rehydrate muscles. The less time there is to rehydrate, the lower the likelihood that the athlete will be capable of becoming optimally hydrated by the beginning of the next exercise session.

At best, athletes consume fluids during exercise at a rate of only up to 70 percent of fluid loss via sweat, but most athletes replace sweat losses at a rate significantly less than this.[52,53] Therefore, it is likely that athletes will need to be adequately rehydrated before the next exercise session begins. In spite of this clear need for fluids, athletes are known to remain in an underhydrated state even when fluids are made available to them.[54] This "voluntary dehydration" suggests that athletes should be placed on a fixed fluid replacement schedule that will decrease the degree to which this dehydration is maintained. A way of encouraging this is to make certain that good-tasting fluids are easily available to the athlete as soon as the exercise session is over.[55]

There is some evidence that commercial sports drinks that contain both carbohydrate and sodium are more effective at restoring water balance than plain water.[56] It appears, however, that to maximize rehydration a level of sodium greater than that provided in most sports drinks is desirable.[57] This added sodium can be obtained through the normal consumption of foods, many of which have added salt (sodium).[58] This is one case where lowering the intake of salt or consuming salt-free foods would not be beneficial.

In general, athletes should follow these rules for fluid consumption following exercise:

• A large volume of fluid (as much as can be tolerated, perhaps a half liter) should be consumed immediately following exercise. This large fluid volume enlarges the stomach and increases the rate at which fluids leave the stomach and enter the small intestine to become absorbed.

• Following the initial consumption of a large fluid volume, athletes should consume approximately a quarter liter of fluid every 15 minutes, to achieve a fluid intake of approximately three liters of fluid in three hours. The larger the athlete and the greater the sweat loss experienced during activity, the greater the amount of fluid that must be consumed.

• Fluids should contain both carbohydrate and sodium, since both are useful in returning the athlete to a well-hydrated state. In addition, the carbohydrate content of the beverage helps in returning stored glycogen (energy) to muscles in preparation for the next exercise session.

• Sports drinks typically provide approximately 10 to 25 millimoles of electrolytes (mainly sodium) per liter of fluid. However, the optimal sodium concentration for fluid retention is approximately 50 millimoles of electrolytes per liter of fluid.[59] Since adding more sodium to fluids may make the fluid unpalatable and cause the athlete to consume less fluid, the athlete should be encouraged to consume some lightly salted snacks (such as pretzels or saltine crackers) during the period immediately following the exercise.

• The loss in body weight that results from exercise should be the key to determining the total amount of fluid that must be replaced before the next exercise session. As a general guide, one pint of *retained* fluid is equal to one pound of body weight. Since not all consumed water is retained, twice as much fluid may need to be consumed than the fluid equivalent to weight loss.

• Fluids and foods containing caffeine and related substances (coffee, tea, colas, chocolate, etc.) should be avoided since they increase urinary water loss.

Summary

There is perhaps no other factor that so clearly impacts on performance than hydration state. Most athletes, regardless of the sport, could gain an *immediate* performance benefit by taking steps to assure that physical activity begins, continues, and ends with body water at an optimal level. To do this, athletes should train themselves to drink fluids on a fixed schedule rather than by relying on thirst as the only stimulus to drinking. Since the thirst mechanism doesn't occur until the athlete has already lost a substantial amount of water (about 1.5 liters), reliance on thirst guarantees that the athlete will perform in an underhydrated state, and performance *will* be negatively affected. Well-formulated sports beverages that contain a small amount of electrolytes (sodium and potassium) and carbohydrate (6 to 7 percent carbohydrate solution is optimal) have been found to encourage fast absorption, so they can replace both needed water and fuel quickly. Athletes should find a good sports beverage that tastes good while they are physically active and consume enough to maintain body weight during exercise. Entering physical activity in a well-hydrated state is important, since improving hydration status while exercising is impossible (water is lost at such a fast rate that the athlete can only hope to *maintain*, but not increase, body water during exercise). This is easiest if the athlete has a good source of water or other fluid easily available. Many athletes carry around a liter bottle of water or sports beverage with them wherever they go. After exercise is completed, the athlete should continue to drink to replace any amount of fluid that was unreplaced during the exercise. In summary, the athlete should drink before, during, and after exercise with the confidence of knowing this strategy is critically important to performance.

3 Assessing Body Composition

Lean as Can Be But All You See Is Fat

Imagine a talented athlete at the peak of her competitive life. This was an Olympian who was just a hair's width behind the best person on the swim team, and someone who was willing to do anything to make that place hers. Of course, everyone has an inherited physique, and this powerhouse clearly had inherited all the qualities (both good and not-so-good) of her genetic donors. She was on the short side of small and had a block house figure. Nevertheless, while swimming her laps, there was no one better to look at: great strokes, perfect flip turns, powerful starts off the blocks, a rocket finish—and it all came together to make her one of the best. However, despite her national and international competitive successes, she still wasn't considered the best this country had to offer, and this ate away at her psyche like nothing else could. When I say that she tried everything in her arsenal to get better, I mean just that. She spent more hours practicing; she became more careful about what she ate; and she began bugging her coach for more ideas on how to improve every part of the stroke, even if the resultant improvement would be incrementally miniscule.

Ultimately, she became so unhappy with herself (mind you, this is one of the top swimmers in the world) that she found fault with her appearance. "If only I were leaner . . . " and "If only I had less fat . . . " were common interjections in her conversations. It was as if everything ultimately boiled down to a simple equation that said, "less fat equals improved speed." But when you have someone who, for her sport, is already in the 10th percentile for body fat percent, it's hard to imagine that having less fat would cause a competitive improvement. (In fact, swimmers may find that the reduction in buoyancy associated with too little fat can actually increase drag and reduce speed.) Nevertheless, she began seeing herself as fat and took the only dramatic action she could think of—dieting to the point of starvation—to make herself seem less fat. An eating disorder, regardless of how it rears its ugly head, is never an attractive proposition. For an athlete trying desperately to do anything to gain a fraction of a second, an eating disorder can be disastrous.

As part of our regular evaluations, we noticed that all the swimmers in the lab were comfortably walking around in their swimsuits or in gym shorts and T-shirts—all of them except the swimmer in question. She had on two sweatshirts, gym pants, and a jacket and was still shivering. We knew right away we had a problem on our hands, but we also knew we had to document what was going on. As we suspected, she had lost weight and was, therefore, "smaller." However, she had lost more weight from her lean body mass (muscle) than from her fat mass, so she was less able to move her body weight than before (strength-to-weight ratio is critically important in all sports). In fact, she lost in muscle the equivalent muscle weight represented in one entire arm. When we spoke to her coach to see if he had any concerns, he immediately blurted out that she had become impossible to work with. Her starts were short, her turns had deteriorated, and she no longer had a killer finish. All the strength and skills that were at the core of her successes had virtually disappeared. Her coach was ready to increase her training schedule (even though she was already spending more hours in the pool and weight room than anyone else) because he couldn't see how she could compete in the next big competition given her state of unreadiness. Of course, there was no way she could continue to do even what she was now doing, so increasing her training schedule would have been impossible.

When we reviewed her diet, it became clear that she was trying to cover up her eating disorder. It would have been impossible for her to have eaten what she reported she ate (barring a clinical malabsorption disorder) and have lost so much weight. When I became convinced that we really had a serious problem on our hands, I took the only action I knew to take. I convinced her coach to remove her from the team until she presented him with a letter, from a psychiatrist trained to work with eating disorders, clearly stating that her continued participation in competitive swimming would not place her at risk for an eating disorder. In other words, if she wanted to come back, she had to change what she was doing, and she had to convince an appropriate medical professional that this change would not be altered if she returned to swimming. This strategy was not easy to initiate, and it was devastating for the athlete. Imagine trying all your life to be on a team, succeeding in getting on that team, and then being taken off the team because you were trying anything (albeit wrongly) to be more competitive.

Fortunately, this story has a happy ending. She did it. She went home, went to counseling, learned what she needed to do, accepted her physique as it was, ate better, trained smarter, got her OK letter from her physician, and became a star. If you've watched swimming competitions, you've seen her swim and succeed.

The body is composed of different components (water, muscle, fat, bone, nerve tissue, tendons, etc.), and each has a different density. From a functional standpoint, tissues are grouped together into those that are mainly fat (*fat mass*), which has little water associated with it, and those that have little fat (fat-free mass), which has a great deal of water associated with it. The fat-free mass is also commonly referred to as *lean mass*, although this is a troubling term for many, because the fat-free mass includes a great deal of water (greater than 65 percent). More recently, because of new techniques and improvements in estimating body composition, bone mass or skeletal mass has been included as a third commonly assessed component of body composition. But for the purpose of this book, the components of body composition generally are referred to as fat mass (the amount of tissue in the body that is mainly fat) and lean mass (the amount of tissue in the body that is mainly free of fat).

The fat mass is composed of *essential fat* and *storage fat*. The essential fat is a required component of the brain, nerves, bone marrow, heart tissue, and cell walls that we cannot live without. Adult females are predicted to have approximately 12 to 15 percent of total body weight as essential fat. The majority of this fat is associated with reproduction and includes the additional fat associated with breast tissue. Because males do not have this reproductive function, essential fat in males is approximately 3 percent of total body weight. Storage fat, on the other hand, is an energy reserve that builds up in fat (adipose) cells underneath the skin (subcutaneous fat) and around the organs (interabdominal fat). It is normal for men and women to have approximately 11 to 15 percent of total body weight from storage fat. Combining the essential fat and storage fat compartments, normal body fat percent for males is approximately 15 percent (3 percent essential; 12 percent storage), while normal body fat percent for females is 26 percent (15 percent essential; 11 percent storage).[1]

Women with extremely low body fat percent are at risk for developing reproductive system problems. This commonly manifests itself as irregular menstrual periods. Oligomenorrhea (infrequent menses) and amenorrhea (cessation of menses) are associated with low estrogen production, which increases the risk of osteoporosis (a bone disease associated with low bone density), and increased fracture risk. It appears that a body fat percent of 17 percent to 22 percent is needed to maintain a normal menstrual cycle in most women.[2] Women who develop an excessively low body fat percent typically exercise excessively for the amount of energy they consume, or have an eating disorder. The "female athlete triad" is a condition that has recently been described as prevalent in many female athletes, and includes the interrelated presence of an eating disorder, amenorrhea, and low bone density.

Lean mass is mainly water and protein, but also includes small levels of minerals and stored carbohydrate (glycogen). The main constituents of the fat-free mass include skeletal muscle, the heart, and other organs. While total body weight is approximately 60 percent water, the water content (by weight) of the fat-free mass is 70 percent. This can be compared to the water content of the fat mass, which is below 10 percent water.[3] Athletes typically have a larger lean mass and a lower fat mass than nonathletes do, so well-hydrated athletes have a higher proportion of total weight that comes from water.

Using the "fat mass-lean mass" model of body composition, the combined weight of fat mass and lean mass equals total body weight. However, weight by itself does not discriminate between the two components, so it is considered to be an inappropriate measure of body composition. Therefore, the statement "My weight is increasing, so I must be getting fat," is common but incorrect. It is quite possible for an athlete to increase the lean (i.e., muscle) mass without increasing the fat mass. Clearly, there would be an increase in weight, but not fat weight. It is also possible for an athlete to maintain weight but experience changes in fat or lean mass. This could be either desirable or undesirable depending on which element is increasing. A high strength-to-weight ratio shows an increase in lean mass (strength) with a maintenance or lowering of fat mass (weight) equaling total weight. This scenario is obviously desirable. However, should an athlete increase the fat mass, strength is lost and the strength relative to weight ratio decreases or islow. Assessing these aspects of body composition has become a standard tool for the evaluation of body changes that occur as a result of time, training, and nutritional factors.

Body composition assessment generally results in obtaining a value referred to as *body fat percent,* or the proportion of total weight that is made up by the fat mass. Let's assume an athlete weighs 150 pounds and has a body fat percent of 20 percent. This means that 30 pounds ($150 \times .20 = 30$) is fat weight and 120 pounds is fat-free (i.e., lean) weight. If this athlete experiences a reduction in body fat percent to 15 percent while maintaining weight, this would mean that 22.5 pounds ($150 \times .15 = 22.5$) is fat weight and 127.5 pounds is lean weight. This increase of 7.5 pounds in lean weight and reduction in fat weight means the athlete is now smaller (pound for pound, lean mass takes up less space than fat mass because it has a higher density), which means the athlete should be able to move more quickly and more efficiently (less drag) than before. However, if this 150-pound athlete were to maintain weight but increase fat mass while reducing the lean mass, potential speed and efficiency of movement would be reduced. Therefore, *weight is a poor measure for predicting athletic success*. This example also emphasizes the importance of looking at changes that occur in both the lean and fat mass, since understanding changes in both compartments is necessary to understand the potential impact on performance.

Purpose of Body Composition Assessment

The purpose of body composition assessment is to determine the athlete's distribution of lean (muscle) mass and fat mass. A high lean-mass-to-fat-mass ratio is often synonymous with a high strength-to-weight ratio, which is typically associated with athletic success. However, there is no single ideal body composition for all athletes in all sports. Each sport has a range of lean mass and fat mass associated with it, and each athlete in a sport has an individual range that is ideal for him or her. Athletes who try to achieve an arbitrary body composition that is not right for them are likely to place themselves at health risk and will not achieve the performance benefits they seek. Therefore, the key to body composition assessment is the establishment of an acceptable range of lean and fat mass for the individual athlete, as well as the monitoring of lean and fat mass over regular time intervals to assure the stability or growth of the lean mass and a proportional maintenance or reduction of the fat mass. Importantly, there should be just as much attention given to changes in lean mass (both in weight of lean mass and proportion of lean mass) as the attention traditionally given to body fat percent.

How Important Is Body Composition to Performance?

Athletic performance is, to a large degree, dependent on the athlete's ability to sustain power (both anaerobically and aerobically) and the athlete's ability to overcome resistance, or drag. Both of these factors are interrelated with the athlete's body composition. Coupled with the common perception of many athletes who compete in sports where appearance is a concern (swimming, diving, gymnastics, skating, etc.), attainment of an "ideal" body composition often becomes a central theme of training. Besides the aesthetic and performance reasons for wanting to achieve an optimal body composition, there may also be safety reasons. An athlete who is carrying excess weight may be more prone to injury when performing difficult skills than the athlete with a more optimal body composition. However, the means athletes sometimes use in an attempt to achieve an optimal body composition are often counterproductive. Diets and excessive training often result in such a severe energy deficit that, while total weight may be reduced, the constituents of weight also change, commonly with a lower muscle mass and a relatively higher fat mass. The resulting higher body fat percentage and lower muscle mass inevitably result in a performance reduction that motivates the athlete to follow regimens that produce even greater energy deficits. This downward energy intake spiral may be the precursor to eating disorders that place the athlete at serious health risk. Therefore, while achieving an optimal body composition is useful for high-level athletic performance, the processes athletes often use to attain an optimal body composition may reduce athletic performance, place them at a higher injury risk, and increase health risks.

The mind-set that many people have that food, regardless of the amount and type, is "fat producing" is unhealthy. A much healthier (and from the point of view of an athlete, more appropriate) mind-set is that food is the provider of energy and the nutrients associated with burning energy. You wouldn't think of not putting fuel in your automobile (you know *for certain* it wouldn't run). You should also imagine putting fuel (food) in your body to make your muscles run is normal and desirable. The key is to know what foods make your muscles run best, and how to deliver the food to keep your high-octane tank full (glycogen storage), while limiting the storage of low-octane fuel (fat).

Body fat percentage should be thought of as having an appropriate range for different sports, and it's OK for athletes to fall anywhere on that sport-specific range. For instance, the seven members of the gold-medal winning 1996 U.S. Gymnastics Team were not the leanest individuals on the 20-member national team. They were, for the most part, right in the middle of the range of body fat percentages for the girls on the national team. Despite this, they were selected through competition to be the girls that represented the United States in the Olympic Games, and they won the team gold medal.

Within some reasonable bounds, having a relatively low body fat percentage may aid athletic performance. It does this by improving the strength-to-weight ratio: for a given weight, more of it is represented by lean mass that is power-producing and less of it by fat mass that represents stored fuel. It also helps by lowering the resistance, or drag, an athlete has as she's going through the air, swimming in water, or skating on ice; the smaller the body profile, the less resistance it is likely to produce.

Less resistance, or drag, is so important for some sports (typically the faster you go the greater the importance of drag reduction) that performance techniques are based on reducing drag. Speed skaters, for instance, spend the entire race bent over to reduce wind resistance. Cyclists wear special streamlined helmets and clothing, position their bodies on the bicycle to reduce drag, and even strategize about the best time to sprint ahead of the cycle in front of them. Going too soon can lead to premature exhaustion because it takes a great deal more energy to go the same speed if you're the one facing wind resistance. A gymnast who weighs 110 pounds and is 5 feet tall with a body fat percentage of 15 percent will have a lower wind resistance (i.e., less drag) tumbling through the air than a gymnast with the same weight and height but with a body fat percentage of 20 percent.

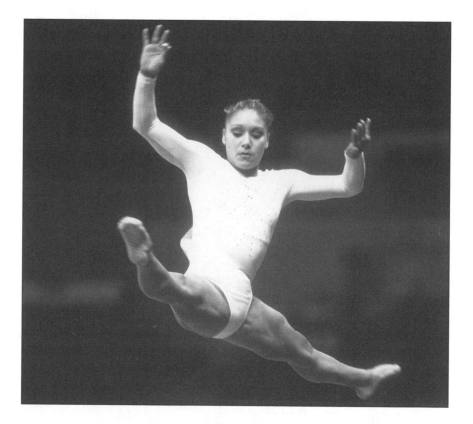

For some sports, however, this may make little or no difference. It's hard to imagine how a power lifter would have a problem with wind resistance, and linemen on football teams are more interested in moving mass than going fast over a distance (although quickness helps). (See table 3.1.)

Table 3.1   Body Fat Fercentage Ranges for Male and Female Athletes in Different Sports

Sport	Body fat percentage (range of average)	
	Males	**Females**
Baseball (age 20–28)	12–16	
Basketball (age 25–27)	7–11	20–27
Cycling	8–9	13–15
Figure skating	9–10	12–13
Football—Defensive backs (age 19.3–20.3)	13–14	
Football—Offensive backs (age 17–24.5)	10–12	
Football—Linebackers (age 17–24.7)	9–12	
Football—Linemen (age 17–24.7)	16–19	
Football—Quarterbacks (age 24.1)	13–14	
Hockey (age 22.5–26.3)	13–15	
Rowing (age 25.6)	5–7	
Racquetball (age 21–25)	8–9	13–14
Speed skating (age 21)	9–11	
Skiing—Alpine (age 16.5–21.8)	9–11	20–21
Skiing—Cross-country (age 20.2–25.6)	7–13	15–22
Skiing—Nordic (age 21.7)	8–9	
Soccer—U.S. Junior (age 17.5)	9–10	
Soccer—U.S. Olympic (age 20.6)	9–10	
Soccer—U.S. Collegiate (age 20.0)	9–11	
Soccer—U.S. National (age 22.5)	9–10	
Swimming—All stroke/distances (age 15.1–21.8)	5–11	26–27
Swimming—Sprints		14–15
Swimming—Middle distance		24–25
Swimming—Distance		17–18
Synchronized swimming (age 20.1)		23–24
Tennis (age 39–42)	15–17	20–21
Track and field—Distance running (age 20–26)	5–7	15–19
Track and field—Middle distance (age 20–25)	6–13	
Track and field—Sprint (age 20–47)	5–17	19–20
Track and field—Cross-country (age 15.6)		15–16
Track and field—Race walking (age 26.7)	7–8	
Track and field—Discus (age 21–28)	16–17	24–26

Sport	Body fat percentage (range of average)	
	Males	**Females**
Track and field—Hurdles (age 20.3)		20–21
Track and field—Shot put (age 21.5–27)	16–20	27–29
Triathlon	7–8	12–13
Volleyball (age 19–26)	11–13	17–22
Weight lifting—Power (age 24.9–26.3)	9–20	
Weight lifting—Olympic (age 25.3)	12–13	
Weight lifting—Bodybuilding (age 25.6–29)	8–14	13–14
Wrestling (age 11.3–27)	4–15	

Note: The values presented are estimates from limited numbers of athletes assessed in different settings using skinfolds or hydrodensitometry and should *not* be considered ideals. The values in this table can be used to compare common body composition values found in different sports.

Adapted from Wilmore and Costill 1988.

In sports where being aerodynamic helps, body composition could make a big difference. The reason for this is something many of us have already experienced: pound for pound, fat takes up more space than lean because it is less dense than lean. People with a high body fat percentage are likely to be able to float better in water than people with a low body fat percentage because the greater amount of fat (which is less dense) makes it easier for them to float. Lean mass is 65 to 75 percent water, while fat mass is essentially anhydrous (has no water). One way to think about the relative densities of water and fat is to think about oil and vinegar salad dressing. The oil always floats to the top because it is less dense than the water-based vinegar.

How Body Composition is Estimated

You can't tell about a person's body composition by weighing them or by looking at them. There are many "thin" people who have lost so much lean mass that they actually have a relatively high body fat percent. There are also many "large" people whom you might assume are obese but who are actually relatively lean. Even with modern equipment and sophisticated equations it is extremely difficult (if not impossible) to accurately measure body fat percentage and to accurately repeat that measure. The most accurate means of measuring fat mass and lean mass—if you lived in a horror story!

(*Don't try this*)—would be to determine the nude weight of a person, put the person in a boiling pot of water, let the fat rise to the top, and then weigh the fat. However, since we can't and don't want to do this, all the other techniques available for measuring body fat percentage are merely estimates of what's really there. Since each technique uses a different means of estimating body composition, cross-comparisons between techniques should *not* be made. For instance, if you had your body composition measured using a skin fold caliper last year, and you used a bioelectrical impedance analysis (BIA) yesterday, it would be misleading to use these values as a means of determining how your body composition has changed over time.

The common methods for assessing body composition include

- hydrostatic weighing (underwater weighing),
- skinfold measures applied to prediction equations,
- bioelectrical impedance analysis (BIA), and
- dual-energy x-ray absorptiometry (DEXA).

Hydrostatic Weighing (Hydrodensitometry)

This is the "classic" means for determining body composition and applies what is known as the "Archimedes Principle."[4] In essence, this principle states that, for an equal weight, lower density objects have a larger surface area and displace more water than higher density objects. From a body composition standpoint, this principle is applied in the following way:

1. The subject is weighed on a standard scale to get a "land weight."
2. Using specialized equipment, the subject's lung volume is estimated (the subject blows into a tube).
3. The subject sits on a chair that is attached to a weight scale.
4. The chair and weight scale are positioned over water and the chair is slowly lowered into the water.
5. When the subject is lowered into the water just below the chin, they are asked to fully exhale and completely lower their head into the water to be completely immersed.
6. While immersed, "underwater weight" is read off the scale that is attached to the chair the subject is sitting on.

Subjects weigh less in water than out of water because body fat (regardless of the amount present) makes the subject more buoyant. The greater the difference between in-water weight and out-of-water weight is a function of how much body fat the subject has. A very obese subject with a high level of body fat would appear light in water relative to land weight. Since lung volume is measured prior to taking the "water weight," there is an adjustment for the buoyancy that can be attributed to the air in the lungs. To minimize the lung-air effect, the subject is asked to exhale prior to full submersion, but there is always some remaining air in the lungs that is referred to as "residual volume."

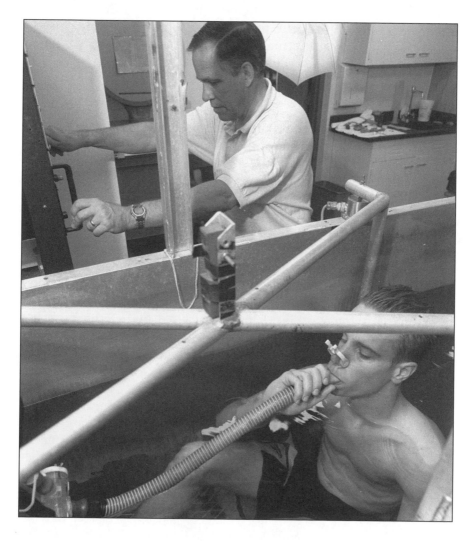

While there is some potential for error with hydrodensitometry related to a person's hydration status, and the residual volume of air in the lungs mentioned earlier, this technique is useful for determining the change in body composition over time if the technicians performing the measurements are good at precisely replicating the measurement procedure. It is also a useful means of determining the body composition of a population, since the errors associated with the technique are likely to average themselves out over many measurements. However, individuals within that population would never be sure if their personal body composition results were accurate. Good laboratories that do research in body composition almost always have invested the several thousand dollars for the equipment needed to accurately do hydrostatic weighing. Importantly, they also invest in making sure they have highly qualified people to take the measurements.

Skinfolds

Skinfold calipers, which vary in cost from free to $500, are used to measure a double thickness of the fat layer under the skin. This fat layer (called subcutaneous fat) is hypothesized to represent approximately 50 percent of a person's total body fat. Therefore, if you can get a good estimate of the subcutaneous fat layer, you should be able to predict the total body fat level. The prediction equations commonly used to determine body composition from skinfolds are based on the body composition determinations derived from hydrodensitometry. It works something like this: You measure a group of people using hydrodensitometry to determine their body fat percentages. Then you measure these same people with a series of skinfolds, which are used in statistics to predict the body fat percentage obtained from hydrodensitometry. If the skinfolds, when applied to the newly created equation, can successfully predict the hydrodensitometry value, then you have a skinfold equation for predicting body fat percentage.

There are a number of different equations available for the general population, and there are also several equations available for athletes. In general, using an equation that is more specific to the person you're measuring yields more accurate results. Also, equations that use more skinfold measurements are generally more accurate. For instance, an equation may require height, weight, age, triceps skinfold, and abdomen skinfold. Another equation may require height, weight, age, and skinfolds at the triceps, subscapular, midaxillary, suprailiac, abdomen, and midthigh sites.

It's important to say a word about the values that are derived from skinfold equations and used to predict body fat percentage. Many of the equations used with athletes are actually meant for the general (i.e., nonathlete) population. Since many athletes are considerably leaner than the average nonathlete, the results that are derived from skinfold equations are unrealistically low. Many athletes come to the lab saying that they have a body fat percentage of 2 percent or 3 percent, and I know immediately that these are estimates from equations that have not been normalized on athletes. It's simply not possible to have a body fat percent that is so low. When athletes think they have such a low body fat percent and are given the true value from a more realistic assessment (using either better, more population-specific equations or a more accurate technique), they don't usually respond positively when they receive the new number (usually somewhere between 8 and 18 percent). It's important for you to remember that, when skinfold equations are used, the single number you get is not going to be perfectly accurate. However, that number can be used as a baseline to determine change over time if the same technique and same equation are used to get the second value. It is completely inappropriate to compare the first value with one that was obtained using a different set of skinfolds and a different equation.

Bioelectrical Impedance Analysis (BIA)

For those of you who know what to do if you're in a swimming pool, and you begin to hear thunder and lightning nearby, you already know the principle behind bioelectrical impedance analysis (BIA). Water is a good conductor of electricity, and most body water is found in the lean mass. Fat, which has almost no water in it, is such a poor conductor of electricity that it actually impedes the electrical flow. BIA equipment comes in two basic forms. In one form, the subject lies down and electrodes are connected to the right wrist and right ankle, which produces an electrical current that runs from the wrist to the ankle. In another form, the subject stands on a platform with bare feet, and an electrical current runs from the right foot, up the right leg, down the left leg, and out the left foot. Regardless of the BIA equipment used, the principle behind the technique is the same. If you know the beginning level of energy (electricity) that enters the system and you can measure the level of energy that exits the system, you know how much of the energy has been impeded in the system. Since muscle, because of the water and electrolytes it contains, is an efficient conductor of electricity, and fat is an efficient insulator of (therefore it impedes) electricity, the greater the impedance, the greater the level of fat. If you start with 100 units of electricity going into your system and 80 units of electricity come out of the system, you have more water and muscle than someone who has 100 units going in and 60 units coming out.

Of course, a number of adjustments to the prediction are necessary. A taller person would have the electrical current running a longer distance, so would automatically have a greater level of impedance. The ratio of weight to height is also important, because it helps to predict the distance the current is running and the composition of the tissues it is running through. Since body composition commonly changes with age (people become less lean and more fat with increasing age), age is also an important predictor of body composition. At the initiation of the adolescent growth spurt, males and females begin to differentiate themselves on body composition, with women having relatively more fat than men. So gender is also an important consideration in this prediction. Therefore, when performing a BIA, the variables age, height, weight, and gender are included in the equation that predicts bodyfat percentage.

While BIA has an excellent theoretical basis for making good body-composition predictions, there are several important protocols that must be followed for the results to be accurate and repeatable. Since the technique is dependent on electrical conductivity through the lean mass, the hydration state of the subject can alter the results. If someone has a BIA measurement taken and is not well hydrated, the electrical current will not be conducted through the lean mass as well, so the subject will appear to have more fat mass than they really have. Therefore, it is critically important that the person having a BIA measurement taken be in a well-hydrated state. It is generally believed that drinking alcohol, exercising, consuming large amounts of coffee, and spending time outside in hot and humid weather within 24 hours of a BIA test leads to sufficient dehydration that the results will not be accurate. Since serious athletes exercise most days, this technique may provide results that show them to have more body fat than they really have. Therefore, athletes who are measured with this technique should do it after a day of rest and should make certain they are well hydrated. An easy hydration check is to see if the urine is clear. The more clear it is, the better hydrated you are.

Dual-Energy X-Ray Absorptiometry (DEXA)

Dual-energy x-ray absorptiometry (DEXA) is the latest, most accurate, and most expensive ($50,000 to $80,000) means of determining body composition, and it is generally considered the current "gold standard" for this purpose. The information you can derive from a full body scan on an athlete is invaluable, including bone density, body fat percentage, lean body mass, fat mass, and the distribution of fat and lean in the arms, body trunk, and legs. DEXA output even provides the differences in lean mass and fat mass between the left and right sides. This information can be particularly important for athletes who wish to develop symmetrical bodies or who, because of the nature of the sport, need to produce the same muscular power in each leg or in each arm.

DEXA works by passing two x-ray beams through the subject and measuring the amount of x-ray that has been absorbed by the tissue it has passed through. One beam is a high-intensity beam and one is a low-intensity beam, so the relative absorbance of each beam is an indication of the density of the tissue it has passed through. The higher the tissue density, the greater the reduction in x-ray intensity. Don't be frightened by all this talk of x-ray beams passing through your body. In fact, the amount of radiation energy that is used with DEXA is extremely small. You would need to have approximately 800 full-body DEXA scans before you got the same amount of radiation received from one standard chest x-ray. In fact, the level of radiation is so low that DEXA is approved by the FDA as a screening device to predict body composition. Usually, x-ray devices are reserved as diagnostic instruments because of the amount of radiation they impart, but not so for DEXA.

The procedure for DEXA, which was originally developed to determine the density of bone, couldn't be easier. The subject lies on the DEXA table for approximately 20 minutes, and the pencil-beam x-rays pass through the subject and are interpreted by a mechanical arm above the subject. Because metal has such a high density, the subject is asked to remove all jewelry and must wear clothing that contains no metal. The resultant value is translated into a density value for bone, lean, and fat tissue. Because the density values are derived from a direct assessment of tissue density, this is as close as we can get to directly assessing tissue density (short of surgery!). If you can find a lab with DEXA, the usual cost for a full-body scan is somewhere between $100 and $250.

Why Does Body Composition Change?

Body composition changes. We can influence that change by taking charge of what we eat and how we exercise. The general rule for lean mass (including bone mass) is "use it or lose it." We're wonderfully adaptive creatures, and we quickly adapt to our environment and our activity. We know, for instance, that astronauts quickly demineralize their bones because the gravity-free environment of outer space eliminates the need for having a strong skeleton. We would do quite well in that environment looking like a jellyfish, and the bones quickly adapt by releasing lots of calcium. The effect of this environment is so strong that astronauts must spend a significant amount of time doing exercise that places stress on the skeleton. Again, we're adaptive creatures, so placing this artificial stress on the bones helps to keep them strong, even in a gravity-free environment. The same thing happens when people are bedridden because of an injury. Both bone and muscle masses are rapidly reduced because they simply aren't needed when you're lying in bed. The important thing to remember about our tissues is that they are alive and will do what's needed to adapt to their current situation. Even bone, which to the casual observer might appear to be a hard, rocklike, unadaptive structure, is actually very much alive and changing itself all the time. Minerals move in and minerals move out, and this process leads to a constant remodeling of bone.

When you consider the influences on body composition, they boil down to the following:

• *Genetic predisposition.* This is everyone's bottom line and, no matter how hard you try, you can't change it. People have different inherited body types, and each type has a different predisposition toward accumulating more or less fat. Endomorphs (large trunk, short fingers, shorter legs) have a predisposition toward higher body fat percentages, and ectomorphs (long legs, long fingers, shorter trunk) have a predisposition toward a slender build with less body fat. What you're born with can't change, so all you can hope to do is optimize what you've been given.

• *Age.* People generally develop a lower lean mass and higher fat mass after the age of 30. However, while this age-related change in body composition is normal, it isn't a mandate. It has been clearly shown that a good diet and regular activity can keep you lean. Since energy metabolism drops about 2 percent for each decade after age 30, it gets progressively more difficult to maintain a desirable weight and body composition. To maintain what you've got, you would have to make either a 2 percent increase in energy expenditure or a 2 percent decrease in energy intake each decade after 30 to match the drop in energy metabolism. While this 2 percent difference seems small, it could make a major difference in your body composition. Consider that the average person consumes about 2,500 calories per day. If you need 2 percent less than this and don't make an adjustment, that represents a 50-calorie error of excess each day. Multiply that over 365 days and it represents 18,250 excess calories per year. Since an excess of 3,500 calories represents a one pound weight gain, in the course of one year this small 50-calorie error would manifest itself as a weight gain of over five pounds. In five years, that's a weight gain of 25 pounds, and in 10 years, that's a weight gain of 50 pounds!

• *Gender.* All other things being equal, women have a higher body fat percentage than men. There's nothing that can be done to alter this, and there is certainly nothing wrong with this. The gender difference is just a manifestation of the different biological expectations of men and women. However, there are *many* women who have a lower body fat percentage than men because they exercise more and eat better. Therefore, despite this baseline difference, doing the right things can help you (regardless of your gender) optimize your body composition for your sport.

• *Type of activity.* Different types of activities place different stresses on the system and, as you would expect, the body responds differently to these stresses. The standard for exercise for reducing body fat percentage is "aerobic" exercise. However, there is good evidence that any type of activity (including anaerobic activity) will reduce the body fat percentage.[5] High-intensity activity (such as that done by sprinters and weight lifters) may increase lean body mass and reduce body fat percentage, so the impact on weight may be minimal. Nevertheless, this shift in body composition is still likely to make the person appear slightly smaller, since, pound for pound, fat weight takes up more space than lean mass weight. Low-intensity activity, on the other hand, appears to reduce body fat percentage with minimal impact on lean body mass, so weight is reduced. When energy expenditure (calories burned) is equivalent, both anaerobic and aerobic activity appear to lower body fat to the same extent.

• *Amount of activity.* Clearly, the more a person exercises, the greater the potential benefits in desirably altering body composition. However, activity must be supported by an adequate intake of energy. Increasing the time of activity without also increasing the amount of energy intake causes a breakdown of muscle mass to support energy needs. There is no question that this would be an undesirable change in body composition for an athlete. In addition, overtraining, although it will not necessarily lead to a reduction in lean body mass, causes an increase in muscle soreness and reduces muscular power and endurance. Therefore, the amount of activity should be carefully balanced with adequate energy intake and with adequate rest to assure maintenance of muscle mass and athletic performance.

• *Nutrition.* Eating too much or too little can both negatively impact body composition. Eating too much, either over the course of a day or at one time, is likely to increase fat storage, and eating too little will lower both lean (muscle) mass and fat mass. In addition to energy intake, there are also nutrients that are important in energy metabolic processes. A failure to consume an adequate level of these nutrients (B-vitamins, zinc, iron, etc.) may reduce your ability to properly burn fuel, thereby limiting your ability to burn fat through exercise.

The Issue of Weight

There is no question that weight is an important issue for athletes because it influences the ease with which they can perform the skills they need to do. However, looking at weight by itself may provide athletes with a misleading picture of what is good or bad about their body composition.

In a number of sports, athletes will increase the time or intensity of a training regimen to improve performance, but then they inappropriately use changes in weight as a marker of success. Imagine a football player who comes to training camp at a weight much higher than the coach is accustomed to seeing in this player. It may well be that the football player worked hard during the off-season to increase muscle mass, and the increase in weight is a result of more muscle. Wouldn't the coach be wrong in telling that player that he has to lose weight? Gymnasts often reach their competitive peak during adolescence, a time when fast growth is the normal biological expectation. In spite of this, gymnasts are sometimes weighed weekly to make certain they are maintaining their weight. Shouldn't all the training they're doing increase their muscle mass and therefore their weight? Shouldn't they be growing and thus increasing their weight? These

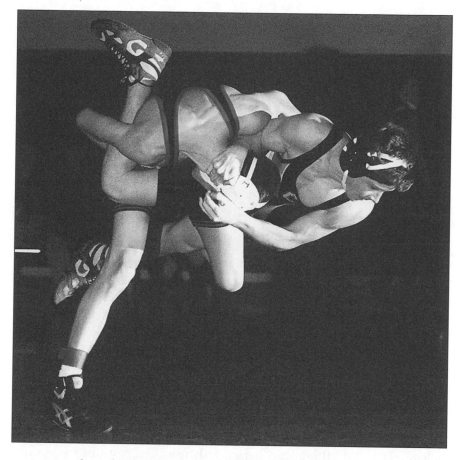

are examples of how weight is often used arbitrarily and wrongly. Tracking the constituents of weight makes much more sense and gives you a much more important idea of whether your body is changing in a desirable way.

Changing body composition is not as straightforward as many people think it is. The most common belief is that dieting is an effective but unpleasant means of weight loss. Logic suggests that a 25-percent reduction in energy intake will lead to a 25-percent reduction in weight. The reality, however, is that energy expenditure following weight loss is less than would be expected by the amount of weight that was lost.[6] This means that the adjustment in energy expenditure to inadequate intake is greater than the mathematical expectation, and leads to a return to the original weight, even on a lower energy intake (i.e., the less you eat, the less you can eat to maintain weight). Logic also suggests that a 25-percent increase in energy intake will lead to a 25-percent increase in weight. In fact, although weight gain does occur, it doesn't appear to increase as much as the increase in energy intake suggests it should. However, when you purposefully overfeed people to gain weight, the amount of weight gain is proportionate to the amount of overfeeding.[7-10] These studies strongly suggest that we have homeostatic mechanisms during periods of energy deficit that help us maintain our weight. This may be a "survival of the species" mechanism that helps humans survive periods of famine. We also appear able to store energy effectively (as fat) during periods of excess. This may also be a "survival of the species" mechanism that enables us to store energy when we are lucky enough to have excess food available.

Since major energy surpluses and deficits appear to activate homeostatic mechanisms, a possible means of making a desired change in weight and body composition is to avoid major energy balance shifts. Exercise should be at the core of any desired body composition change (i.e., an increase in lean mass and a decrease in fat mass, coupled with a small decrease in weight). But such a change might be easier to achieve if the energy deficit and energy surplus created are never too large during the day. See figure 3.1 for example, what can happen to body composition with three different eating patterns. Energy surpluses and deficits are represented, respectively, by variations above and below zero (0) energy-balance line. In the figure, when the line moves above zero, the athlete has consumed more energy than was expended. When the line moves below zero, the athlete has expended more energy than was consumed. Eating pattern 1 represents an athlete eating small meals frequently, and never has energy surpluses or deficits that exceed 400 calories. Eating pattern 2 represents infrequent eating with excess calories consumed at each meal. Eating pattern 3 represents an athlete who spends the majority of the day in an energy deficit state from not eating enough when the energy is needed. When this happens the body will break down muscle tissue for energy. At the end of the day, a very large meal brings the athlete into energy balance, but much of this meal will be stored as fat. Within any one given day, energy balance ($\pm$400 calories) is important for both performance and body composition.

Since the standard three-meal-a-day schedule forces athletes to consume a large amount of energy at each meal to obtain the necessary energy, staying in energy balance is easier on a six-meal pattern. Frequent consumption of small meals to maintain a steady

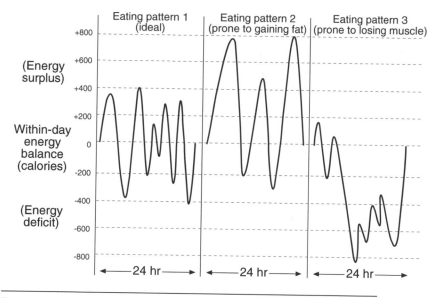

Figure 3.1   Relationship of eating patterns to body composition changes.

energy flow can be an important strategy in making the desired changes. Chapter 7 discusses the importance of meal timing.

Common Issues With Body Composition Assessment

Body composition assessment has become an important part of athlete assessment. The amount of muscle and fat that an athlete has can be predictive of performance, and bone mass assessment is important for understanding if developmental problems exist or if the athlete will face current or future risk for fracture. A periodic assessment of body composition also helps the athlete understand if the training regimen is causing the kinds of physical changes that are being sought. However, there are some important things to keep in mind when assessing body composition.

Desirable Body Composition Change Is Possible

You can change body composition by making changes in your diet and exercise, but these two should be considered together when making changes. Making dramatic changes in either direction is likely to cause unpredictable problems in your body composition. If you are increasing your training regimen, it is necessary to increase your energy intake to support the increase in energy expenditure. Putting yourself in a severe energy deficit state by increasing exercise and maintaining or lowering energy intake is likely to lower metabolic rate, increase fat storage, and also cause a breakdown of muscle to support energy needs. Eating too much is also likely to increase fat storage. It's best to maintain energy intake throughout the day, so athletes should be careful about consuming enough energy to support exercise, rather than making up for an energy deficit at the end of the day.

Keeping Information Private

Athletes often compare body composition values with other athletes, but this comparison is not meaningful and may drive an athlete to change body composition in a way that negatively impacts on both performance and health. Health professionals involved in obtaining body composition data should be sensitive to the confidentiality of this information. They should also explain to each athlete that differences in height, age, and gender are likely to result in differences in body composition, without necessarily any differences in performance. Strategies for achieving privacy and helping the athlete put the information in the proper context include the following:

- Obtain body composition values with only one athlete at a time, to limit the chance that the data will be shared.
- Give athletes information on body composition using phrases such as "within the desirable range" rather than a raw value, such as saying, "your body fat level is 18 percent."
- Provide athletes with information on how they have changed between assessments, rather than offering the current value.
- Increase the focus on muscle mass, and decrease the focus on body fat.
- Use body composition values as a means of helping to explain changes in objectively measured performance outcomes.

Comparing Body Composition Results Obtained From Different Methods

Different methods for assessing body composition produce different standard results. Therefore, it is inappropriate to compare the results from one method with the results of another. If athletes are being evaluated to determine body composition change over time (an appropriate use of body composition assessment), this comparison should only be made if the same method has been used for the entire assessment period. For instance, the difference in two DEXA scans taken several months apart provides valuable information on how body composition has changed in an individual, as does the difference in two skinfold assessments. However, the difference between body composition values from a DEXA scan and skinfold equation is not useful in determining change. Even within methods, the same prediction equations should be used to determine if an athlete's body composition has changed between measurements.

Seeking an Arbitrarily Low Level of Body Fat

Most athletes would like their body fat level to be as low as possible. However, athletes often try to seek a body fat level that is arbitrarily low (so low that it has nothing to do with the norms in the sport or their own body fat predisposition), and this can increase the frequency of illness, increase the risk of injury, lengthen the time the athlete needs before returning to training following an injury, reduce performance, and increase the risk of an eating disorder. Body composition values should be thought of as numbers on a continuum that are usual for a sport. If an athlete falls anywhere on that continuum, it is likely that factors other than body composition (training, skills acquisition, etc.) will be the major predictors of performance success.

Seeking arbitrarily low body fat levels and/or weight is a particular problem for athletes in sports where making weight is a common expectation. Wrestlers, in particular, make dangerous efforts—sometimes leading to death—to lower body fat levels and weight in order to be more competitive. Read more about this subject in the section on wrestling in chapter 9, "Power Sports."

Excessive Frequency of Body Composition Assessment

Athletes who are assessed frequently (frequent weight and/or skinfolds taken) are fearful of the outcome, since the results are often (and inappropriately) used punitively. Real changes in body composition occur slowly, so there is little need to assess athletes weekly, biweekly, or even monthly. Assessing body composition two to four times each year is an appropriate frequency to determine and monitor body composition change. In some isolated circumstances when an athlete has been injured or is suffering from a disease, such as malabsorption, fever, diarrhea, or anorexia, it is reasonable for a physician to recommend a more frequent assessment rate to control for changes in lean mass. Coaches who have traditionally obtained weight and/or body composition values weekly, biweekly, or monthly should shift their focus to a more frequent assessment of objective performance-related measures.

Summary

The assessment of body composition can be a useful tool in helping the athlete and coach understand the changes that are occurring as a result of training and nutritional factors. Health professionals involved in obtaining body composition data should focus on using the same technique with the same prediction equations to derive valid comparative data over time. Care should be taken that body composition values are used constructively as part of the athlete's total training plan. Ideally, the emphasis should be on a periodic (biyearly or quarterly) monitoring of the athlete's body composition to determine change of both the lean and fat mass. Many athletes are sensitive about body fat, so care should be taken to use body composition values in a way that enables their constructive use in the athlete's general training plan.

4 Training With Supplements

To Creatine or Not to Creatine

If there is a single, prominent ergogenic aid that virtually everyone is either taking or is willing to take, it's creatine. When I go around the country talking about sports nutrition, the first and most frequently asked question is "Should I take creatine?" Interestingly enough, these people are *already* taking creatine, and what they really want is a confirmation that what they're doing is right. That's the way it goes with so many supposedly "ergogenic" products. Many athletes are in such a hurry to improve that they're willing to try almost anything, even before we know if it works. The interesting thing is that the placebo effect in nutrition is so powerful that when athletes *believe* something works (even if they're taking a sugar pill), they may actually derive a measurable benefit. This is a story about exactly such an athlete.

We were doing a double-blind pretest, posttest study on creatine monohydrate (the supplemental form of creatine) on a team of world-class female athletes. On their first visit to the lab, we performed a Wingate test to measure anaerobic power and anaerobic endurance by using resistance on a laboratory bicycle (called an ergometer). The athletes were randomly selected to be either in the control group (fruit juice) or in the experimental group (fruit juice with creatine). We did a triangle test (a standard testing method for assessing taste) to make certain no one could tell the difference between the creatine and non-creatine beverages. Since this was a double-blind test, neither the athlete nor anyone in direct contact with the athletes knew who was in which group. (The key for who was in which group was secretly and closely held by a graduate student.) Thus neither the athletes nor the researchers could influence the results. We basically did what we had to do to assure that the results we obtained were "real."

After the first Wingate test, the athletes were put on a protocol of either a glass of plain fruit juice four times each day (in addition to everything else they were eating) or, for the experimental group, a glass of fruit juice that contained 2.5 grams of creatine monohydrate. We kept this protocol up for three days while the athletes participated in an intensive training camp. At the end of the three days, we again performed a Wingate test to see if the creatine intake explained any differences in either anaerobic power or anaerobic endurance.

Sally, from her very first drink of fruit juice, was certain she was in the creatine group. She said she felt more light on her feet, faster, and had more energy. I, of course, had no idea whether she was or wasn't and told her we'd have to wait to the end of the experiment to find out. She persisted in telling everyone within earshot that she was in the creatine group, and that she thought that stuff was great! On the second round of Wingate tests, Sally really *did* do better. After we had completed the experiment, she was the first in line waiting to confirm that she had, indeed, been taking creatine over the last several days. As you may have guessed by now, Sally wasn't in the creatine group. While we found that the creatine group was generally better able to maintain anaerobic power and anaerobic endurance after three days of an intense training camp, we didn't find that there was any absolute improvement in either power or endurance. And, of course, there were individuals in the control group who did better without creatine and individuals in the experimental group who did worse with creatine. You can see the problem. Humans are different, and the way they react to different substances is different. Sometimes the *belief* that something will help really does, as it did with Sally. The ideal circumstance, and what scientists are dedicated to doing, is to find what *really* works so athletes can derive a double benefit from a nutritional intervention. Athletes would gain the biological benefit from the ergogenic aid, and they would also gain from the belief that it really works.

The term ergogenic aids is used to refer to substances that make claims to be performance enhancing. Some of these substances are defined as nutritional ergogenic aids because they work by entering a well-established nutritional metabolic pathway, or because they consist of one or more known nutrients. For instance, taking extra carbohydrate to improve performance makes carbohydrate a nutritional ergogenic aid. Also, taking creatine monohydrate to improve sprint performance makes creatine a nutritional ergogenic aid because creatine is a normal constituent of food; consuming it causes creatine to enter a known metabolic pathway.[1,2,3,4] Non-nutritional ergogenic aids represent products (often of unknown origin because producers don't clearly specify what they consist of) that are neither nutrients nor other substances with nutritional properties. The best-known non-nutritional ergogenic aids are anabolic steroids.

In most cases, the claims for performance enhancement attributed to ergogenic aids exceed reality. Since many of the products are considered foods, nutrients, or nutrient based, there are few controls for government agencies to police the claims made for them. The only truly credible sources of information come from published scientific works and the newly formed Office of Dietary Supplements of the National Institutes of Health. Where improvements are seen, it is often due to a placebo effect: People believe it will help, so it actually helps even though there is no biochemical basis for the improvement. In other cases, improvements occur because the product is providing a chemical missing from the foods that an athlete commonly consumes. For instance, protein powders or amino acid powders are often taken by bodybuilders to aid in the enlargement of muscle mass. However, studies clearly indicate that the rate of protein usage by the body is well below the level consumed by those who take these protein powders. This means that the body's limit for using protein to build muscle and maintain tissues is much lower than the amount of protein that is commonly being consumed through food and protein supplements. The upper limit for protein usage is below 2 grams per kilogram of body weight, and those who take protein supplements often are taking more than 4 grams of protein per kilogram of body weight. The excess protein is burned as a fuel or stored as fat, but it can't be used to build more muscle. It is also known that bodybuilders often have an inadequate level of energy intake (they don't eat enough), making it difficult for them to support their larger muscle mass.[5]

The reason the extra protein helps (if, in fact, it does) is more likely because it is used as an energy substrate (burned as calories) than because of its potential tissue-building effect. In fact, bodybuilders would do much better by consuming 300 extra calories from carbohydrate than by taking the extra calories as protein powders—and it would also be much cheaper!

There are numerous ergogenic aids, ranging from known nutrients to supposed nutrients, (such as vitamin B-15, which has no official definition, varies in content by manufacturer, and is not a recognized vitamin), to herbs with no known chemical content or known active ingredient. There is so much misinformation in the marketplace and in the locker room about these products that the buyer should beware. Rather than focusing on a magic bullet to improve performance, athletes should take a realistic approach and consume a balanced intake of foods that provides sufficient energy and nutrients to support growth, activity, and tissue maintenance. This chapter discusses some of the more common ergogenic aids.

Carbohydrate (Glycogen) Loading

Since carbohydrate is typically the limiting energy substrate (that is, it will run out before fat or protein runs out) in exercise, starting exercise with more of it in the tissues should aid exercise endurance. In high-intensity exercise, carbohydrate is the primary fuel used by the muscles. In low-intensity but long-duration exercise, fat may be the primary fuel, but fat requires carbohydrates to burn completely.[6] In either case, when carbohydrates (glycogen stores and blood glucose) are depleted, exercise performance is dramatically reduced.[7,8] The basis behind carbohydrate loading is to put as much carbohydrate in the tissues as they can hold.

The traditional or classical regimen for carbohydrate loading (referred to as the Astrand regimen for the person who first described it) achieves maximal muscle glycogen stores by first completely depleting the muscles of glycogen. This is followed by a phase in which muscle glycogen is restored to maximal levels. This regimen is no longer recommended because of the dangers associated with glycogen depletion, which include irregular heartbeats and a sudden loss of blood pressure. There have also been deaths reported in the literature that have been attributed to the glycogen depletion of this technique. The Astrand regimen was followed for approximately one week in preparation for a competition:

- Seven days before the competition the athlete performs exhaustive exercise and consumes a low-carbohydrate diet (0 to 10 percent carbohydrate) to deplete carbohydrate stores.
- After the depletion phase, the athlete tapers exercise to almost nothing and consumes a high-carbohydrate diet (80 percent carbohydrate) to replenish carbohydrate stores.

While this type of regimen has been shown to be useful for supersaturating tissues with glycogen, the depletion phase is dangerous.[9,10] Athletes have found serious disturbances in heart rhythm and glycose metabolism. *Therefore, this regimen is NOT recommended.*

The recommended method for carbohydrate loading is commonly referred to as the "Sherman/Costill Method." This method was developed after the Astrand method by Sherman and Costill and was found to be safer than the Astrand method, but equally effective in maximizing glycogen storage. This approach is based on maintaining carbohydrate stores at all times and tries to avoid carbohydrate depletion. The athlete should do the following:

• Consume a diet that is 55 to 65 percent carbohydrate daily. On this regimen, the carbohydrate intake should be increased slightly to 60 to 70 percent carbohydrate in preparation for competition.
• Taper down exercise gradually over seven days prior to the competition, with the goal of not exercising on the day before the competition. During this tapering phase, a high-carbohydrate intake is maintained.

This method is just as useful in supersaturating the tissues with glycogen (stored carbohydrate) as the Astrand regimen, but it avoids the difficulties associated with carbohydrate depletion.[11]

Not all sports and activities are suitable for carbohydrate loading. It is important to remember that, for every gram of stored glycogen, the body stores approximately three grams of water. If the tissues are packed full with glycogen and water, the athlete is likely to experience some degree of muscle stiffness. In sports where flexibility is important, carbohydrate loading may cause difficulties. See table 4.1 for a list of activities that are considered appropriate for and may benefit from carbohydrate loading.

The type of carbohydrate does appear to make a difference. Glucose polymer products (including commercially available sports gels and polycose) and maltodextrins (which are found in numerous sports beverages) are easily digested into glucose and appear to be

Table 4.1 Activities That May Benefit From Carbohydrate Loading

Clear benefit	Less clear benefit
Marathon	Gymnastics
Triathlon	Baseball
Cross-country skiing	Middle-distance/short-distance running
Cycling (long-distance)	Weight lifting
Swimming (long-distance)	Sprinting
Any endurance event lasting more than 90 minutes	Rowing (short distance)
Practice sessions lasting longer than 2 hours	

Note: High carbohydrate intakes are recommended for all sports and activities. The tapering of activity may not be needed in the sports/activities on the right column.

Adapted from Bucci 1993.

more effective in glycogen production than other carbohydrates. However, starches from pasta, bread, rice, and other cereals are also effective at maximizing glycogen storage.[12,13]

Creatine Monohydrate

Phosphocreatine serves as a storage depot for maintaining adenosine triphosphate (ATP) levels during high-intensity activities, such as sprinting, that can quickly deplete ATP. (Note: ATP is the high-energy fuel used by cells.) Creatine is a compound made from three amino acids that joins with phosphorus to make phosphocreatine. It is believed, therefore, that saturating muscles with creatine will enhance our ability to maintain the high-energy compound ATP and delay fatigue in high-intensity activity.[14] We can synthesize creatine in the liver from the amino acids arginine, glycine, and methionine, and we can also obtain creatine from foods, mainly meats. However, normal cooking can easily reduce the creatine level of foods. Given the ever-increasing importance of fully cooking meat products to reduce the chance of bacterial infection, the amount of dietary creatine is likely to be small.

Many athletes are now taking daily creatine supplements, and there is some limited evidence that creatine supplements (commonly in the form called "creatine monohydrate") may enhance anaerobic power and anaerobic endurance.[15,16,17] While creatine is synthesized by the body from three amino acids, the creatine monohydrate supplement is the commercially synthesized form of creatine. It is possible, however, that the benefit derived from taking creatine monohydrate may be due to the inadequate energy (caloric) intake commonly seen in athletes.[18] As previously mentioned, inadequate energy intake is one of the major problems that athletes face. It is possible that athletes with an adequate energy intake would not benefit from these supplements, although this has never been adequately tested.

If an athlete does take creatine monohydrate, the daily total should be between 10 and 28 grams that are divided into four doses over the day. For instance, if the goal is to take 10 grams per day, individual doses should be 2.5 grams four times daily. The smaller the athlete, the smaller the daily dose should be.

There is evidence that taking daily creatine supplements causes a saturation of creatine in muscle tissue after five days.[19] Therefore, creatine should not be taken for longer than five days. There should also be an approximately five-day break in supplementation before supple-

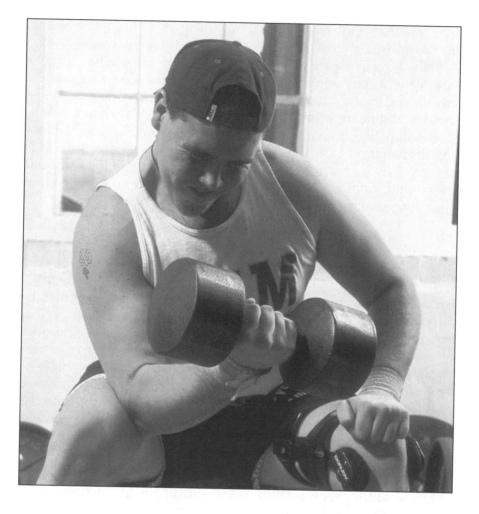

ments are resumed. Some studies suggest that taking creatine supplements five days per month is adequate to saturate muscle tissue.[20,21]

Athletes should know that the long-term safety of creatine monohydrate supplementation has never been tested on children, adolescents, or adults. In one recent article by two British researchers, creatine supplementation was linked to renal (kidney) damage.[22] In this article, the scientists found that the athlete with renal damage had been taking oral creatine supplements to prepare for the soccer season. He had not been exceeding the recommended doses, but once he stopped the supplements, renal function recovered. There is also evidence that creatine storage in muscle causes a retention of water with a concomitant increase in weight.[23] These potential problems should give athletes a reason to be vigilant about whether creatine supplementation is appropriate for them. Before an athlete tries creatine supplementation, it may be prudent to first be certain that an adequate level of energy (calories) is being consumed.

There is no evidence to suggest that creatine supplementation is unsafe for healthy adults, nor is there no information on its safety if taken over long periods of time, or by children. Therefore, even though creatine supplementation may be beneficial for short, repetitive bouts of high-intensity exercise, athletes should be careful about supplementation until more information on long-term effects is known. A reasonable approach would be to consume sufficient energy and, within that context, periodically consume foods that are good sources of protein and creatine (meat and fish).

Glycerol

Glycerol (or glycerine) is a three-carbon simple lipid that is metabolized like carbohydrate. It is the three-carbon unit that holds dietary fatty acids together to form triglycerides. Glycerol is a powerful humectant and has the ability to hold a high level of water. A number of endurance athletes use glycerol as a means of superhydration because of this capacity to hold water, as well as glycerol's ability to be easily metabolized for energy. Adding a little glycerol to water enables the athlete to store more water and, in doing so, may aid the athlete in endurance competitions that take place in hot and humid environments. Refer to chapter 2 "Staying Hydrated" for more information about superhydration.

Formula for Adding Glycerol to Water for Superhydration

To make a glycerol beverage, use 1 gram glycerol and 21.4 milliliters water per kilogram of body weight.[24]

1. Drink the entire glycerol-added fluid portion, except 16 ounces, using typical fluid consumption protocol, within two hours before exercise.

2. Reserve 16 ounces of the glycerol-added fluid to drink about 30 minutes before exercise.

3. Drink additional pure water or a sports beverage as necessary to make urine clear prior to race.

4. Continue to drink a sports beverage at every opportunity during the race. Usual intake should approach 3 to 6 ounces every 10 minutes.

Storing additional water in your body *will* make you feel stiff. Many athletes complain that at the beginning of any race for which they have added glycerol to their water they feel, at least initially, stiff and sluggish. However, a number of them claim that the benefits of having extra water at the *end* of the race far outweighs the feeling of sluggishness at the beginning of the race. While other athletes are dehydrated and overheating, these athletes claim that they feel more fresh when it counts the most.

A word of caution: While a number of endurance athletes use glycerol in water to enhance their hydration state, this product has never been adequately tested for safety. Since it is a normal component of the diet and is easily metabolized, it is unlikely that glycerol itself would cause any difficulty. However, it is unclear how much additional stress there is on the cardiovascular system when additional water is stored in the system.

Bicarbonate (Sodium Bicarbonate or Bicarbonate of Soda)

Researchers have theorized that sodium bicarbonate buffers the acidity (lactic acid) created by anaerobic metabolism, allowing for prolonged maintenance of force or power.[25] Since many activities involve mainly anaerobic metabolic processes, it would appear that some athletes could derive a benefit from sodium bicarbonate consumption. Study results, however, are mixed and generally indicate that well-hydrated athletes do not derive a performance benefit.

It is possible that the sodium in the sodium bicarbonate is more useful than the bicarbonate (the acid buffer). Sodium is an electrolyte that helps to increase or maintain blood volume, creating a larger buffering space (more fluid) for muscles to excrete the extra acidity created by high-intensity activity. For instance, think of sugar as the acid produced from anaerobic activity and a glass of water as blood volume, and you can see what might happen. If the glass of water is half full, and you put a cube of sugar in it, the concentration of sugar would be higher than if you put the same amount of sugar in a full glass of water. Nevertheless, the negative side effects from taking sodium bicarbonate, including the potential for severe gastrointestinal distress and nausea, should give athletes reason to be cautious before taking this potential ergogenic aid.

Proteins and Amino Acids

Amino acids are the building blocks of proteins. Putting amino acids together in different sequences and numbers results in proteins of different characteristics. For instance, the protein in hair has a sequence of amino acids and the protein in muscle has another sequence of amino acids. When you break proteins apart, what results is a pool of amino acids that constitute the protein. In this context, you can almost speak of protein supplements and amino acid supplements as being essentially the same.

Many athletes take protein supplements and believe this helps them build muscles. However, assessments of their diets indicate that the protein supplement is simply providing the calories needed to support the larger muscle mass desired. It would be easier, cheaper, and safer to simply eat more food that is high in carbohydrates. Studies are in general agreement that humans cannot use more than 1.5 grams of protein per kilogram of body weight.[26,27] You can think of the protein requirement as being directly related to the amount of fat-free mass the person has, plus a very small amount that

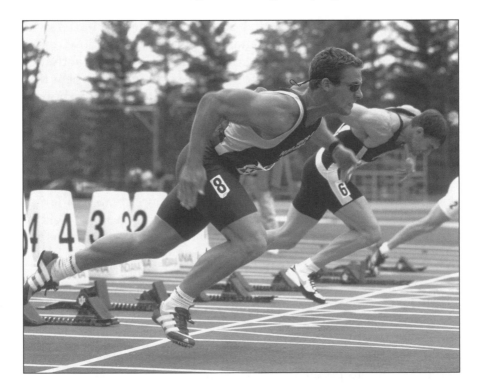

is used to supply energy. Taken together, this amounts to a requirement range for athletes that is between 1.0 to 1.5 grams per kilogram of body weight. Having more than this simply means the protein will be burned as energy or stored as fat. Burning protein as energy is undesirable because it creates a great deal of nitrogenous waste (ammonia, urea, etc.) that is toxic and must be excreted. This urinary excretion causes an increase in water loss and increases the chance for dehydration.

Since the vast majority of athletes already consume 1.5 grams of protein per kilogram of body weight without consuming protein or amino acid powders, there is little reason to supplement with these products. Instead, athletes should increase total energy intake, mainly from carbohydrates, to support the larger muscle mass they seek. If protein is needed, it is much less expensive to eat poultry or fish. These products also have the added benefit of providing other important nutrients, including iron and zinc, which are often low in the diets of athletes.

Caffeine

Caffeine, one of several methylxanthines found in coffee, tea, cola, chocolate, and a variety of other foods and beverages (see table 4.2), has been shown to help endurance-type performance in those who are *unaccustomed* to consuming caffeinated products.[28] In a number of studies, it was found that caffeine ingestion increased the "free fatty acid" (FFA) concentration in plasma significantly.[29] The increased availability of FFA enhances the ability to use these fats as a fuel in endurance-type low-intensity activities. Since humans adapt to caffeine intake, frequent and regular consumption results in a reduced dose effect. In other words, the more you have, the more you must have to achieve the same effect.

There are no studies demonstrating that caffeine is useful in power or speed-type events, such as weightlifting, sprinting, or gymnastics. Also, because of the potential ergogenic properties that caffeine imparts in endurance-type events, such as long-distance running, the International Olympic Committee (IOC) has placed limits on its use (no more than 12 micrograms per liter of urinary caffeine). This level of caffeine excreted in the urine can be reached by drinking 8 cups of coffee in a time span of 12 hours (see table 4.2 for other items containing caffeine). As you can see, a combination of foods and

Table 4.2   Caffeine Content* of Common Beverages and Foods

Caffeine-containing food products	Caffeine content (mg)
Soft drinks (12 oz, or 1 can)	
Coca-Cola	45
Dr. Pepper	40
Jolt	75
Mellow Yellow	53
Mountain Dew	54
Mr. Pibb	41
Pepsi Cola	38
Coffee (1 cup, or 8 oz)	
Brewed, drip method	130
Brewed, percolator method	94
Decaffeinated	3
Instant	74
Tea (1 cup, or 8 oz)	
Brewed (imported tea)	96
Brewed (U.S. brand tea)	64
Iced tea	47
Instant	48
Chocolate brownie (1.25 oz)	8
Chocolate cake (1 medium slice)	14
Chocolate candy (1 oz)	8
Chocolate ice cream (2/3 cup, or 6 oz)	5
Chocolate milk (1 cup, or 8 oz)	8
Chocolate pudding (1/2 cup, or 4 oz)	6

*The United States Olympic Committee considers urinary caffeine levels greater than 12 micrograms per milliliter as doping, making caffeine a banned substance at this level. As a guide, two cups of coffee typically produces a urinary caffeine level of 3 to 6 micrograms per milliliter and two colas produces a urinary caffeine level of 1.5 to 3 micrograms per millileter. Consumption of products more highly concentrated in caffeine will result in higher levels of urinary caffeine excretion.

products can also exceed the IOC caffeine limits. For instance, three cups of coffee plus two No-Doze plus three colas could provide enough caffeine to cause the urinary excretion of caffeine to exceed the acceptable limit. Caffeine is a diuretic (causes an increase in urinary output) that may exacerbate the state of dehydration. This fact, plus the lack of evidence for a benefit in high-intensity sports, including gymnastics, sprinting, bodybuilding, and weight lifting, should discourage athletes from increasing caffeine consumption to achieve performance enhancement.

Carnitine (Typically L-Carnitine)

The theory behind taking carnitine supplements is sound. L-carnitine is a common name for beta-hydroxy-butyrate, which was first discovered in muscles in the early 1900s. It is mainly involved with transporting long-chain fatty acids that reside inside cells into the mitochondria of the cells, where they are metabolized. Carnitine increases blood flow by improving fatty acid oxidation in the artery wall, and it detoxifies ammonia, a by-product of protein breakdown that is associated with early fatigue.[30] We synthesize carnitine from the amino acids lysine and methionine, and it is found in abundant quantities in all meats and dairy products, so a deficiency is unlikely. If there is a deficiency, it is most likely to be found in vegetarians who avoid consumption of dairy products. With an adequate intake of meats or dairy products, there is little reason to take this expensive supplement. While never tested, it is possible that vegetarians, who consume no dairy products and have a marginal protein intake, might benefit from L-carnitine supplementation, if they are involved in high-intensity exercise.

Studies of carnitine generally show no benefit for low-intensity endurance activities. Some studies, however, have demonstrated a benefit in high-intensity activities when taken either just before the activity or for several days. The typical dose is between one to two grams per day. *But the safety of L-carnitine supplementation has not been adequately tested.* The type of carnitine taken is also important. There are reports that DL-carnitine supplementation (a less expensive form of carnitine) may cause muscle weakness. Therefore, if an athlete insists on taking this supplement, only the L-carnitine form should be considered.

Omega-3 Fatty Acids

These fatty acids, commonly found in cold-water fish, may be useful in reducing muscle soreness. They may have several other effects including the following:[31]

- Improved delivery of oxygen and nutrients to muscles and other tissues.
- Improved aerobic metabolism due to better delivery of oxygen.

- Higher release of somatotropin (growth hormone) in response to normal stimuli (exercise, sleep, hunger). This may have an anabolic effect and may improve muscular recovery.
- Reduced inflammation of tissues that results from muscular fatigue and overexertion allowing for faster recovery.

Omega-3 fatty acids are available as over-the-counter supplements. You can also increase your regular consumption of cold-water fish such as salmon, herring, and sardines to obtain these fatty acids.

Medium-Chain Triglycerides

Medium-chain triglycerides (MCT) are found in coconut oil and palm kernel oil, which are among the most saturated fatty acids in human nutrition. Medium-chain triglycerides have carbon lengths of 6 to 12 carbon atoms, while the majority of the triglycerides consumed have considerably longer carbon chains. This difference, however, allows MCT oils to be absorbed and metabolized differently than other fats. The liver readily takes them up where they can be rapidly oxidized for cellular energy.[32] In addition, MCT oils do not require L-carnitine to deliver energy to cell mitochondria for metabolism (other fats require L-carnitine).[33] MCT oils have several properties that may be useful for athletes. These include the following:[31]

- Quick source of energy.
- Aids in mobilizing body fat stores for energy.
- Increases the metabolic rate.
- Spares lean body mass (muscle).

MCT oils have been used for many years as a source of energy for those on enteral (tube) feedings, and they have a long history of safety. They are widely available in drugstores and health food stores.

Ginseng

Ginseng has been used for centuries in Asian cultures to reduce fatigue. In a limited number of studies, components of ginseng have been shown to spare glycogen usage and increase the oxidation of fatty acids.[31] Exercised animals that have been injected with a ginseng extract have shown reduced fatigue.[34] However, human studies that have evaluated various doses of ginseng root for periods of up to two months have shown no clear ergogenic benefit. There is only limited evidence that providing a supplement of ginseng extract may improve endurance performance by improving oxygen delivery to the muslces.

Summary

There is an almost never-ending array of products that advertise themselves as having ergogenic properties available to athletes. For the most part, there is little evidence that well-nourished athletes derive any benefits from consumption of these products. On the other hand, those selling the products certainly derive a great deal of benefit. Athletes should carefully consider the adequacy of their own diets before attempting to use ergogenic aids. These products are expensive, and few of them have ever been adequately tested for safety.

If you choose to use an ergogenic aid, proceed cautiously. Call an appropriately credentialed health professional to get as much information on the product as possible. When you take it for the first time, observe carefully whether you experience any gastrointestinal upset, and try to document how you feel. Most of these ergogenic aids are powerful chemicals that are easily handled if taken in the small amounts commonly provided by the foods we eat. However, when they are taken in the large bolus doses often prescribed to achieve an ergogenic benefit, the impact on your system may be entirely different and unexpected.

Of all the ergogenic aids I have mentioned, it is very clear that carbohydrates hold the greatest promise for improving both endurance and power performance. Before trying anything else, try consuming a high, regular amount of carbohydrates with plenty of fluids. The ergogenesis you experience from this is likely to be real.

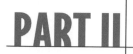

PART II

Tailoring Nutrition to Your Training

5 Eating for Anaerobic Power

Protein for Breakfast, Lunch, and Dinner

One of my favorite graduate students of all time was a young man who took up competitive bodybuilding after he completed his undergraduate biology degree and several years before he entered our graduate program in sports nutrition. When I first saw him, I knew I didn't want to make him angry, but I came to find out that his muscular appearance did not reflect his personality. He had arms the size of my neck, and his legs were the size of my waist, but he was gentle, caring, and very, very bright. When I asked him why he wanted a graduate degree in sports nutrition, he knew exactly why. He was tired of getting information on how to train and how to eat from people who were unqualified, and he wanted to be the purveyor of good information rather than the recipient of bad information.

He took all his core requirements (nutritional biochemistry, nutrition and metabolism, research design, etc.) and finally became eligible to take my class in advanced sports nutrition. During his entire time in graduate school, he was training and competing as a bodybuilder, but he occasionally shared that his successes were not what they should have been. I noticed in class that he was almost always tired and that he was always eating something. He did this discreetly enough, so it didn't disturb anyone. Besides, I'm such an advocate of snacking behavior that I was actually pleased to see an athlete find ways to take in enough energy.

We came to a point in class when we were discussing the various nutritional protocols that might work for different sports, and I asked our bodybuilder if he wouldn't mind sharing what he did to build muscle and stay competitive in the sport. He said he found that the critical thing was to "eat protein all the time, and eat lots of it." Even though this was the standard for so many athletes in the sport (albeit a bad one), I was stunned by his answer. How could someone so educated go down this protein path? His statement, of course, initiated a discussion on whether this was an appropriate strategy and what was happening, metabolically speaking, with all that protein. What came out in the discussion boiled down to this: he knew that eating too much protein could cause difficulties with hydration (getting rid of all that extra metabolic waste from protein causes an increased water loss) and that it wasn't the best fuel for his muscles, but whenever he tried eating carbohydrates instead of protein he started losing weight—and that wasn't something this bodybuilder could afford to do. As it turns out, what he was eating all the time was steak, roasts, and chicken (fried and otherwise), which also has a good deal of fat associated with it. All of this protein *and* fat (fat is a highly concentrated form of energy) helped him maintain his caloric requirement and weight, but wasn't the best combination for muscle function. However, when he tried eating more carbohydrate and less protein, his total energy intake dropped because he was eating almost no fat. I made it a class project to find a way that he could eat the right foods *and* take in enough total energy to maintain (and even build) his muscle mass. The result was lots of fluids with a balanced diet heavy on carbohydrates (about 60 percent of calories), moderate in protein (about 15 percent of calories), and moderately low in fat (about 25 percent of calories), consumed six times per day.

About one year after he graduated, he came back to say hello, and he showed me one enormous trophy with his name on it. He said his change of food intake gave him so much more "energy" that he was able to train harder and longer, and he felt better all the time. Imagine that. Following the science really does work.

Different sports place different demands on the energy system. Some sports require quick bursts of activity, some require steady continuous movement with occasional periods of fast activity, while others require that muscles work slowly and continuously for hours. Each type of activity places unique demands on the muscles and on the fuels that muscles demand.

There are clear metabolic differences in activities that require endurance and activities that require power. Power activities mandate that the athlete have the ability to explode off a starting block, jump high distances, throw a heavy weight, or push someone of equal size backwards. The better the power athlete can do some of these things, the more successful the athlete is. Getting power athletes to train muscles for these activities is critical for competitive success, and this training regimen must be supported by proper nutrition, or all that hard work will be fruitless.

Energy Demands

Power activities are dependent on the conditioning of the fast-twitch muscle fibers. These fibers have unique characteristics that help to explain the basis for the nutritional recommendations for power athletes. Fast-twitch, or Type IIB fibers, have the capacity to produce a tremendous amount of power, as well as a high capacity to store glycogen (stored carbohydrate), but they have a low capacity to store triglycerides (fats). The intermediate fast-twitch muscle fibers (Type IIA) also produce a tremendous amount of power, but these muscle fibers can be trained to behave more like the Type I slow-twitch fibers that are characteristic of endurance athletes. The type of training that is done, therefore, is important because it can influence the behavior of the muscle fibers. Power athletes want *all* the fibers capable of producing a high level of power to produce that power. If there is a lot of aerobic conditioning in the training regimen of the power athlete, the Type IIA fibers will lose some of their power potential because they are behaving more like endurance fibers (see table 5.1). Interestingly, there is evidence that the intermediate fast-twitch fibers will revert to their genetic baseline (more like Type IIB than Type I) rather quickly if the aerobic training ceases. To summarize, slow-twitch muscle fibers have a tremendous capacity to store and burn fats, and fast-twitch muscle fibers have a tremendous capacity to store and burn glycogen. The intermediate fibers can be trained to behave like either slow-twitch or fast-twitch fibers, but at their baseline, are more like fast-twitch fibers.

Table 5.1 Characteristics of Different Muscle Fiber Types

Muscle fiber	Type I (slow-twitch)	Type IIA (intermediate fast-twitch)	Type IIB (pure fast-twitch)
Glycolytic capacity (ability to burn glycogen)	Low	Moderate	High
Oxidative capacity (ability to use oxygen in energy reactions)	High	Moderate	Low
Contraction speed (ability to produce power)	Slow	Fast	Fast
Glycogen storage (ability to hold glycogen for energy reactions)	Moderate-High	Moderate-High	Moderate-High
Triglyceride storage (ability to hold fat for energy reactions)	High	Moderate	Low
Capillary supply (blood flow into the fibers)	Good	Moderate	Poor

Adapted, by permission, from B. Saltin, J. Henriksson, E. Nygaard, 1979, "Muscle fiber types and their characteristics," *Ann NY Acad Sci* 301:3-29.

In general, sudden high-speed activity that is not long lasting (such as the gymnastics vault or a 50- to 100-meter sprint) demands fuel that is already in the muscles in a ready-to-go or almost-ready-to-go state. Muscles can't hold too much of this type of fuel, so there is a limit to how long muscles can go using this type of system—the phosphagen system. For a well-nourished athlete, the phosphagen system may provide enough fuel for the first five to eight seconds. Of course, that's not enough time for most events, so muscles also have the ability to quickly convert stored glycogen into useable fuel *without oxygen*. However, since the fuel is being burned without oxygen, there's a lot of "smoke" in this type of system that limits how long an athlete can go anaerobically. Most scientists believe that the anaerobic maximum (i.e., the amount of time an athlete can work at absolute full tilt) is 1.5 minutes. When you combine the phosphagen system with the anaerobic system, both of which are used when an athlete is going as hard and fast as possible, you've got a limit on activity of slightly over a minute and a half of continuous movement before the athlete stops.

That's certainly not long enough for a basketball player or a soccer player, but, fortunately, we have another system (aerobic metabolism) that allows us to burn fuel with oxygen, and for a long time. However, this system works best when you're able to provide enough oxygen to the working muscles for the work they're doing. The faster they work, the more fuel that's burned, and the more oxygen they need to burn the fuel. When the muscles work hard and fast enough so that you can't provide enough oxygen, then we start to burn some fuel without oxygen. Do enough anaerobic work and the system stops because of the byproducts produced. The secret to all of this is to become sufficiently well-conditioned so that you can provide a lot of oxygen to your muscles when you need to. That limits the amount of anaerobic muscular work you'll need to do and, importantly, delays fatigue. Of course, having the right fuels available to the muscles is also important, since none of the systems work well if they don't have the fuel they need. For instance, everyone has lots of stored fat (even the most lean people around have a lot of fat available for fuel), and fat is an excellent fuel for aerobic work. However, for fats to burn cleanly, carbohydrates are also necessary. If you run out of carbohydrate fuel, you lose your ability to burn fats effectively and muscular fatigue sets in.

To summarize, we have two basic means for getting energy from the food we eat. We can get energy anaerobically (without oxygen) and we can get energy aerobically (with oxygen). Anaerobic energy pathways are typically used with very high-intensity activities of short duration, while aerobic energy pathways are typically used with activities of lower intensity but longer duration. Let's take a closer look at these fuel systems that we have available to us.

Phosphagen System (Creatine Phosphate)

Enough energy can be released anaerobically from the phosphates in adenosine triphosphate (ATP) and creatine phosphate (CP) to support high-intensity exercise for up to eight seconds. This system, referred to as the phosphagen system because of the immediate availability of high-energy phosphate, is the basis for the popularity of a widely used ergogenic aid—creatine monohydrate (see chapter 4). This system is, to a large extent, dependent on creatine phosphate to quickly provide a high-energy phosphate molecule to form ATP, which is the ultimate source of energy for muscular work. In theory, if you have more creatine in the tissues, you can increase the amount of creatine phosphate available for forming ATP. With more ATP, you can do more extremely high-intensity work. There are a number of sports that rely heavily (if not exclusively) on this phosphagen system. These sports include shot put, long jump, triple jump, discus, gymnastics vault, and short sprints. In addition, other sports that have quick bursts of activity intermingled in the activity (such as football, volleyball, and hockey) are also reliant on this energy pathway. In some of these sports, the ability to do repeat high-intensity moves often determines the winner. For instance, the high jumper, long jumper, and pole-vaulter all need two or three stellar efforts with the hope that one of them will be good enough to win. These repeated bouts of high-intensity work place a tremendous reliance on the phosphagen system. The athlete who has the ability to store more creatine may be at an advantage in these activities. With improved creatine storage, it is possible that the athlete would retain much of the power produced on the first attempt in the second and third attempts.

Assuming that your total energy and protein intake is adequate, your body can manufacture the creatine it needs for multiple quick bursts of high-intensity activity. To improve the storage of ATP-CP in the muscles, athletes must practice activities that focus on this system (i.e., activities that last no more than eight seconds, that are high-intensity, and that are repeated multiple times during an exercise session). This type of training, by itself, is not sufficient to improve short-duration, high-intensity performance. At the same time consuming sufficient energy and protein, by itself, is also not sufficient to improve short-duration, high-intensity performance. However, when both proper training and proper nutrition are combined, the athlete can experience very real gains in short-duration, high-intensity performance.

Anaerobic Metabolism (Glycolysis)

This energy pathway is typically used during high-intensity exercise that exceeds the athlete's ability to provide sufficient oxygen for the work being done. When exercise is this intense, the predominant source of energy is stored muscle glycogen (the storage form of glucose/carbohydrate). When the stored glycogen runs out, the athlete performing this type of high-intensity activity fatigues quickly and the exercise stops. Typically, anaerobic metabolism provides only a small proportion of the total energy used by muscles. Nevertheless, it is important because it can provide energy quickly, and helps to fill the energy gap between the initiation of exercise and the time it takes for aerobic energy metabolism to take over. If someone tries to maintain a high-intensity (i.e., anaerobic) activity, the fuel for this will run out after approximately 1.5 minutes, and the athlete will become quickly fatigued. This 1.5 minutes is the limit that a human being can work if in an anaerobic exercise mode, and a period of rest must follow (typically 3 to 5 minutes) to allow time for muscles to become replenished with energy (glycogen and phosphocreatine). There are some sports that are intentionally limited to 1.5 minutes because of the realization that humans simply can't go longer than this at full tilt. For example, the floor routine in gymnastics lasts up to 1.5 minutes. If you've ever seen a gymnast practice the floor routine, it would be unthinkable for the gymnast to repeat a routine without taking a break. It simply wouldn't be possible, because the muscles have been depleted of the all-important energy needed for that type of high-intensity work. In fact, when you view a gymnastics training session, which often lasts four to five hours, much of the time is spent standing around. This "standing-around" time is important for letting the muscles get ready to do the next round of highly intense work.

Some sports are predominantly aerobic, but may rely on the anaerobic energy pathway to make the difference between winning and losing. The long-distance runner that has managed to go most of the distance while preserving some muscle glycogen, still has the energy reserves to finish the race with a strong (anaerobic) "kick." The ability to do this at the end of the race may be the only difference between first place and those who follow. For runners running short-distance races, for swimmers in short races, and for hockey players skating at full bore at the end of a game to go for a winning score, this anaerobic pathway is the key to success—and carbohydrate makes it happen.

Power athletes are performing power activities that use mainly the phosphocreatine and glycolytic anaerobic systems. To a large degree, this helps to explain what power athletes need to be eating. The limited storage of fats in these fibers means that they don't metabolize fats as an energy substrate. This is confirmed by the fact that they also have a low oxidative capacity, which means that they can't use oxygen well enough to burn fats completely. To make matters worse, these fast-twitch fibers have a relatively poor capillary (blood) supply, so it is difficult to get nutrients into the fibers and to get metabolic

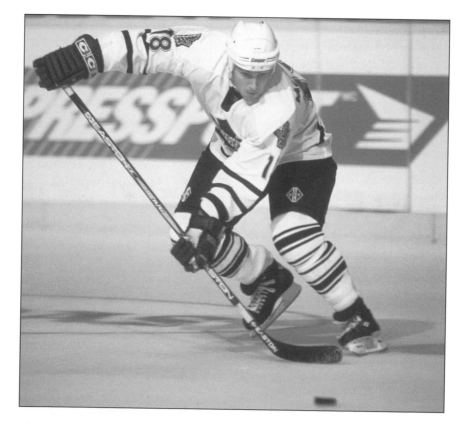

by-products out of the fibers. This is one of the reasons that purely anaerobic (high-intensity, power) activities never go beyond 1.5 to 2.0 minutes. Because fuel can't easily get into the muscles, the athlete needs a recovery break of two to five minutes to allow the muscles to recover. The recovery phase allows the muscles to be refueled and cleaned by letting toxic metabolic by-products out (see table 5.2).

Due to a heavy dependence on fast-twitch fibers to do mainly high-intensity anaerobic work, power athletes find it more difficult, to a great extent, to burn fat as an energy substrate than athletes doing aerobic activities. This translates into a higher potential for gaining (fat) weight. Power athletes continue to burn some limited amounts of fat, but high-intensity anaerobic activity dramatically favors carbohydrate (glycogen) over fat as a fuel because of the kind of muscle fibers that are bring used. This clear preference for glycogen fuel is important, since many power athletes have competitive seasons where activity is high and off-seasons where activity drops. These alterations in activity patterns often translate into wide modulations in weight and body fat percent. It is not uncommon to hear of football players who have been fined for showing up at preseason training camp too fat. When power athletes stop their intensive in-season training but maintain their high-calorie, relatively high-fat diets, a sufficient difference in energy balance occurs that causes inevitable increases in body fat.

Table 5.2 Characteristics of the Three Major Energy Systems

System	Fuel	Oxygen required	Speed of energy provision	Relative energy (ATP) produced
Anaerobic (without oxygen via PC)	Phosphocreatine	No	Fastest	Little; limited
Anaerobic (without oxygen via glycolysis)	Glycogen (carbohydrate)	No	Fast	Little; limited
Aerobic (with oxygen)	Glycogen, fats, proteins	Yes	Slow	Much; unlimited (assuming adequate provision of energy substrates)

Note: PC = phosphocreatine; ATP = adenosine triphosphate

Fast-twitch muscle fibers and anaerobic activity have such a low capacity to burn fats that power athletes could easily consider themselves to be at a fat-eating disadvantage. However, so many power athletes require a large mass, that it becomes inevitable that they consume a substantial amount of fat to meet their tremendous energy requirements. Linemen on football teams commonly report having energy intakes that exceed 5,000 calories per day! On a high-carbohydrate, low-fat intake, an athlete would have to spend much of the day eating to meet these energy demands. Fats, which are more than twice as concentrated in energy as carbohydrates (9 calories/gram vs. 4 calories/gram), help these athletes meet their energy requirements without spending all day in the kitchen. In-season exercise patterns help these athletes burn the consumed calories, but maintaining these diets off-season almost guarantees a significant fat gain. Besides the poor competitive shape this results in, there is good evidence that all the weight cycling that many power athletes experience (either from trying to make weight or from dietary or exercise errors) makes them become obese after they retire from the sport. There is also evidence that weight fluctuations are associated with more frequent illnesses and earlier mortality.[1,2]

Building Lean (Muscle) Mass

Power athletes are usually looking for ways to increase lean body (muscle) mass. The greater the mass, the greater the *potential* for increasing strength and power. There are many techniques employed for increasing muscle mass, including resistance training, consumption of more energy (calories), and the intake of products that claim to enhance muscle development. Some of these techniques and products work, while others do not. Athletes should carefully evaluate the adequacy of their diets before embarking on a regimen of costly and unproven supplements that are meant to enhance muscular development, muscular strength, or both.

Building muscle mass has been the tradition for centuries with power athletes. The Greek Olympic wrestling champion of the sixth century, Milo of Crotona, was famous for doing progressive resistance training and eating an enormously high protein intake: he carried a growing calf the length of the stadium each day, and after four years of carrying it, he ate the calf. It was estimated that Milo had an average meat (beef) intake of 20 pounds per day![3,4]

When I view the eating behaviors of power athletes, I wonder if much has changed since the time of Milo. Surveys suggest that power athletes have tremendously high meat intakes and supplement all this protein with additional protein powders, protein shakes, and amino acids. There is clear evidence that competitive weight lifters need about 1.5 grams of protein per kilogram of body weight. However, surveys suggest that the protein intake of lifters is up to four grams per kilogram of body weight.[5] The question is: does all this protein intake work? The answer is: not as well as they think it does. Since protein provided at a level above 1.5 grams per kilogram of body weight is likely to be stored as fat or burned as a fuel, there is no anabolic or ergogenic advantage to high levels of high protein intake. Whether the excess protein is stored or burned, there is an increased need to excrete the nitrogen associated with protein, and this causes a greater urinary output that can lead to dehydration. In fact, many athletes claim they lose weight on a high protein intake, but this is likely to be due to the high level of body water that is lost rather than from the loss of fat.

Nutrients That Control Muscle Development

It is well established that resistance training stimulates muscle development, and that the level of muscle development may be influenced by the circulating level of human growth hormone (HGH), insulin, testosterone, and other anabolic hormones.[6,7,8,9] In as much as nutrition may impact on the availability of these substances, it seems reasonable to believe that specific nutrients may play a role in muscle development. However, it is also reasonable to believe that nutrient intake would *not* influence the body's production of these substances if their levels are already normal. In other words, in the absence of a specific nutrient deficiency, it is difficult to believe that taking more of a nutrient would alter the production of muscle-building hormones. Again, more than enough is not better than enough. Once you've provided what the cells need, providing more doesn't help. In fact, studies are mixed and inconclusive on whether increasing the specific nutrient intake of a well-nourished subject alters the hormonal milieu.

Individual amino acids have been widely tested to determine if their intake might change the production of HGH in athletes. In fact, amino acid mixtures are the largest category of supplements used by bodybuilders.[10] While some earlier studies have shown that increasing the consumption (via supplement) of the amino acid ornithine may increase HGH production, there is more recent evidence that there is no significant increase in HGH from taking, either individually or in various combinations, the amino acids arginine, lysine, ornithine, and tyrosine.[11,12,13,14,15] In addition, there is evidence that taking a broad-range supplement containing all 20 amino acids has *no* effect on either HGH or testosterone production.[16]

Two studies in the 1980s suggested that taking one gram of the amino acid ornithine and one gram of the amino acid arginine each day would help to reduce body fat and would increase lean body mass and strength if taken in conjunction with a strength training program.[17,18] Food supplement vendors have used this study to claim that these amino acids stimulate HGH and increase muscle mass.[19] However, recent studies that have used more appropriate statistical designs and procedures (incorporating a double-blind protocol where neither the subjects nor the researcher knows what subjects are receiving the nutrient and what subjects are receiving the placebo,

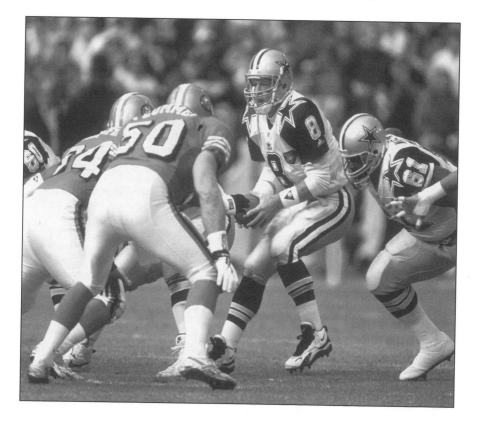

so the outcome cannot be influenced) indicate that oral supplementation of these amino acids has *no* impact on strength or endurance.[20,21]

When a molecule or two of ornithine is attached to a molecule of alpha-ketoglutarate, the resultant molecule (called OKG for ornithine alpha-ketoglutarate) is said to have a muscle-building affect. Although a report in the 1980s, indicated that an increased insulin production was the result of OKG administration, there are no available scientific reports to confirm that OKG actually stimulates muscle development or enhances strength.[22,23] There are several other nutrients and substances that may have a controlling effect on muscular development. See table 5.3 for a summary of these substances.

Table 5.3   Nutrients/Substances That May Have a Controlling Effect on Muscular Development

Substance	What it is	How it works
Choline	An amine that is part of phospholipids common in plant and animal foods. It is a precursor to acetylcholine (a common neurotransmitter) and lecithin (an emulsifying agent important in fat absorption and transport).	It is suggested that choline supplementation increases strength and aids in the loss of body fat, but there is no evidence to support either of these actions.
Creatine	A nitrogenous substance found in meat and synthesized in the body from three amino acids. Combines quickly with phosphate to form phosphocreatine, a high-energy compound stored in muscle.	There is evidence of a significant increase in lean body mass following six days of supplementation with creatine (25 grams/day). It is unclear whether this increase in mass is due to a greater production of muscle proteins (unlikely) or due to a greater retention of water in the muscles (likely). More scientific evidence is needed to confirm that creatine increases muscle mass and increases performance on repeated bouts of short, high-intensity activity.
Glandulars	These are extracts from animal glands (pituitary, thymus, adrenal, and testes).	It is suggested that the glandulars impart the same effect as the effect of the gland it has been derived from (e.g., testes extract enhances testosterone production). However, these extracts are degraded in the extraction and digestion process, so they are inactive. There is no evidence to support their purported action.

Substance	What it is	How it works
Inosine	A nucleotide that helps in the formation of purines such as adenine.	It is suggested that the formation of adenine stimulates a greater production of adenosine, which is part of the high-energy compound adenosine triphosphate (ATP). There is no evidence to support this.
Yohimbine	A nitrogenous alkaloid found in the bark of the yohimbe tree. It increases the serum levels of norepinephrine (adrenaline). It is used in the treatment of obesity and impotence.	It is suggested that yohimbine increases serum testosterone levels, but there is no evidence to support that it has an anabolic effect.

Adapted from Williams 1993.

The single most important factor in muscle development is assuring that the athlete has sufficient energy intake to support a larger mass. If an the athlete has an appropriate energy distribution (about 60 percent from carbohydrate, 15 percent from protein, 25 percent from fat), approximately 3,500 calories are equivalent to one pound. Therefore, for an athlete to gain one pound of muscle mass in one week, an excess of 3,500 calories needs to be consumed during that week. Divided out over seven days, that's an excess of 500 calories each day. It is impossible to increase muscle mass by adding noncalorie-providing supplements to an existing intake. Therefore, when athletes are in a weight-stable state, it is important for them to take stock of the amount and type of food that they consume to maintain that weight. Once determined, then an additional amount of energy is required to support a larger mass.

There is sufficient evidence to support a protein intake for athletes that is approximately double that for nonathletes. This increase in requirement is due to an increase in muscle damage, some protein losses in the urine, and some breakdown of protein in normal energy metabolic cycles, all of which occur for normal regular exercise.[24] The Recommended Dietary Allowance (RDA) for protein for adult nonathletes is 0.8 grams of protein per kilogram of body weight, and the recommended intake for athletes is approximately 1.5 grams of protein per kilogram of body weight. This difference is because athletes have a higher lean body (muscle) mass that requires more protein to sustain it. However, there is almost no survey evidence to suggest that athletes have protein intakes below 1.5 grams per kilogram. In fact, surveys show that the protein intake of athletes is commonly double (approximately 3 grams per kilogram) the recommended level. Athletes taking protein or amino acid supplements often have protein intakes that exceed 4 grams per kilogram. The one exception to this is athletes who are following vegetarian eating patterns. These vegetarian athletes tend to meet the RDA for protein, but consume less than the level commonly recommended for athletes.[25]

Given the generally high intake of protein that athletes currently have, it makes little sense to consume more protein to support a larger muscle mass. Nevertheless, if more protein is consumed it will clearly be used to support energy requirements rather than to support tissue and hormone synthesis. In fact, it is likely that the protein intake consumed by many athletes is misinterpreted as being important for enlarging muscle mass. This excess protein is burned as energy, allowing the body to better meet the energy demands of a larger mass. Without this extra energy, the resultant energy deficit makes it difficult for the athlete to enlarge the muscle mass. It is the general consensus of studies that the extra 500 calories consumed to aid in the enlargement of muscle mass should be mainly from carbohydrates, since this is a more efficient energy source and, unlike protein, one that does not increase metabolic waste that must be excreted.

The nitrogenous wastes that are created from burning protein as an energy source results in increased urinary output, which increases the risk of dehydration. Some athletes believe that protein supplements are better or more effective in supporting lean mass than foods that are high in protein. Good food sources of protein, such as meat, fish, poultry, dairy products, and legumes in combination with cereals are all excellent. There is no evidence that taking supplementary protein is better than eating these foods. As an added benefit, these foods typically contain a great deal of zinc and iron, both of which tend to be low in the diets of many athletes and which are critically important for working muscles.[26,27,28]

It is common for athletes to take multivitamin and multimineral supplements, but there is *no* evidence that these supplements enhance performance in sports that require power.[29,30] Despite the lack of scientific evidence to support taking supplemental doses of vitamins, there is a common belief among power athletes that a number of these vitamins enhance strength. The vitamins and minerals sold to enhance strength include vitamin B-12, vitamins C, E, and beta-carotene (antioxidants), chromium, boron, and magnesium.

Vitamin B-12

The theory behind vitamin B-12 is that it is essential for the synthesis of DNA, and having more DNA enhances muscular development. However, there is no evidence that vitamin B-12 or B-12 derivatives have any beneficial impact on muscular development or on improvements in strength.

Antioxidants

The antioxidant vitamins (C, E, and beta-carotene) may speed recovery time for sore muscles. If this is found to be true, there may be a real benefit to taking antioxidants (which are easily obtained by consuming fresh fruits and vegetables) at the initiation of a strength-training program. It is during this phase that muscles more easily become sore, so the benefit (if there is one) would be greatest at this time.

Chromium

Chromium is essential for the effective metabolism of glucose and is the key component in a compound called "glucose tolerance factor," or GTF. Chromium enhances the effectiveness of insulin and is marketed as a substance that can enlarge muscles, improve strength, and lower body fat. Typically, chromium is marketed in the "chromium picolinate" form (chromium attached to a picolinate carrier). Recent evidence suggests that chromium picolinate is ineffective in doing any of the things it is supposed to do.[31,32]

Boron

Boron is an important mineral that may help prevent the bone disease osteoporosis. In 1992, a study on boron-deprived postmenopausal women reported that boron supplements doubled their serum testosterone levels.[33] However, this study showed that continued intake of boron did not further enhance serum testosterone, and supplementation of males had no impact on testosterone, at all. Another study on bodybuilders indicated that boron supplementation had no impact on serum testosterone, lean body mass, and strength.[34]

Magnesium

Magnesium is the second most predominant (after potassium) intermuscular electrolyte, and it has a number of important functions related to protein synthesis and muscular contractions. It appears that magnesium supplementation is more useful in untrained individuals who are initiating a training program than in athletes who are already well trained. In one study, it was found that both untrained males and female who were in a seven-week weight training session had important increases in muscular power as a result of magnesium supplementation.[35]

Fats and Fat Derivatives

Fat intake may be important (critical for some athletes) as a means of obtaining sufficient energy to maintain a high body mass. A number of fat derivatives are marketed, however, because of their supposed positive impact on energy metabolism, or because they are chemically similar to hormones that enhance muscular development. For instance, some plant sterols (called phytosterols) are similar to the hormone testosterone.[36] However, there is limited evidence that any of these fat-derivative functions work to enhance muscle mass or athletic performance. The major fat-derivative products marketed to athletes include medium-chain triglycerides (MCT oil), omega-3 fatty acids (O-3FAs), gamma oryzanol, and smilax. See table 5.4 for a summary of their functions.

Table 5.4 **Fat Derivatives That Are Advertised as Enhancing Muscle Development and Strength**

Substance	What it is	How it works
Medium-chain triglycerides (MCT oil)	MCT oil represents short-carbon-chain fats that are easily absorbed and metabolized. They have been used in clinical environments for many years as a means of providing sufficient energy to patients receiving tube feedings.	There is no evidence that MCT oil enhances muscle mass development or improves weight gain (or loss) in strength trained athletes.
Omega-3 fatty acids (O-3FAs)	O-3FAs are found in the oil of cold-water fish and are known to lower blood viscosity and red cell stickiness. They are also known to reduce tissue inflammation.	These fatty acids may be metabolized into prostaglandin EI, which stimulates the production of human growth hormone. There is no substantive evidence that this occurs in strength trained athletes to a degree that an improvement can be measured.

Substance	What it is	How it works
Gamma oryzanol	This is a plant sterol derived from rice bran oil.	This substance and the related substance ferulic acid are advertised as being capable of increasing testosterone and human growth hormone levels. While there is some evidence that gamma oryzanol influences the metabolism of fats, there is no evidence that it produces an ergogenic effect in humans. There is some animal evidence that taking these substances actually *reduces* testosterone production.
Smilax	This is a plant sterol commonly extracted from sarsaparilla root. This has been used in folk medicine for many years.	This substance is advertised as being capable of stimulating testosterone production, increasing muscle mass, and increasing muscular strength. There are no data to support these claims.

Adapted from Williams 1993.

Summary

Power and strength are critical components for athletes doing quick, short-duration, high-intensity activities. While also important for athletes involved in longer-duration activities (the "kick" at the end of a marathon often determines the winner), they are not the issue of central importance. The development and maintenance of a large and strong muscle mass are important in developing power, and proper nutritional strategies can aid the athlete in obtaining the muscle mass they seek. A key nutritional element in building and maintaining muscle mass is the acquisition of sufficient energy to support the mass. Although consuming large amounts of protein can do this, consumption of additional carbohydrate is less expensive and more effective. In fact, power athletes are even more dependent on carbohydrates than endurance athletes because the muscle fibers they use don't have the capacity to burn fats effectively. Power athletes often make the mistake of thinking that protein is the key to their success. Not only is this erroneous thinking, but it's potentially dangerous as there are also problems associated with excessive protein consumption. For instance, excess protein intake is inevitably associated with an increase in dehydration because of the increased requirement to excrete more metabolic (nitrogenous) waste.

Supplementation of vitamins, minerals, protein products, and fat analogues has not been found to be successful in improving power, muscle mass, or athletic performance in power athletes. While the risk of taking these products is likely to be low, there are insufficient data to know for certain if these products are, indeed, safe when taken in the amounts and duration prescribed by the manufacturers of these products. A more sensible approach is to consume a balanced and varied diet that is high in carbohydrates (60 to 70 percent of calories), moderate in protein (12 to 15 percent of calories), and low in fat (18 to 25 percent of calories). This intake has the benefit of providing the minerals and vitamins needed for supporting athletic performance, and will provide the best source of energy for your muscles to work efficiently. There is no question about the safety of consuming a varied diet that is high in carbohydrates.

6 Eating for Aerobic Power

Feeling Better Means You'll Do Better

The single most common eating error I see in the endurance athletes I work with is that they do their morning run *before* they have anything to eat. Then they come back—feeling queasy—and fill the tank. If anyone has a car that lets you fill up *after* the trip, please let me know!

When Jack, a duathlon (bike and run) champion, came through my lab (Laboratory for Elite Athlete Performance at Georgia State University) and shared his daily training regimen with the staff, we hardly flinched. He was doing exactly what he had been taught to do, and what everyone he trained with was also doing. You get up, get your gear on, and go for your morning workout. When something like this is so common, it's inevitable that we'll get strange looks when we say that this strategy keeps them from benefiting from their morning training. Of course, the athlete has *many* reasons for doing this, not the least of which is that he doesn't feel good exercising with food in his stomach. This is absolutely true, since *no one* feels good exercising with food bouncing around in his or her stomach, but this doesn't change the fact that you need energy to do work. So when Jack said this, we were prepared with the math: "You use x amount of energy per hour when you sleep. Your liver stores x amount of energy, which is used to maintain blood sugar during the night so your lungs and heart will keep working. The amount of energy left in the liver when you get up is, based on your rate of utilization and liver storage capacity, zero. The body creates glucose to maintain blood sugar when the liver is empty. The sugar it creates is made mainly from protein (i.e., muscles). When you exercise with no sugar in the liver you break down the very muscles you're trying to improve with the exercise. Therefore, you don't benefit from the exercise, and the improvement in endurance you're seeking won't come."

The reaction to this information is also universally consistent: "Oh my! What do I do?" When we talked with Jack about the best strategy for *him*, we wanted to know what juice he likes to drink—one that gives him no stomach upset. That's the starting point. We ask that he try drinking half a glass of juice before the run. This is fairly quickly absorbed and is useful in maintaining blood sugar. After he tries that for awhile, we suggest that he add half a piece of dry toast (no butter, no marmalade) with the half glass of juice. Ultimately, we want him to work up to one glass of juice and one piece of toast *before* the morning workout.

When Jack came back six months later, he said he couldn't believe how much better he was feeling and doing and how much more "energy" he had. He attributed this improvement to having the small "breakfast" before his morning workout. I might add that he ate the rest of his rather enormous breakfast after he returned from the workout. The interesting thing about his response to his new regimen was that he didn't realize he could feel better, since he had no sensation of feeling "bad" when we first talked. Of course, when you do something enough, you think the way you feel is "'normal" and expected. Feeling better after following a sound strategy is just an added bonus, because it makes you want to continue what you're doing. And when you feel better, you'll do better as well.

Endurance athletes are involved in events where there is continuous movement for longer than 20 minutes. Some endurance sports combine periods of slow, continuous movement with periods of fast, quick bursts of movement (soccer, tennis, etc.), and other endurance sports require continuous movement over long distances or time periods (marathon, cross-country skiing, triathlon, etc.). In both types of activity, there is a premium on supplying sufficient energy and fluid to assure that the athlete does not become exhausted from the activity or become overheated from the continuous energy burn. A failure to supply sufficient energy of the right type will lead to early fatigue and poor athletic performance. The goal for the endurance athlete is, therefore, to establish a workable strategy for supplying sufficient energy and fluids before and during practice and competition to sustain muscular work for a long duration and at the highest possible intensity.

The majority of endurance activity takes place at an intensity that allows fats to contribute a high proportion of the fuel for muscular work. Since there is an almost inexhaustible supply of fat in even the leanest athlete, supplying fats before and during physical activity is not a concern and would not be a goal. However, carbohydrate is involved in the complete combustion of fats, and since the storage capacity for carbohydrates is relatively low and easily depleted, the goal for endurance athletes is to find a way to supply enough carbohydrates to last for the duration of the activity. Therefore, while power athletes must consume sufficient energy to maintain or enlarge the muscle mass, endurance athletes must consume sufficient energy (as carbohydrate) to maintain muscular work over long time periods.

Aerobic metabolism is the energy system of greatest importance for endurance athletes. In this energy pathway, oxygen is used to help transfer phosphorus into new ATP molecules. Unlike anaerobic metabolism, this energy pathway can use protein, fat, and carbohydrate for fuel by converting pieces of these energy substrates into a compound called acetyl CoA (acetyl coenzyme A). Glucose is converted to pyruvic acid (an anaerobic, energy-releasing process), and this pyruvic acid can either be converted into acetyl CoA with the help of oxygen, or it can be converted to an energy storage product called lactic acid. Of course, if too much lactic acid builds up, the muscle will fatigue and activity will stop (the problem with doing exclusively anaerobic work). However, the lactic acid can easily be reconverted to pyruvic acid to be used as a fuel aerobically.

Aerobic metabolism occurs in the mitochondria of cells, where the vast majority of all ATP is produced from the entering acetyl CoA. Fats can be converted to acetyl CoA through a process called the beta oxidative metabolic pathway. This pathway is very oxygen dependent, which means that fats can only be burned aerobically.

The ability of an athlete to achieve a steady state of oxygen uptake into the cells is a function of how well an athlete is aerobically conditioned. An athlete that frequently trains aerobically is likely to reach a steady state faster than one who does not train aerobically. For a well-conditioned person, it can take five minutes before enough oxygen is in the system to support aerobic metabolism at a steady state. The first five minutes of activity are supported by a combination of anaerobic and aerobic metabolism. Achievement of a fast steady state is therefore important because that diminishes the amount of time an athlete is obtaining energy via anaerobic pathways. This places a heavy burden on the most limited fuel—carbohydrates. In theory, once an athlete reaches a level of oxygen uptake that matches oxygen requirement for the given level of exertion, the exercise could go on for as long as the body's carbohydrate level and fluids did not reach a critical state. For instance, a long-distance runner who is in a steady state could continue running provided the runner replaced the carbohydrate and fluids that are used in the activity. Therefore, endurance is enhanced with a periodic intake of carbohydrate and fluid *during* the activity.

Athletes with different levels of conditioning are likely to achieve steady state at different levels of exercise intensity. If you're well conditioned, you might be able to maintain a steady state at a high enough level of exercise intensity to easily win a race. In other words, you can go really fast but still provide enough oxygen to your cells to satisfy your aerobic needs. At the 1996 Centennial Olympic Games in Atlanta, Georgia, the winner of the marathon ran over 26 miles at a speed that averaged just over a 5-minute-per-mile pace—an unbelievably fast pace! However, if you're not well conditioned aerobically, you may only be able to run at a 10-minutes-per-mile pace and maintain a steady state. Each person has his or her own pace that allows maintenance of a steady state. Exceeding that pace causes a greater proportion of the muscular work to rely on anaerobic metabolism, with an associated increase in the reliance on carbohydrate fuel. Since there is a limited storage of carbohydrate fuel, the fuel tank runs dry more quickly, and the person becomes exhausted faster.

Energy Demands

The energy demands of endurance athletes are enormous. It has been estimated that cross-country skiers use approximately 4,000 calories during a 50-kilometer race and use even more energy (up to 8,000 calories per day) when in intensive training.[1] It has been recommended that, as a general rule, athletes should consume at least 45 calories per kilogram of body weight per day if training for at least 1.5 hours per day.[2] A survey of triathletes determined that they consumed approximately 60 calories per kilogram per day when training 19 hours per week, but only 37 to 40 calories per kilogram when training 11 hours per week.[3] It has been estimated that a 25-year-old female marathoner weighing 125 pounds and running 10 miles at a six-minute-per-mile pace in the morning and eight miles of interval training in the afternoon would require 3,000 calories for the activity, plus 1,331 calories to cover the needs of "resting energy expenditure"[4] (see table 6.1)[7a]. Resting energy expenditure represents the baseline amount of energy a person uses while at rest. A consistent failure to supply this 4,331 calories would lead to weight loss in people who are already extremely lean.[5]

Fluids

As athletes exercise, there is an inevitable loss of body water through sweat. This cooling system, plus the normal urinary water loss, may amount to over 10 liters (about 11 quarts) of daily water loss when exercising in a warm environment.[6] In a hot and humid environment, water losses may exceed three liters per hour but may be less than 0.5 liters per hour in cool and dry environments.[7] Despite the high rates of sweat losses experienced by athletes, most athletes replace only 50 percent of the water that is lost, a behavior that inevitably leads to

Table 6.1   Resting Energy Expenditure* Calculation in Athletes

	Formula
Age	**Males**
10-18	(17.5 x body weight in kilograms[†]) + 651
18-30	(15.3 x body weight in kilograms[†]) + 679
30-60	(11.6 x body weight in kilograms[†]) + 879
	Females
10-18	(12.2 x body weight in kilograms[†]) + 746
18-30	(14.7 x body weight in kilograms[†]) + 496
30-60	(8.7 x body weight in kilograms[†]) + 829

*Resting energy expenditure (REE) represents the energy needed to maintain the lean mass, as well as the energy needed to carry on normal body functions, when the body is at rest. When REE is added to the cost of energy for an activity and the amount of energy that it takes to digest and metabolize food (called the thermic effect of food), you can predict the total energy requirement.

[†]To calculate weight in kilograms, take weight in pounds and divide by 2.2. (e.g., a 100-pound person weighs 45.5 kilograms).

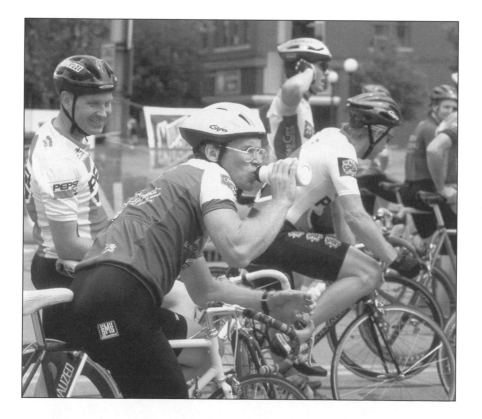

progressive dehydration and a decline in performance.[8] Research has clearly demonstrated that even a slight dehydration (2 percent of body weight) causes a measurable decrease in athletic performance.[9,10] Therefore, when athletes take steps to satisfy fluid requirements, they are helping to guarantee optimal athletic performance (see chapter 2, "Staying Hydrated").

Carbohydrate

Athletes require carbohydrate during both high-intensity and lower-intensity activities. When carbohydrate stores are depleted, the athlete quickly becomes fatigued and performance drops dramatically. However, since the storage level of carbohydrate is relatively low when compared to fat stores, athletes must make a conscious effort to replace carbohydrate at every opportunity. Having high levels of stored carbohydrate (glycogen) and consuming carbohydrate during activities that last one hour or more are well-established techniques for optimizing athletic endurance. Consuming carbohydrate during activity helps to maintain blood sugar (glucose) and insulin, which encourages sugar uptake by working muscles.[11] This helps to increase the muscular metabolism of carbohydrates and also helps to assure that carbohydrates are not depleted during activity. In a study of cyclists doing endurance work, those who consumed a carbohydrate-containing beverage during the exercise were able to exercise an additional hour when compared to cyclists who consumed only water.[12] In general, athletes are encouraged to consume approximately 9 to 10 grams (35 to 40 calories) of carbohydrate per kilogram of body weight each day (see table 6.2). This amounts to about 600 grams (2,400 calories) of daily carbohydrate intake for a 150-pound athlete. The general recommendation is that athletes should consume foods that provide at least 60 percent of the total consumed energy (calories) as carbohydrate.[13]

There is evidence that the *concentration* of carbohydrate consumed early during endurance running may influence the degree to which the athlete gets gastrointestinal (GI) discomfort. It was found that a 5.5 percent (13 grams of carbohydrate per 8 ounces of fluid) carbohydrate solution produced the same (relatively low) level of GI distress as plain water. A 6.9 percent (16 grams of carbohydrate per 8 ounces of fluid) solution, on the other hand, doubled the incidence of distress when athletes were asked to perform the same exercise. In addition, only the 5.5 percent carbohydrate solution imparted a significant improvement in performance.[14] There were similar results in a study

**Table 6.2   Carbohydrate Intake Recommendations
for Athletes**

Body weight (pounds)	Grams of carbohydrate	Calories of carbohydrate
100	400	1,600
125	500	2,000
150	600	2,400
175	700	2,800
200	800	3,200
225	900	3,800

Adapted from Murray and Horswill 1998.

of marathon running performance. Marathoners, who run over 26 miles, were asked to consume either water, a 5.5 percent carbohydrate solution, or a 6.9 percent carbohydrate solution on three different occasions.[15] The fastest times were recorded when they consumed the 5.5 percent carbohydrate solution, while consuming the 6.9 percent solution resulted in times that were similar to consuming plain water. Therefore, the classic nutritional paradigm holds true here as well: "More than enough is not better than enough." Although athletes have a tremendous need for carbohydrate, trying to provide too much too fast causes difficulties and may detract from performance.

The *type* of carbohydrate may also make a difference in endurance performance and gastrointestinal distress. In one study, 6-percent solutions of different types of sugars (glucose, fructose, and sucrose) were compared during 105 minutes of cycling exercise. (See table 6.3 for an explanation of different carbohydrates.) While consumption of glucose and sucrose resulted in positive outcomes, the consumption of the fructose solution resulted in more GI distress, a greater drop in blood volume, a greater increase in stress hormone response, and measurably poorer exercise performance.[16] When Gatorade, a 6-percent carbohydrate and electrolyte beverage (containing glucose and sucrose as the source of carbohydrate), is consumed during high-intensity activity, it has been found to blunt the increase in the stress hormones angiotestin-I, ACTH, and cortisol when compared to water.[17] Therefore, it appears clear that having a carbohydrate-containing beverage during exercise is a very good thing to do.

Resynthesis of glycogen following activity is also important, since glycogen reserves are severely depleted following activity lasting

Table 6.3   Different Types of Carbohydrates

Fructose	Also called "fruit sugar" since it is prevalent in fruit and honey. It is the sweetest tasting of the sugars (i.e., for the same amount, fructose tastes sweeter than glucose or sucrose). Fructose is not easily put into solution with water, so it tends to drop to the bottom of the container if not mixed. Try putting honey in water to see this effect.
Glucose	This is the primary energy source for the body. Because it is so important, we can convert all other sugars to glucose, and we can make glucose from the breakdown of amino acids (proteins). Glucose is also referred to as *dextrose*.
Glucose polymers	This is a starch made up of *many* units of glucose. When digested, many units of glucose become quickly available.
Maltodextrins	These are polymers that have at least five glucose units attached together. Maltodextrins have a relatively low sweetness level when compared to other sugars, so they are not widely used, even though they have the capacity to provide many glucose units quickly.
Maltose	This is a sugar composed of two molecules of glucose and is commonly found in grain (malt) products. While maltose is a quick source of glucose, its relatively low sweetness keeps it from being widely used.
Sucrose	This sugar is composed of equal parts of glucose and fructose. Because it is composed of two sugars, it must be broken up into its component parts to be used for energy. The glucose is immediately available for energy, while the fructose must be converted to glucose in the liver to be used as energy. Sucrose is also called *table sugar* and is commonly found in sugar beets and sugar cane. Because of its easy solubility in water and its sweet taste, sucrose is a common sugar in beverages.

one hour or longer. The efficiency of glycogen resynthesis is dependent on several factors, including[18]

- the timing of the carbohydrate intake,
- the amount of carbohydrate consumed,
- the type of carbohydrate consumed, and
- the degree to which muscle has been damaged during the exercise (damaged muscle is slower to resynthesize glycogen than healthy muscle).

Foods containing carbohydrates that enter the blood quickly (i.e., high glycemic index foods) are better able to resynthesize liver and muscle glycogen than foods low on the glycemic index scale (see table 6.4).

The general recommendation is to consume approximately 200 calories of carbohydrate every two hours following exercise, with the first 200 calories being provided as soon after exercise as possible.[19]

Table 6.4 Glycemic Index of Foods

Foods	Glycemic index
Glucose	100
Maltose (grain sugar)	95
Carrots	92
Honey	87
Cornflakes cereal	80
Whole-wheat bread	72
White rice	72
Potatoes	70
Shredded wheat	67
Bananas	62
Sucrose (table sugar)	59
Sweet corn	59
Potato chips	51
Peas	51
Oatmeal	49
Orange juice	46
Baked beans	40
Apples	39
Yogurt	36
Ice cream	36
Whole milk	34
Fructose (fruit sugar)	20
Peanuts	13

Note: Foods with higher glycemic values produce a faster rise in blood sugar (glucose) than foods with lower values. Nothing produces a faster rise in blood glucose than pure glucose, with a glycemic index of 100. It is generally considered better to have a slow and steady rise in blood glucose rather than a sudden rise in blood glucose. Therefore, foods with a glycemic index below 75 are preferable for usual consumption.

Adapted from Foster-Powell and Miller 1995.

Building Energy and Fluid Reserves to Support Endurance Activities

The importance of building and maintaining energy reserves to support endurance activity is well established. In virtually every study that has examined athletes with high glycogen reserves versus those with lower reserves, those with higher reserves consistently have better endurance and perform better athletically. It is *very* clear that endurance athletes who begin competition with more stored carbohydrate have more available at the end of the competition, and this difference alone may be enough to determine the winner. In addition, athletes who are better hydrated during competition perform better than those who are less well hydrated.

Having optimal carbohydrate and fluid intake doesn't happen automatically. It is something that must occur with foresight and planning. To make the right plans, athletes should consider the opportunities they have available in the following four different blocks of time:

- *Before competition/practice.* This is the period immediately preceding (three to six hours before) competition and/or practice.
- *During competition/practice.* The competition and/or practice itself.
- *After competition/practice.* The period immediately following (up to two hours after) competition and/or practice.
- *General daily considerations.* The remaining portion of the day not considered above.

Before Competition/Practice

When carbohydrates are consumed prior to exercise, there is improved performance.[20] The general recommendation is for athletes to consume between 800 to 1,200 calories during the hours that precede competition and/or practice.[21]

Foods consumed prior to competition should be foods that have been consumed without difficulty prior to training. Trying to improve carbohydrate status before a competition by trying out new foods, gels, or sports drinks is an almost guaranteed formula for competitive disaster. Rehearse what you intend to do for competition during practice to make certain your body responds well to it. Competition is not a time for experimentation.

Consumption of fluids prior to competition is also important, and since glycogen storage requires additional fluids (three grams of fluid for each gram of glycogen stored), carbohydrate consumption should always take place with substantial fluid intake. Since it is common for athletes to drink only when thirsty, a conscious effort should be made to consume fluids even when not thirsty. If you know you have difficulty taking in enough fluids because you don't think about it or because of a lack of fluid available, try beginning each day with a two-liter water bottle that you carry with you (backpacks work nicely) every day. Getting and staying well hydrated may be the single most important thing you can do to assure good athletic performance. Since it is almost impossible to adequately replace all fluids lost during training and/or competition, it is useful for athletes to enter the exercise in a well-hydrated state.

It is impossible to become well hydrated during exercise if you enter the exercise poorly hydrated to begin with. Assuming that ample fluids have been consumed during the day leading up to the precompetition/practice period, athletes should consume an additional 16 ounces of fluid approximately two hours before the exercise begins. After this, fluids should be consumed every 15 to 30 minutes to maintain the hydration state leading into the exercise. It is also recommended that 8 to 16 ounces of fluid be consumed during the 30 minutes prior to exercise. You will know if you've adequately hydrated yourself by checking on the color of your urine. Dark urine suggests that you are not well hydrated, while clear urine suggests that you are. Using sports beverages prior to exercise is useful because they provide the two things athletes need most: carbohydrates and fluids. The American College of Sports Medicine position on fluids states that[22]

- the fluid consumed should be flavored and sweetened to encourage fluid intake;
- to help maintain training intensity, the fluid should contain carbohydrate; and
- to stimulate rapid and complete rehydration, the beverage should contain sodium chloride (salt).

Sports beverages that meet these criteria are particularly useful in helping to deliver both carbohydrates and fluids to athletes.

During Competition/Practice

In events, such as 10-kilometer races and marathons, where fluids are available at regular intervals, the athlete should take full advantage of each fluid station and consume fluids. Since water is constantly being lost, frequent and regular consumption of fluids helps to maintain the body's water level. Since most athletes consume less water than they need, techniques for assuring hydration during activity have been studied. The following recommendations have been suggested:[23]

- Make certain that fluid is always nearby, since accessibility helps to assure better fluid intake.
- All athletes should have their own bottle from which to drink, and this bottle should be with them whenever they exercise or are at a competition.
- Coaches should design practices that enable athletes to drink frequently.
- The coaching staff should be aware of those athletes with high sweat rates to make certain they consume more fluids than those with lower sweat rates.
- Help athletes learn to drink frequently by considering this to be part of the training regimen.

To understand how much fluid an athlete needs to consume during practice and competition, a log should be maintained with the amount of fluid consumed and the beginning and ending weight of the athletes. If an athlete consumes 32 ounces during practice and weighs 2 pounds less at the end of practice than at the beginning, this athlete should learn to consume an additional 32 ounces of fluid during the practice (1 pound = 16 ounces of fluid).

Consumption of fluids that contain carbohydrates is important during exercise, and properly designed sports beverages can aid in providing both fluids and carbohydrates quickly. The ideal sports beverage should have the following characteristics:

- Cool beverages are tolerated best.
- A carbohydrate solution of between 5 and 6 percent delivers both the carbohydrate and the fluid quickly. A higher carbohydrate concentration slows delivery to the muscles by delaying gastric emptying and may increase the risk of gut upset.

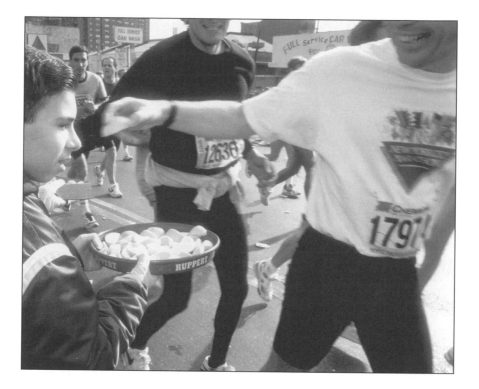

- A small amount of sodium helps drive the desire to drink, and in so doing helps to assure that the athlete stays better hydrated. Sodium may also aid in getting the water and carbohydrate absorbed more quickly, as well as help to maintain blood volume. Maintenance of blood volume is an important predictor of athletic performance. There is some evidence that hyponatremia (low blood sodium), which results from large losses of sodium in sweat that goes unreplaced, occurs in endurance and ultra-endurance events. [24] This is a rare but serious condition that may result in seizures, comas, or death.

- The beverage should taste good to the athlete. The taste sensation may be altered during exercise, so there is no guarantee that a fluid you enjoy drinking at dinner will taste good to you while exercising. Make sure an athlete tries different flavors *during exercise* to determine what is best liked.

- The carbohydrate should be from a combination of glucose and sucrose. Beverages containing predominantly fructose increase the risk of creating gut upset.

- Noncarbonated sports drinks are preferred over carbonated drinks during endurance exercise.[25]

Consumption of carbohydrates in solid and liquid forms both results in the same performance outcomes, so athletes in some sports may choose to consume carbohydrate foods rather than carbohydrate beverages.[26] Cyclists who go long distances, for instance, often consume bananas and carbohydrate gels to support their carbohydrate requirement. It appears as if the consumption of 45 to 75 grams of carbohydrate per hour (180 to 300 calories from carbohydrate per hour) helps to improve athletic performance.[27] This amount of carbohydrate can be found in approximately one quart of sports beverage with a 6 percent carbohydrate concentration.

After Competition/Practice

While you may think you've done everything you need to do once your exercise is over—except shower—it is clear that drinking more fluids and consuming more carbohydrates *after* the exercise or competition is important. Doing this will help you replenish your glycogen stores and get you ready for the next day of exercise. The best glycogen replenishment occurs if you consume high glycemic index carbohydrates (see table 6.4) immediately following exercise, and continue consuming carbohydrates (via snacks) until the next meal.[28]

General Daily Considerations

The before-exercise, during-exercise, and after-exercise periods are meant to provide carbohydrates and fluids to support the activity, but what you do the rest of the time helps to assure that the before-, during-, and after-exercise strategies actually work. Obviously, the consumption of carbohydrates and fluids during these periods doesn't provide all the nutrients and minerals an athlete needs to support health and activity. For this reason, it is imperative that what you eat the rest of the time provides a balance of nutrients that can keep you healthy. It is *very* true that healthy athletes are better athletes. A good basic strategy to follow for your regular meal times is to distribute foods as indicated on the Food Guide Pyramid. This guide encourages the consumption of a wide variety of foods that are high in complex carbohydrates, moderate in protein, and low in fats and sugars. This type of food distribution is perfect for athletes and will help to assure that all necessary nutrients are consumed.

There is nothing an athlete can do just before competition to correct a nutrient deficiency and help performance. If your intake of iron is consistently low, and you develop iron deficiency anemia, it could take six months on a good diet and iron supplements to bring your iron level up to a point where performance won't be negatively impacted. If you've got a nutrient deficiency, doing everything right before, during, and after exercise still won't have you performing up to your conditioned ability. So eat well and eat wisely when you've got the chance and, of course, drink plenty of fluids.

Other Nutritional Recommendations

There are several rules of nutrition that apply here. Among them is the idea of the need to consume a wide variety of foods to assure that the body is exposed to all of the essential nutrients. On the backside of this rule, there is another benefit. By consuming a wide variety of foods, athletes can avoid being exposed to any potentially toxic substances that are more prevalent in some foods. Therefore, eating a wide variety of foods is a good nutritional rule to live by. Another rule is the idea that it is possible to eat too much of something, even if you think it's good for you. Learning to balance your diet through variety will help ensure your body of both proper maintenance and adequate nutrient intake.

Protein

Endurance athletes actually require slightly more protein than power athletes, even though it's usually the power athletes who take more protein and amino acid supplements. While most endurance athletes appear to consume at least the Recommended Dietary Allowance for protein (0.8 grams of protein per kilogram of body weight, as established by the Food and Nutrition Board of the National Research Council), the estimated requirement for endurance athletes is about double this level (1.5 grams per kilogram).[29] With the exception of vegetarians, most endurance athletes appear to consume this level of protein from food alone.[30]

Consumption of excess protein has always been a concern for athletes, since many of the products marketed for improvement of athletic performance are some form of protein supplement or amino acid powder preparation. There have been several studies suggesting that consistently high protein intakes (above 1.6 grams per kilogram) may contribute to kidney disease or exacerbate an existing kidney problem. In addition, since high protein diets are almost inevitably also high fat and high cholesterol diets, there is concern that those with a genetic predisposition to heart disease would be negatively impacted. Of course, if excess protein is derived from supplements, it may be low in fat but these carry their own set of difficulties. For instance, it is difficult to be sure that the supplement is of high quality. In addition, any amount of protein that exceeds the requirement is likely to increase water loss and increase the risk of dehydration, regardless of whether it comes from food or supplements.

There is little reason for *any* athlete, no matter the sport, to consume a level of protein that exceeds 1.5 to 2.0 grams per kilogram of body weight. In general, this amounts to between 12 and 15 percent of total calories consumed. For athletes on high protein intakes, protein consumption is often more than three grams per kilogram of body weight, or 30 percent of total calories consumed. By any measure, this is excessive. Since high protein intakes commonly result in either the excess protein being stored as fat or, if there is a general energy intake inadequacy, being burned for fuel, the nitrogenous waste products must be removed. This excess urea excretion causes a greater urinary volume to be produced, increasing the chance for dehydration. Since staying well hydrated is of central importance to athletic performance, having a diet that induces dehydration must be considered counterproductive. It is likely that this extra water loss is at least partially responsible for the weight losses seen in people who consume high-protein, low-carbohydrate diets. While the weight loss may appear desirable, the negative impact this has on endurance should cause you to think carefully about whether this type of intake is for you. (It shouldn't be!)

Fat

While the high-protein, high-fat, low-carbohydrate diet (40 percent carbohydrate, 30 percent protein, and 30 percent fat) has reared its ugly head once again (it seems to return with a new name every 10 to 20 years), it is no better now than it was when it was first introduced. There is *nothing* in the science or experience to suggest that this type of intake is useful for any athlete. For endurance athletes, all the literature makes it amply clear that the higher the carbohydrate intake, the better the performance. Therefore, for endurance athletes, this type of intake must be considered a disaster for athletic performance. When these diets rear their heads, I sometimes

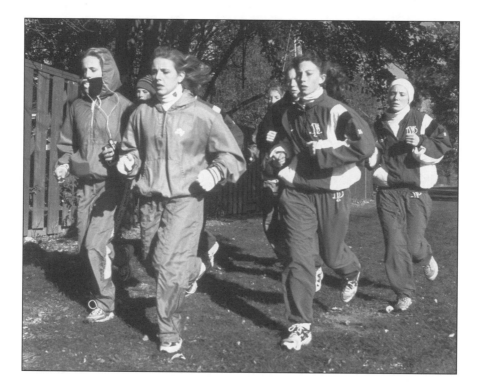

wonder if they've been secretly introduced by some country or group that wants to win a competitive edge in competition.

Vitamins

Vitamin supplements for otherwise well-nourished athletes do not improve athletic performance. However, athletes who know they don't eat a good balanced diet may benefit from taking a low-level (50 to 100 percent of the RDA) multivitamin, multimineral supplement. B-vitamins are critically important for endurance activities, but athletes consuming high-carbohydrate diets (60 to 70 percent carbohydrate or a minimum of 30 calories per kilogram of body weight) are virtually assured of obtaining sufficient B-vitamins from the foods they consume. The B-vitamins work together, so taking a single B-vitamin does little or no good. In one study, niacin (vitamin B-3) was added to a carbohydrate-containing sports beverage to determine if it would enhance exercise endurance during long-range cycling. The findings indicate that, because niacin inhibited the release and utilization of free fatty acids, the muscles became more reliant on glycogen, resulting in earlier fatigue.[31]

There is also some limited evidence that taking antioxidant vitamins (vitamins C, E, and Beta-carotene) may reduce the time muscles remain sore following an intensive workout or competition. However, regular consumption of high-carbohydrate foods, such as fresh fruits and vegetables, helps to assure that plenty of antioxidant vitamins are presented to the tissues.

Minerals

While the mineral needs of athletes are covered more completely in chapter 1, "Balancing Essential Nutrients," it warrants mentioning here that the oxygen-carrying capacity of endurance athletes is important. If an athlete's iron status is compromised, oxygen-carrying capacity will drop and so will performance. Zinc is also an important mineral in numerous enzymes involved in oxidative energy metabolism. The best dietary source for iron and zinc is meat (beef, poultry, pork, lamb, etc.). For endurance athletes who do not consume meat, there is a natural concern that both their iron and zinc status may be a problem. To be safe, these nonmeat-eating athletes should have yearly blood tests to assure that iron status and zinc status are within acceptable bounds. If not, supplements of these minerals, as recommended by a physician, may be warranted.

Another mineral of concern is calcium, because strong bones help reduce the incidence of musculoskeletal problems, such as stress fractures, in athletes. Because endurance athletes do the same anatomical motion hundreds and thousands of times, weak, poorly mineralized bones may be at increased risk of developing stress fractures at points where the bones continually receive stress. Since estrogen helps bones become mineralized in women, female athletes who don't have menstrual periods are at risk for developing weak bones. For these women, it is even more important that they take plenty of calcium and lots of sunshine (vitamin D) to help compensate the problem of inadequate estrogen.

Summary

In general, athletes with long training schedules should focus on the consumption of diets that are high in carbohydrate and should develop a drinking habit that frequently delivers fluids to the body. While fats constitute a major proportion of burned energy for endurance (aerobic) activities, the storage capacity for fat is relatively high for even the most lean athletes. The storage capacity for carbohydrates, however, is limited. Since fats require some carbohydrate to be completely burned, the limited storage capacity for carbohydrate can limit the body's ability to burn fat during exercise. To overcome this limitation, athletes should be constantly vigilant to keep body stores of carbohydrate at maximal levels before activity begins and should replace carbohydrate during activity through whatever means are available. A failure to supply sufficient carbohydrate before and during endurance activity will significantly reduce athletic performance. See table 6.5 for the recommended nutrient intake for athletes training 90 minutes or more each day.

Table 6.5 Recommended Nutrient Intakes for Endurance Athletes

Total energy intake	Calculated as 1.6 to 2.4 times the resting energy expenditure (see table 6.1 for formulas used to calculate resting energy expenditure). Higher values are used for athletes who do endurance work at higher intensities.
Fluid	16 ounces of fluid 2 hours prior to exercise. Additional 8 to 16 ounces of fluid during the 30 minutes prior to exercise. Do not delay drinking, even if not thirsty. Drink fluids every 10 to 15 minutes to replace water loss via sweat and to prevent dehydration. If the activity prevents regular, frequent fluid intake, drink as much as can be tolerated during natural breaks in the activity. Drink enough following the activity to return body weight to normal prior to next day's activity.
Carbohydrate	Greater than 60 percent of total caloric intake should come from carbohydrates. This should amount to 500 to 600 grams of carbohydrate per day (equivalent to 2,000 to 2,400 calories of carbohydrate per day). Carbohydrate intake should be at least 4 to 5 grams of carbohydrate per pound of body weight per day. (A 100-pound athlete would consume 500 grams of carbohydrate or 2,000 calories of carbohydrate each day. A 200-pound athlete would consume double this amount.)
Fat	Fat intake should remain as low as possible, never exceeding 30 percent of total calories from fat. Most athletes should have a fat intake of between 20 to 25 percent of total calories. Higher levels of fat intake are only useful if endurance athletes are incapable of consuming sufficient energy from carbohydrates to sustain desirable weight.

(continued)

Table 6.5 *(continued)*

Protein	Endurance athletes require approximately 1.6 grams of protein per kilogram of body weight per day. (This level generally translates into 10 to 15 percent of total calories as protein.) The best sources of protein include meats (beef, chicken, fish, pork) and dairy products (eggs, milk, cheese). However, protein is also present in grains, cereals, and legumes.
Minerals	Iron, zinc, and calcium are of concern for all athletes. Iron and calcium may be of particular concern for female athletes. Vegetarian athletes are at increased risk of inadequate iron, zinc, and calcium intakes. For female and vegetarian athletes, iron, zinc and calcium supplements may be warranted. Heavy sweating causes increased losses of sodium, chloride, and (perhaps) potassium. Consumption of a wide variety of foods, including meats and dairy products, helps to assure an adequate intake of iron, zinc, calcium, sodium, chloride, and potassium.
Vitamins	Fortified grains and cereals are an excellent means of obtaining sufficient B-vitamins, which are necessary for the metabolism of energy. The supplemental intake of antioxidants should not exceed the level recommended by the U.S. Olympic Committee (33,340 IU of beta-carotene; 1,000 mg of vitamin C; 400 IU of vitamin E).

Adapted from Murray and Horswill 1998.

7 Timing of Meals and Snacks

Timing Is Everything

There was a talented gymnast at a National Team training camp who could do the skills well enough to make it onto the National Team three years in a row, but she just couldn't break into the top level to compete at the key competitions. She was eager to talk with me when she heard I was the new nutritionist for the team, and she found her way to see me during the first possible rotation. I wasn't ready for what she said as she introduced herself to me: "I'm tired of being called bubble butt, but I can't do anything about it—and believe me, I've tried *everything*!" It was true that she was genetically predisposed to carrying a bit more fat around the hips than other places, but it was also clear to me that 99.9 percent of all women on the planet would like to look as fit and as athletic as she did. However, in the world of gymnastics, she clearly was carrying more fat than most.

We talked at length about what she had done in the past to lower her body fat, and she told me about past discussions she had had with exercise physiologists and nutritionists—each one putting her on a different exercise regimen and evaluating her dietary adequacy over and over again. It was at this point that she said something very interesting to me. She explained that at her last visit to the nutritionist, she was told that her total daily caloric intake was almost a perfect match for her daily caloric expenditure. That was even more frustrating for her, since she imagined that having a perfect diet should lead to a perfect physique. I wondered, was her diet really perfect?

I started asking her some questions about her daily schedule and when she ate her meals, and it became almost immediately clear that the calories were right, but they weren't right at the right time. She was "backloading" her food intake because her daily schedule was so busy. This is something that *many* athletes do because they all have incredibly busy schedules. Instead of spreading out their calories throughout the day, they eat a little bit during the day and eat a huge amount in the evening (i.e., backload) to take in the energy they need. (Backloading food intake is a bit like getting into your car in the morning and noticing that the gas tank is completely empty, then saying to the car, "Well, take me to my meeting now, and I'll fill you up once we get there." It just doesn't work that way.) We talked about whether it would be possible to spread out the food and drink throughout the day to avoid hunger and thirst, and to make certain there was enough of the right fuel (i.e., carbohydrate) in the system to train productively. We worked out a strategy for moving a bagel from here to there, and consuming more sports beverage during practice but having less at night, and she agreed to give it a try. (After all, she had tried *everything* else!)

When someone calls you on the phone, you can usually tell if they have a smile on their face while they're talking. Well, she called me about a month after the training camp with a big smile on her face and said she'd never felt stronger and her jeans had never fit better. I was happy for her and said we could talk again at an upcoming competition in two weeks. When we met again, it was as if I was looking at a different person. She was smiling, feeling good, and wasn't carrying around the "bubble-butt" label on her forehead. I took her weight and was surprised that she was about five pounds heavier, and I couldn't have been more happy. For the first time in a long while, her muscles were responding to her hard training because there was enough fuel around at the time the fuel was needed. So, she looked smaller, weighed more, had less fat, and was performing better. She was eating the same foods in the same amounts, but eating them when she needed them the most. Timing is everything.

It is interesting that the question most frequently asked when I speak to athletes has to do with what to eat before competition. Although this is important, it is of relatively small importance when compared to how the athlete eats most of the time. You can't properly prepare for a competition by eating some pancakes several hours before you place your feet in the starting blocks. It takes consistent and long-term effort in conditioning and good nutrition. There is no way that an athlete with iron deficiency can magically cure the condition by consuming some red meat the day before the event. It may take six months on a proper diet to get to a state of normal iron status. Therefore, the first and most important step in preparing for competition is to *consistently eat enough energy and nutrients to support your needs*. A failure to do this will inevitably lead to a poor competition outcome, no matter what you do just before the competition.

In addition to consuming enough energy and nutrients, it's equally important to *eat the foods at the times the body can benefit the most from them*. The timing of meals is also important for making certain that the muscles have enough energy and nutrients to grow and get stronger during training sessions, rather than get burned for energy because the athlete hasn't eaten enough. Put simply, it's important to *get enough and get it on time*. This isn't easy to do, because athletes have terribly hectic schedules, and it takes strategic thinking and good scheduling to make certain food is consumed when it's needed. While careful meal planning may not seem as important as having a well-developed training plan, they should be thought of as being equally important. They should also be thought of *together* to make certain the training plan can be properly supported with the foods that are consumed.

If the general food intake is supportive of the training plan, what should an athlete do differently for the days leading up to a competition? The sequence of events for the seven days prior to competition has three major goals:

1. The athlete should gradually become rested. This may be a problem for many athletes and coaches, since athletes (either with or without the encouragement of the coach) often *increase* the training schedule during the week leading up to a competition. This *overtraining* is a big problem and may increase the risks of getting sick or getting injured. It certainly doesn't help the athlete do their best at the upcoming competition.

2. The athlete should gradually build up muscle glycogen (energy) stores. The main purpose of gradually reducing the intensity and duration of training sessions before the competition is to be sure that the athlete can begin the competition with full muscle glycogen stores. The storage capacity for glycogen is relatively small, and athletes are heavily reliant on stored glycogen for muscular work (it's the limiting fuel for muscular work, regardless of the type of exercise the athlete is doing). Therefore, it's important to eat plenty of carbohydrates and reduce work so glycogen stores are full going into the competition.

3. The athlete should become well hydrated. When athletes work hard it is difficult (if not impossible) to maintain an optimal hydration state. It takes time to return lost body water, and athletes should give themselves the time to do so by reducing the training intensity and duration—and drinking plenty of fluids. An additional benefit to becoming well hydrated is that glycogen storage is enhanced. The gradual tapering of training during the seven days prior to competition makes it easier for the athlete to start the competition in a well-hydrated and optimally energized state.

There are, of course, many sports where athletes don't have the luxury of tapering activity on a seven-day cycle. Basketball players play several games each week during the season, baseball players play nearly every day, and hockey players often have a game twice a week. While these and other athletes don't have schedules that permit seven-day activity tapering, the principles behind tapered activity, glycogen storage, and optimal hydration should be remembered and, when possible, adhered to. For athletes with daily schedules that eliminate the possibility of tapering, consumption of high-carbohydrate diets and maintenance of optimal hydration become even more important components of athletic performance. Athletes with these schedules should have an eating and drinking plan that is as solid as the training and competition plan. Make an eating and drinking schedule, and stick with it.

All too often athletes prepare for a big competition by *increasing* their training regimen as the competition draws nearer. This is a big mistake. Coaches working in high-skill sports, such as figure skating and gymnastics, commonly ask their athletes to do multiple run-throughs of the routines the day before competition, just to be sure the athlete can do them. Well, if you can't be sure the athlete can do the routine by then, then you're just reducing the chance the athlete will do it right during competition, because they enter the competition exhausted *and* insecure. The message this sends to the athlete (i.e., "I don't believe you're ready, and we're going to keep practicing until you get it right") is also counterproductive. There is nothing more confidence building for athletes than entering the competition well rested and knowing the coach is secure in their ability to do a good job. This is true whether the athlete is a professional or a T-ball player in little league baseball.

Seven-Day Taper

The following tables provide an example of how these principles can be put to work. They illustrate what and how athletes might eat if they typically train twice daily. You'll notice that the food is spread out over six smaller meals rather than two or three larger ones. You'll also notice that the caloric level of the meals does not emphasize dinner at the end of the day. While dinner is important, the training takes place *before* dinner, so there has to be ample energy provided when the athlete needs it the most. Breakfast comes *before* the morning workout because, by the time the athlete wakes up, blood sugar is marginal and the liver is virtually depleted of energy, so maintaining blood sugar is virtually impossible. Having some food to eat prior to the morning workout helps to assure that the muscles will benefit from the training and helps to keep the athlete feeling better. *Nobody* feels good with low blood sugar.

These tables also suggest that foods should be consumed long enough before the training session so that the athlete feels no discomfort from training while there is food in the stomach. In addition, you'll notice that there are always some carbohydrates provided immediately after a workout. This helps to assure an effective replenishment of the glycogen that was used up during the training. Waiting to eat too long after the training can diminish the efficiency with which muscle glycogen is replaced.

Seven Days Before Competition

This is the day for a complete, total, and exhaustive workout. All the skills are practiced completely and repetitively, and the athlete spends a good deal of time practicing his or her weakest area. If a basketball player has trouble making foul shots during the game, then a good deal of time should be spent shooting from the foul line *after* all the other practice regimens have been followed. He or she should get a feel for what it's like when they feel a bit tired, just like in a game. In other words, seven days before the competition is not a time for being timid about the workout. Give your body a sufficiently good workout so that you know you've really gone through it. (See table 7.1 for a sample competition-minus-7-days.)

Table 7.1 Sample Exercise and Eating Schedule for Competition-Minus-7-Days

Time of day	Activity	Food
7:00 A.M. to 8:00 A.M.	• Light breakfast (*before* getting dressed for workout) • Dress for A.M. workout	• 2 slices white bread toast • 1 cup fruit juice • 1 cup sports beverage [Average 300 calories]
8:00 A.M. to 9:30 A.M.	• Stretch (30 minutes) • 1 hour vigorous run, bike, or equipment-based activity	• 1 cup sports beverage during stretch (sipped over 30 minutes) • 16 ounces sports beverage during 1 hour activity (sipped at the rate of 4 ounces every 15 minutes) [About 150 calories]

(continued)

Table 7.1 *(continued)*

Time of day	Activity	Food
9:30 A.M. to 10:00 A.M.	• Postexercise breakfast (*before* getting washed and dressed)	• 1 boiled egg • 4 slices of toast with 2 tablespoons of jam • 1 fresh orange • 1 bowl (1 cup) of whole-grain cereal with 6 ounces of 1% milk • 12 ounces fruit juice [About 900 calories]
10:00 A.M. to 12:30 P.M.	• Shower and dress • Relaxed activities (read, walk, light work around the house, desk work, etc.)	• Sip on 12 ounces of fluids (any kind *except* those containing caffeine or alcohol) [About 75 calories if a sports beverage]
12:30 P.M. to 1:00 P.M.	• Lunch	• Large bowl (2.5 cups) of pasta with marinara sauce • 3 slices of French bread • 12 ounces of fruit juice [About 1,200 calories]
1:00 P.M. to 2:45 P.M.	• Postlunch relaxation (read, desk work, slow walking, driving, etc.)	• Sip on 12 ounces of water [0 calories]
2:45 P.M. to 3:30 P.M.	• Preparation for afternoon workout (get dressed for exercise, etc.)	• Sip on 12 ounces of sports beverage [About 75 calories]
3:30 P.M. to 7:00 P.M.	• Late-afternoon workout • Practice skills • Work on conditioning • Work on endurance • Work up a sweat!	• Sip on 16 ounces of sports beverage per hour (4 ounces each 15 minutes) • Take your nude weight prior to exercise and after exercise to see if you have consumed an appropriate amount of fluid. For each pound of weight loss, you should have consumed an additional 16 ounces of beverage. [About 350 calories]
7:00 P.M. to 7:30 P.M.	• Post-exercise nutritional replenishment	• 1 banana • 12 ounces of sports beverage • 2 slices of bread [About 315 Calories]

Time of day	Activity	Food
7:30 P.M. to 8:00 P.M.	• Shower and dress	• Don't drink the shower water unless you're really thirsty!
8:00 P.M. to 9:00 P.M.	• Dinner	• Large baked potato • Broccoli (1 spear) • Small lean steak (4 ounces) • Orange juice (1 cup) • Rice pudding (1 cup) [About 1,050 calories]
9:00 P.M. to 10:00 P.M.	• Relaxation activities	• 1 cup of water or sports beverage (sipped) [About 75 calories if a sports beverage]
10:00 P.M. to 7:00 A.M.	• Sleep, glorious sleep!	• No eating or drinking permitted!

Intake totals: 4,500 calories
79% of calories from carbohydrate
11% of calories from protein
10% of calories from fat

Note: The food intake in this example would meet the needs of a 190-pound (86.4-kilogram) athlete with a **very intensive** exercise schedule. In this example, the energy requirement for competition-minus-7-days is estimated as **50 calories per kilogram of body weight.** Importantly, it is high in fluids, high in carbohydrates, low in fat, and moderate in protein. This type of intake supports glycogen (energy) storage in the muscles and liver. Athletes weighing less than this would consume proportionately less food, while maintaining the same frequency of intake.

During this workout, all the protocols discussed earlier in this book should be followed. It's important to drink plenty of carbohydrate-containing fluids during the workout (see chapter 2). It's also important to follow the workout with plenty of carbohydrates. Consuming at least 400 calories from carbohydrate immediately following the training regimen is desirable, followed by at least 800 calories during the next several hours. This is your first attempt at getting your muscles to replace the glycogen that has been lost during the workout.

Six Days Before Competition

This represents the first day of tapered exercise but with maintenance of a high-carbohydrate intake with plenty of fluids. Since activity is reduced, total energy intake should also be reduced to match needs.

Activity can be reduced in total time spent in training, or by reducing the intensity of the activities in training. For instance, a weight lifter could do fewer repetitions or could do the same repetitions with less weight. Regardless of the technique followed, competition-minus-6-days should provide a training schedule that is not as exhaustive as competition-minus-7-days (see table 7.2).

Table 7.2 Sample Exercise and Eating Schedule for Competition-Minus-6-Days

Time of day	Activity	Food
7:00 A.M. to 8:00 A.M.	• Light breakfast (*before* getting dressed for workout) • Dress for A.M. workout	• 1 slice white bread toast • 1 cup fruit juice • 1 cup sports beverage [Average 230 calories]
8:00 A.M. to 9:30 A.M.	• Stretch (30 minutes) • 1 hour vigorous run, bike, or equipment-based activity	• 1 cup sports beverage during stretch (sipped over 30 minutes) • 12 ounces sports beverage during 1 hour activity (sipped at the rate of 4 ounces every 15 minutes) [About 125 calories]
9:30 A.M. to 10:00 A.M.	• Postexercise breakfast (*before* getting washed and dressed)	• 1 boiled egg • 2 slices of toast with 2 tablespoons of jam • 1 fresh orange • 1 bowl (1 cup) of whole-grain cereal with 6 ounces of 1% milk • 8 ounces fruit juice [About 690 calories]
10:00 A.M. to 12:30 P.M.	• Shower and dress • Relaxed activities (read, walk, light work around the house, desk work, etc.)	• Sip on 12 ounces of fluids (any kind *except* those containing caffeine or alcohol) [About 75 calories if a sports beverage]
12:30 P.M. to 1:00 P.M.	• Lunch	• Large bowl (2.5 cups) of pasta with marinara sauce • 2 slices of French bread • 8 ounces of fruit juice [About 1,000 calories]
1:00 P.M. to 2:45 P.M.	• Postlunch relaxation (read, desk work, slow walking, driving, etc.)	• Sip on 12 ounces of water [0 calories]

Time of day	Activity	Food
2:45 P.M. to 3:30 P.M.	• Preparation for afternoon workout (get dressed for exercise, etc.) • Stretch (at least 30 minutes)	• Sip on 12 ounces of sports beverage [About 75 calories]
3:30 P.M. to 7:00 P.M.	• Late-afternoon workout • Practice skills • **Lower the conditioning/ endurance training intensity from the day before.** • Should be an invigorating, but not exhaustive, training regimen	• Sip on 16 ounces of sports beverage per hour (4 ounces each 15 minutes) • Take your nude weight prior to exercise and after exercise to see if you have consumed an appropriate amount of fluid. For each pound of weight loss, you should have consumed an additional 16 ounces of beverage. [About 350 calories]
7:00 P.M. to 7:30 P.M.	• Postexercise nutritional replenishment	• 1 banana • 8 ounces of sports beverage • 2 slices of bread [About 290 calories]
7:30 P.M. to 8:00 P.M.	• Shower and dress	• Don't drink the shower water unless you're really thirsty!
8:00 P.M. to 9:00 P.M.	• Dinner	• Large baked potato • Broccoli (1 stalk) • Small lean steak (4 ounces) • Orange juice (1 cup) • Rice pudding (1 cup) [About 1,050 calories]
9:00 P.M. to 10:00 P.M.	• Relaxation activities	• 1 cup of water (sipped)
10:00 P.M. to 7:00 A.M.	• Sleep, glorious sleep!	• No eating or drinking permitted!

Intake totals:

3,900 calories
78.5% of calories from carbohydrate
11.3% of calories from protein
10.2% of calories from fat

Note: The food intake in this example would meet the needs of a 190-pound (86.4-kilogram) athlete with an **intensive exercise schedule.** The energy requirement for competition-minus-6-days is estimated as **45 calories per kilogram of body weight.** Importantly, it is high in fluids, high in carbohydrates, low in fat, and moderate in protein. This type of intake supports glycogen (energy) storage in the muscles and liver. Athletes weighing less than this would consume proportionately less food, while maintaining the same frequency of intake.

Five Days Before Competition

This represents the second day of reduced exercise intensity and duration but with a consistent maintenance of a high-carbohydrate and fluid intake. Since activity is reduced, total energy intake should also be reduced to match needs. This day, competition-minus-5-days, is characterized by activity that is discernibly less than the athlete is accustomed to doing. (See table 7.3 for a sample of an eating and training schedule.)

Table 7.3   Sample Exercise and Eating Schedule for Competition-Minus-5-Days

Time of day	Activity	Food
7:00 A.M. to 8:00 A.M.	• Light breakfast (*before* getting dressed for workout) • Dress for A.M. workout	• 1 slice white bread toast • 1 cup sports beverage • NO FRUIT JUICE [Average 115 calories]
8:00 A.M. to 9:30 A.M.	• Stretch (30 minutes) • 1 hour moderate-intensity run, bike, or equipment-based activity	• 1 cup sports beverage during stretch (sipped over 30 minutes) • 12 ounces sports beverage during 1 hour activity (4 ounces sipped every 15 minutes) [About 125 calories]
9:30 A.M. to 10:00 A.M.	• Postexercise breakfast (*before* getting washed and dressed)	• 1 boiled egg • 2 slices of toast with 1 teaspoon of jam • 1 fresh orange • 1 bowl (1 cup) of whole-grain cereal with 6 ounces of 1% milk • 4 ounces (1/2 cup) fruit juice [About 600 calories]
10:00 A.M. to 12:30 P.M.	• Shower and dress • Relaxed activities (read, walk, light work around the house, desk work, etc.)	• Sip on 12 ounces of water
12:30 P.M. to 1:00 P.M.	• Lunch	• Large bowl (2.5 cups) of pasta with marinara sauce • 2 slices of French bread • 4 ounces of fruit juice [About 925 calories]
1:00 P.M. to 2:45 P.M.	• Postlunch relaxation (read, desk work, slow walking, driving, etc.)	• Sip on 12 ounces of water

Time of day	Activity	Food
2:45 P.M. to 3:30 P.M.	• Preparation for afternoon workout (get dressed for exercise, etc.) • Stretch (at least 30 minutes)	• Sip on 12 ounces of water
3:30 P.M. to 6:30 P.M.	• Late-afternoon workout • Practice skills • Both time and intensity of training are reduced.	• Sip on 16 ounces of sports beverage per hour (4 ounces each 15 minutes) • Take your nude weight prior to exercise and after exercise to see if you have consumed an appropriate amount of fluid. For each pound of weight loss, you should have consumed an additional 16 ounces of beverage. [About 350 calories]
6:30 P.M. to 7:30 P.M.	• Postexercise nutritional replenishment	• 1 banana • 12 ounces of sports beverage • 1 slice of bread [About 250 calories]
7:30 P.M. to 8:00 P.M.	• Shower and dress	• Don't drink the shower water unless you're really thirsty!
8:00 P.M. to 9:00 P.M.	• Dinner	• Medium baked potato • Broccoli (1 stalk) • Small lean steak (4 ounces) • 1 glass water • Rice pudding (1 cup) [About 850 calories]
9:00 P.M. to 10:00 P.M.	• Relaxation activities	• 1 cup of water (sipped)
10:00 P.M. to 7:00 A.M.	• Sleep, glorious sleep!	• No eating or drinking permitted!

Intake totals:

3,200 calories
75.61% of calories from carbohydrate
12.54% of calories from protein
11.85% of calories from fat

Note: The food intake in this example would meet the needs of a 190-pound (86.4-kilogram) athlete with a **moderate exercise schedule.** The energy requirement for competition-minus-5-days is estimated as **40 calories per kilogram of body weight.** Importantly, it is high in fluids, high in carbohydrates, low in fat, and moderate in protein. This type of intake supports glycogen (energy) storage in the muscles and liver. Athletes weighing less than this would consume proportionately less food, while maintaining the same frequency of intake.

Four Days Before Competition

This is a good time for making your final strategic plans for the competition. Your training regimen should focus on key *elements* of the special skills you have, but with an emphasis on practicing skills in a way that keeps you from becoming exhausted. As with the previous days, you should maintain a high carbohydrate and fluid intake to support your needs.

This is also a good time to have a little extra protein, up to 2 grams/ kilogram, to make certain all your tissue repair needs are covered, and to have some extra protein to support the manufacture of creatine. For the 190-pound athlete in this example, 2 grams of protein per kilogram of body weight amounts to 173 grams of protein. The earlier examples provided 1.26 grams of protein per kilogram of body weight, an amount that is well within the general requirements for athletes (1.0 to 2.0 grams per day). Therefore, providing a little extra protein merely provides some assurance that protein intake is not a limiting factor in performance.

Three Days Before Competition

Three days before competition is similar to four days before competition, with a continued emphasis on low- to moderate-intensity exercise, a high-carbohydrate intake, a low-fat intake, and a slightly greater emphasis (up to 2.0 grams per kilogram) on protein. Other activities during the day should also be reduced, with more time made available for both physical and psychological relaxation. The athlete should absolutely avoid becoming overheated or exhausted from any activity. Use table 7.4 as a sample exercise and eating schedule for competition-minus-4- and competition-minus-3-days.

Table 7.4 Sample Exercise and Eating Schedule for Competition Minus-4-Days and Minus-3-Days

Time of day	Activity	Food
7:00 A.M. to 8:00 A.M.	• Light breakfast (*before* getting dressed for workout) • Dress for A.M. workout	• 1 slice white bread toast • 1 cup sports beverage [Average 115 calories]
8:00 A.M. to 9:30 A.M.	• Stretch (30 minutes) • 1 hour low-to-moderate-intensity run, bike, or equipment-based activity	• 1 cup sports beverage during stretch (sipped over 30 minutes) • 12 ounces sports beverage during 1 hour activity (4 ounces sipped every 15 minutes) [About 125 calories]

Time of day	Activity	Food
9:30 A.M. to 10:00 A.M.	• Postexercise breakfast (*before* getting washed and dressed)	• 2 boiled eggs • 2 slices of toast with 1 teaspoon of jam • 1 fresh orange • 1 bowl (1 cup) of whole-grain cereal with 6 ounces of 1% milk [About 530 calories]
10:00 A.M. to 12:30 P.M.	• Shower and dress • Relaxed activities (read, walk, light work around the house, desk work, etc.)	• Sip on 12 ounces of water
12:30 P.M. to 1:00 P.M.	• Lunch	• Medium bowl (1.5 cups) of pasta with marinara sauce • 2 slices of French bread • 1 banana (in place of 4 ounces of fruit juice) [About 800 calories]
1:00 P.M. to 2:45 P.M.	• Postlunch relaxation (read, deskwork, slow walking, driving, etc.)	• Sip on 12 ounces of water
2:45 P.M. to 3:30 P.M.	• Preparation for afternoon workout (get dressed for exercise, etc.) • Stretch (at least 30 minutes)	• Sip on 12 ounces of water
3:30 P.M. to 5:30 P.M.	• Late-afternoon workout • Practice skills • Both time and intensity of training are reduced.	• Sip on 16 ounces of sports beverage per hour (4 ounces each 15 minutes) • Take your nude weight prior to exercise and after exercise to see if you have consumed an appropriate amount of fluid. For each pound of weight loss, you should have consumed an additional 16 ounces of beverage. [About 350 calories]
5:30 P.M. to 7:30 P.M.	• Postexercise nutritional replenishment	• 1 banana • 12 ounces of sports beverage • Omit bread [About 175 calories]

(continued)

Table 7.4 (continued)

Time of day	Activity	Food
7:30 P.M. to 8:00 P.M.	• Shower and dress	• Don't drink the shower water unless you're really thirsty!
8:00 P.M. to 9:00 P.M.	• Dinner	• Medium baked potato • Broccoli (1 stalk) • Medium lean steak (4 ounces) • 1 glass water • Rice pudding (1 cup) [About 800 calories]
9:00 P.M. to 10:00 P.M.	• Relaxation activities	• 1 cup of water (sipped)
10:00 P.M. to 7:00 A.M.	• Sleep, glorious sleep!	• No eating or drinking permitted!

Intake totals:
3,000 calories
65.0% of calories from carbohydrate
20.0% of calories from protein
15.0% of calories from fat

Note: The food intake in this example would meet the needs of a 190-pound (86.4-kilogram) athlete with a **light-to-moderate-exercise schedule.** The energy requirement for competition-minus-4-days and minus-3-days is estimated as **35 calories per kilogram of body weight.** Importantly, it is high in fluids, high in carbohydrates, low in fat, and **moderately high** in protein. This type of intake supports glycogen (energy) storage in the muscles and liver. Athletes weighing less than this would consume proportionately less food, while maintaining the same frequency of intake.

Two Days Before Competition

This is an excellent time to get more rest, and a good way to do that is to eliminate the morning training schedule. The afternoon training should be reduced to no more than 1.5 hours, with a moderate-to-low intensity. The focus should be on reviewing skills and reinforcing the mental strategy it will take to compete effectively. Of course, carbohydrate and fluid intake should remain high. See table 7.5 for a sample exercise and eating schedule for competition-minus-2-days.

One Day Before Competition

This day should be characterized by plenty of rest (both physical and mental) and relaxation. Athletes and coaches should be restrained from running through multiple full routines, a full-speed run, or a full "game intensity" practice. Walking parts of the course, getting

Table 7.5 Sample Exercise and Eating Schedule for Competition–Minus–2–Days

Time of day	Activity	Food
<--- Sleep Late! No Morning Exercise --->		
9:30 A.M. to 10:00 A.M.	• Postexercise breakfast (*before* getting washed and dressed)	• 2 boiled eggs • 2 slices of toast with 1 teaspoon of jam • 1 fresh orange or banana • 1 bowl (1 cup) of whole-grain cereal with 6 ounces of 1% milk • 1 slice white bread toast • 1 cup sports beverage [About 650 calories]
10:00 A.M. to 12:30 P.M.	• Shower and dress • Relaxed activities (read, walk, light work around the house, desk work, etc.)	• Sip on 12 ounces of water
12:30 P.M. to 1:00 P.M.	• Lunch	• Medium bowl (1.5 cups) of pasta with marinara sauce • 2 slices of French bread • 1 banana [About 800 calories]
1:00 P.M. to 2:45 P.M.	• Postlunch relaxation (read, deskwork, slow walking, driving, etc.)	• Sip on 12 ounces of water
2:45 P.M. to 3:30 P.M.	• Preparation for afternoon workout (get dressed for exercise, etc.) • Stretch (at least 30 minutes)	• Sip on 12 ounces of water
3:30 P.M. to 5:00 P.M.	• Late-afternoon workout • Practice skills • Both time and intensity of training are reduced.	• Sip on 16 ounces of sports beverage per hour (4 ounces each 15 minutes) • Take your nude weight prior to exercise and after exercise to see if you have consumed an appropriate amount of fluid. For each pound of weight loss, you should have consumed an additional 16 ounces of beverage. [About 350 calories]

(continued)

Table 7.5 *(continued)*

Time of day	Activity	Food
5:00 P.M. to 7:30 P.M.	• Postexercise nutritional replenishment	• 1 banana • 12 ounces of sports beverage [About 175 calories]
7:30 P.M. to 8:00 P.M.	• Shower and dress	• Don't drink the shower water unless you're really thirsty!
8:00 P.M. to 9:00 P.M.	• Dinner	• Medium baked potato • Broccoli (1 stalk) • Medium lean steak (4 ounces) • 1 glass water • Rice pudding (1 cup) [About 800 calories]
9:00 P.M. to 10:00 P.M.	• Relaxation activities	• 1 cup of water (sipped)
10:00 P.M. to 7:00 A.M.	• Sleep, glorious sleep!	• No eating or drinking permitted!

Intake totals: 2,800 calories
65.0% of calories from carbohydrate
20.0% of calories from protein
15.0% of calories from fat

Note: The food intake in this example would meet the needs of a 190-pound (86.4-kilogram) athlete with a **light-to-moderate-exercise schedule.** The energy requirement for competition-minus-2-days is estimated as **35 calories per kilogram of body weight.** Notice that the activity and food amounts in bold have changed from the previous day's schedule. Importantly, it is high in fluids, high in carbohydrates, low in fat, and **moderately high in protein** (approximately 1.8 grams of protein per kilogram of body weight to assure tissue maintenance and repair needs are met). This type of intake supports glycogen (energy) storage in the muscles and liver. Athletes weighing less than this would consume proportionately less food, while maintaining the same frequency of intake.

familiar with the competition venue, or watching films of your opponents are OK activities, but only if you know they won't make you anxious and unable to relax. Sport psychologists I have worked with have indicated that it's probably better to watch films of your own successful competitions rather than to watch films of what your opponent(s) are going to do. By one day before competition, you should have already been briefed long ago about who you're competing against and what strategy to follow.

This is almost your last chance to make certain your glycogen stores are at peak values, and you should maintain a steady fluid intake to assure optimal hydration going into the next day's activities (see table 7.6). The carbohydrates you consume should be those high in starch and relatively low in fiber. Pasta, bread, rice, fruits (without seeds or skins) are excellent choices. Vegetables and legumes tend to have lots of fiber and may produce gas (causing you to become uncomfortable and bloated). Vegetables in the cabbage family (cabbage, brussels sprouts, kohlrabi, etc.) are particularly notorious for their gas-creating capabilities.

Table 7.6   Sample Exercise and Eating Schedule for Competition-Minus-1-Day

Time of day	Activity	Food
<--- Sleep Late! No Morning Exercise --->		
9:30 A.M. to 10:00 A.M.	• Breakfast *[Note:* Avoid eating high-fiber cereals if they cause you to bloat or give you gas. If this occurs, puffed rice or cornflakes may be good alternatives.]	• 2 boiled eggs • 2 slices of toast with 1 teaspoon of jam • 1 fresh orange or banana • 1 bowl (1 cup) of cereal with 6 ounces of 1% milk • 1 slice white bread toast • 1 cup sports beverage [About 650 calories]
10:00 A.M. to 12:30 P.M.	• Shower and dress • Relaxed activities (read, walk, light work around the house, desk work, etc.)	• Sip on 12 ounces of water
12:30 P.M. to 1:00 P.M.	• Lunch	• Medium bowl (1.5 cups) of Spanish rice • 2 slices of French bread • 1 banana [About 800 calories]
1:00 P.M. to 2:45 P.M.	• Postlunch relaxation (read, desk work, slow walking, driving, etc.)	• Sip on 12 ounces of water
2:45 P.M. to 3:30 P.M.	• Preparation for afternoon workout (get dressed for exercise, etc.) • Stretch (at least 30 minutes)	• Sip on 12 ounces of water

(continued)

Table 7.6   *(continued)*

Time of day	Activity	Food
3:30 P.M. to 5:00 P.M.	• Late-afternoon workout should be very mild. Walking around your neighborhood or becoming familiar with the competition venue are good activities. • Both time and intensity of training are low.	• Sip on 16 ounces of sports beverage per hour (4 ounces each 15 minutes) • Take your nude weight prior to exercise and after exercise to see if you have consumed an appropriate amount of fluid. For each pound of weight loss, you should have consumed an additional 16 ounces of beverage. [About 350 calories]
5:00 P.M. to 7:30 P.M.	• Postactivity nutritional replenishment	• 1 banana • 12 ounces of sports beverage [About 175 calories]
7:30 P.M. to 8:00 P.M.	• Shower and dress	• Have fluids available in a bottle to sip on to avoid thirst.
8:00 P.M. to 9:00 P.M.	• Dinner *[Note:* **Avoid eating high-fiber vegetables that could cause bloating and gas. Cabbage, broccoli, cauliflower, and raw spinach are particularly known for being gas causing.]**	• Medium baked potato (do not eat the skin) • Cooked carrots (3/4 cup) • Medium chicken breast without skin (baked) • 1 glass water • Rice pudding (1 cup) [About 800 calories]
9:00 P.M. to 10:00 P.M.	• Relaxation activities	• 1 cup of water (sipped)
10:00 P.M. to 7:00 A.M.	• Sleep, glorious sleep!	• No eating or drinking permitted!

Intake totals: 2,800 calories
65.0% of calories from carbohydrate
20.0% of calories from protein
15.0% of calories from fat

Note: The food intake in this example would meet the needs of a 190-pound (86.4-kilogram) athlete with a **light activity schedule.** The energy requirement for competition-minus-1-day is estimated as **35 calories per kilogram of body weight.** Importantly, it is high in fluids, high in carbohydrates, low in fat, and **moderately high in protein** (approximately 1.8 grams of protein per kilogram of body weight to assure tissue maintenance and repair needs are met). This type of intake supports glycogen (energy) storage in the muscles and liver. Athletes weighing less than this would consume proportionately less food, while maintaining the same frequency of intake.

Competition Day

This is the day you've been waiting for, so don't do anything that will destroy all your hard work. It is particularly important that you don't do anything you're not accustomed to doing or eat anything you've never tasted. You should have a checklist already prepared of what you'll need and where it is. Competition day is not when you want to go running around the house screaming, "Where did I put my running shoes!" Leave nothing to chance and have a backup plan if you think you need one.

Eating and drinking appropriately on competition day are important, so make certain you have the right foods and drinks immediately available (don't leave it to chance). Take charge of knowing what you need and take charge of getting it. Imagine drinking sports beverage X during practice all year, then getting up the morning of the competition to find out that your spouse couldn't find sports beverage X at the store, so he bought sports beverage Y instead. Avoid being put in any situation that will cause you stress on competition day.

Early Morning Competition

If the competition is early in the morning, you should get up two to three hours *before* the competition. If you know you have difficulty getting up early in the morning, you should practice doing it for several days before the competition. You should give yourself enough time to eat some carbohydrates, drink some fluids, and get to the competition. Finish eating at least 1.5 hours before the start of your competition (assuming you are eating mainly starchy carbohydrates). Different athletes process foods differently, so know what your best time differential is between eating and the competition. If you know you feel best when you finish eating two hours prior to competition, you should follow this time differential. If you're part of a team and eat as a team, make whatever minor adjustments you need to make so that you're certain you've optimized your schedule to suit what works for you. Once you're finished eating, keep sipping on sports beverages the *entire* time leading up to the competition. Don't put yourself in a position where you're rushed. When that happens, the food inevitably gets the short end of what you should do, and then you suffer for that mistake (either through poor endurance or GI distress) during the entire competition.

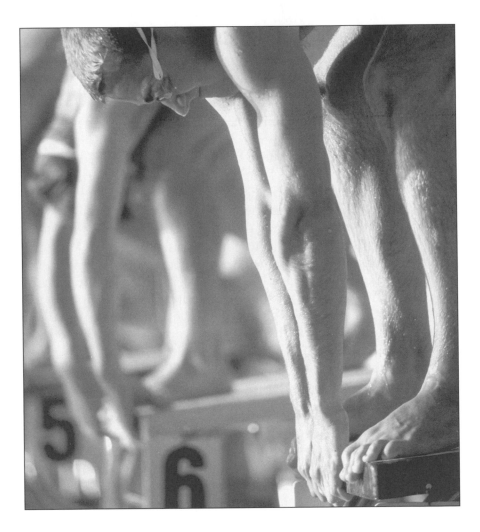

Late-Morning or Early-Afternoon Competition

This is a time when people are feeling tired and hungry because the food they ate for breakfast has stopped providing energy by this time. Therefore, it's important to remember to have something to eat every 2.5 to 3.5 hours. If you're not accustomed to this eating pattern, you should do whatever you can to learn to eat this way. For an 11:00 A.M. competition, you might wake up and have breakfast at 6:30 A.M., and eat again at 9:00 A.M. After your 9:00 A.M. meal, you should initiate your constant fluid-sipping protocol until competition time. For an early-afternoon competition (at 1:00 P.M.), you can have your last meal at 10:30 A.M., and begin your fluid-sipping protocol until the competition begins. Going into competition hungry is a sure formula for failure.

Midafternoon or Early-Evening Competition

This is a tough time to compete, especially if it's an outdoor sport and it's hot. This is also a bad time because athletes typically go off schedule with a midafternoon competition. The best thing to do is to spend the morning eating and drinking as usual (Breakfast, mid-morning snack, lunch), and then begin the countdown to the competition by having some starchy carbohydrates (a banana, some toast or crackers, etc.) and some fluids about 1.5 to 2.0 hours before the competition starts. The fluid-sipping protocol should then be initiated until competition time. The excitement of the competition can make athletes forget they're hungry, when they really are. Therefore, it's a good idea to have a well-rehearsed eating, snacking and drinking schedule, and stick to it.

Late-Evening Competition

This is a difficult time to compete, because your body wants to sleep, but the competition is keeping it awake. Therefore, sleeping late and eating something every 2.5 to 3.0 hours will help to keep your energy level up until it's time to compete. Keep checking your hydration state by seeing if your urine is basically clear. Remember, a successful late-evening competition is sweet and will help you get a good and restful night's sleep!

Summary

The main idea behind getting ready for competition is to set your body up so that it has a full tank of both carbohydrate (as glycogen) and fluid. The muscles and psyche should both be well rested, and the athlete should be getting clear messages of confidence from the coach. Getting sufficient rest prior to competition can't be overemphasized. When athletes are involved in sports where competitions occur frequently, getting sufficient rest between competitions is critical. A colleague of mine once responded to a question from a sports reporter about whether it was bad for an athlete to have sex before competition by saying, "Having sex is not a problem, it's the going out late at night looking for it that's the problem." There's a lot of truth in this, because anything that keeps you from getting a good night's sleep and being well rested will cause difficulties in competition. The keys to good preparation for competition include the following:

1. Get plenty of rest.
2. Begin tapering down physical activity six to seven days prior to competition.
3. Eat enough carbohydrates to maximize glycogen stores.
4. Drink sufficient fluids to maximize fluid stores.
5. Eat frequently, approximately once every three hours, to maintain blood glucose and muscle glycogen levels, and to *feel* good.
6. Consume enough energy *before* activity to assure there's enough fuel in the system to support the activity and to avoid burning muscle as a fuel.
7. Practice the eating and drinking schedule of your competition day in advance, so you know what makes you feel good.
8. Don't do *anything* on competition day that you haven't practiced doing before hand.
9. Be ready with *everything* you'll need (sports beverages, snacks, etc.) long before the competition day arrives.

8 Eating on the Road

Should I Bring Some Cans of Tuna Fish?

It's not often that an athlete really takes to heart the information they receive from their coach, their parents, or their nutritionist. However, some elite athletes are so motivated to succeed that they become a bit compulsive about taking advice from those they trust. This was the case with Nicole, a gymnast training in the same gym as some of the best gymnasts in the country. She had vainly tried for a number of years to make the national team and, finally, from sheer will and hard work she made it! Not only that, but she was getting ready to go on her first international trip with three of her teammates to represent her country. It's hard to imagine anything more exciting, and she was going to make the best of it.

One evening, at about 11:00 P.M., my wife Deborah answered the phone and told me it was a young gymnast wanting to speak with me. I commonly get calls at home from athletes I work with but never so late at night. I figured it must be some emergency, so there was more than a touch of nervousness in my voice when I said hello. It was Nicole, the evening before her flight to Bulgaria for the competition. I, of course, asked what the problem was. To my surprise, Nicole said, "There's no problem. I just need some advice." She wanted to know a little bit about Bulgaria. Was the water safe to drink? Is the food safe to eat? Is the food similar to what she's accustomed to eating? Do people get sick when they travel there? Can she brush her teeth with the tap water? What are the bathrooms like? Can she get Cheerios with skim milk for breakfast? (After all, that's all she really likes for breakfast . . .) The questions were coming fast and furiously, and I couldn't get a response in edgewise. She was having the "traveling for competition jitters," and what she really wanted was someone to tell her that, with a little care, everything would be all right.

As it turns out, I've heard from a number of people that the treatment of our athletes in Bulgaria has always been excellent, and the food is clean and delicious. I shared that information with Nicole, but also asked her what she would miss the most if she couldn't get it there to eat. She said Cheerios and water-packed tuna fish (something she really liked to have for lunch). Believe it or not, these are items that you can get virtually anywhere in Europe. But this conversation was about feeling secure. I said, "You absolutely should bring some Cheerios, a few cans of water-packed tuna fish, a box of crackers, and five bottles of water with you, just to be safe." Nicole couldn't have been more thankful for this advice, and she was extremely happy she called. It was, she said, good to know what to bring along.

About a month later, I saw Nicole at a national team training camp, and she rushed up to me to tell me about how great the trip to Bulgaria was. She felt she did great and had no problems with food at all. I told her I couldn't have been more pleased and was glad she brought some food with her. She said she didn't touch any of it the whole trip, because the food there was great! She now eats fresh fruit, some cheese, and some bread for breakfast, just like the Bulgarians do. "After all, it's so much better than plain old cereal," she said. I was happy that she had a good international experience (after all, that's one of the benefits of being a great athlete), but reminded her that competition was not a time to experiment with new foods. So, I said with a smile, bring that can of tuna fish with you whenever you go on an international trip!

Nicole's been on several international trips now, and every time I see her she tells me she *still* hasn't opened that can of tuna fish, but she likes knowing it's with her. That's the idea. After all, it's good to feel you're in familiar territory, even if you're not.

Serious athletes will inevitably find themselves competing away from home, often in faraway lands where the foods are unfamiliar. Whether the athlete travels to the southern part of the state, to the next state, or to a foreign state, planning ahead is a key to making certain the athlete will perform up to his or her trained capabilities. Sadly, few athletes take serious measures to minimize the negative physical and psychological impact of traveling long distances. Having a plan that will assure the availability of the right kinds of foods at the right time is critical when you compete at home, and it is no less critical when you compete away from home. Perhaps the biggest mistake an athlete can make when traveling to a competition is to assume that what they need to eat will be there waiting for them. Make no such assumption. If you don't take care of your training and eating plan, no one else will either.

In addition to the issue of food, there is the issue of adaptation. It takes time to adapt to a new location, and you should give yourself enough time for your body to make the changes it needs by getting to your destination early enough. Acclimatization is particularly important if the athlete is traveling to a location that is hotter than where the training normally occurs. Physiological adjustments to heat take 7 to 14 days, and without adequate heat adaptation performance will clearly be affected.[1] Whether it's food or time, planning ahead is the key to success.

General Guidelines for "Eating on the Road"

Most of the guidelines that follow require advance planning. When you get ready for a trip, it's assumed that you'll check to make sure you have your uniform and athletic shoes packed (although I've heard stories!). It's just as important that you've given some thought to where, when, and how you'll eat to satisfy your needs. The worst thing that can happen to you while traveling is to become hungry or thirsty and not have anything to eat or drink. Plan to see that this doesn't happen. Try the following general tips for eating on the road:[2]

• *Bring your own snacks.* Fresh fruits, fruit juices, crackers, low-fat rice and pasta salads, and low-fat energy bars are nutritious and easy to carry (see table 8.1).

• *Watch out for hidden fats.* Creamy soups, bread-type flaky pastries, mayonnaise-based salad dressings, and sauces in sandwiches add unnecessary fat to the food. There are, however, good alternatives. Consuming clear, broth-based soups instead of creamy soups may

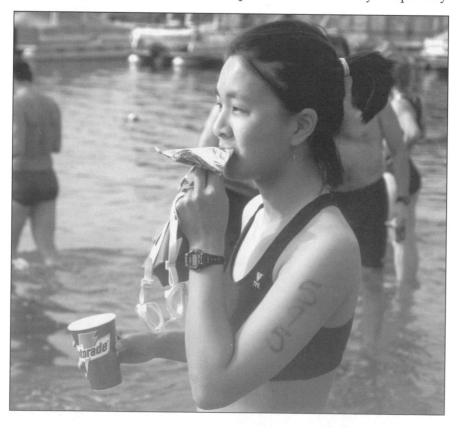

provide all the nutrients but with considerably less fat. Using lemon-juice based salad dressing rather than mayonnaise-type dressing lowers the fat and makes it possible to eat more salad.

• *Consume grilled, baked, boiled, and broiled foods rather than fried or sautéed foods.* You must *ask* for it the way you want it. Make no assumptions about how it will be prepared by the way the food is described on the menu. When possible, request lower-fat dairy products and lower-fat salad dressings.

• *Order "a la carte" to get exactly what you want.* Full dinners often don't fit with the way a serious athlete should be eating. For instance, the grilled fish may be exactly what you want, but the full dinner may come with mashed potatoes that are soaked in gravy, broccoli that is covered with cheese sauce, and a piece of apple pie with ice cream. The serious athlete would be better with broiled fish, a plain baked potato, broccoli with lemon juice, and fresh fruit for dessert.

• *If you travel by air, tell the travel agent you'd like to eat vegetarian.* There's a greater chance you'll have foods that are higher in carbohy-drates and lower in fat. However, you have to give the airlines fair warning of your special dietary requirements, so make certain the airlines are notified at least 24 hours in advance of the flight.

• *If you travel by air, bring something to drink on the plane with you.* Air travel is one of the most dehydrating experiences a person can have. Because of this, passengers often contract sore throats and other upper respiratory illnesses. As a preventative measure, keep sipping on fluids during the flight to keep your mouth and throat moist. As there may be a significant delay between the time you take off and when you receive your first drink. Drink bottled water or sports beverages.

Table 8.1   Snacks to Take With You for "Eating on the Road"

Milk products	Cheese wedges, string cheese, yogurt
Meats and protein foods	Beef sticks, peanut butter sandwiches, hard-cooked eggs, nuts
Fruits and vegetables	Dried apricots, apples, banana chips, raisins, fruit-filled cookies
Grains	Low-fat granola, breadsticks, bagels, crackers, bran muffins, soft pretzels
Fluids	Sports drinks, fruit juices, bottled water

© 1993, The American Dietetic Association. "*Sports Nutrition: a Guide for the Professional Working With Active People.*" Used with permission.

• *If you're changing time zones, get on the local schedule as soon as possible.* Have dinner when the local population is eating rather than at the time you eat at home. You'll still have difficulty getting your eating pattern on track because travel and changing time zones are tiring and disorienting. To make certain you're completely ready to compete, try to arrive at the competition site early.

Minimizing Jet Lag

Leaving enough time to adjust to long-distance travel is important. Even the most seasoned travelers suffer from jet lag, and most of them don't have to run, jump, hit, or kick faster, higher, or harder than they ever had before. Jet lag can make you feel ill, will lower your appetite, and can keep you from getting a good night's sleep.[3] Jet lag can come in two forms: (1) travel involving small but consecutive trips, causing multiple shifts in usual eating patterns; and (2) travel involving one large trip that crosses multiple time zones, causing a major change in eating and sleeping behaviors. You should never put off eating when you become hungry, so have some snacks with you that can take away hunger until you find a place and a time to eat a regular meal. The following recommendations may help to alleviate the effects of jet lag:[4]

1. For small, consecutive time-zone changes (called phase shifts):
   • *Eat meals at regular times after arriving at the new destination.* This will help you get on the local schedule quickly and aid your adjustment to the new time zone.
   • *Drink plenty of liquids.* Plane cabins are notoriously dry, and dehydration is the cause of many complaints, including headaches and mild constipation.
   • *Alternate light meals with heavy meals before the flights.* The stress of travel may increase protein requirements slightly, so eat a high-protein breakfast and a low-protein, high-carbohydrate dinner following the phase shift.
   • *Avoid caffeine until the end of the flight.* Caffeine is a diuretic that can increase water loss in an environment that is already dehydrating. Consume fluids that will help you maintain hydration state (water, sports beverages, fruit juices, etc.).
   • *Avoid alcohol during and after the flight.* Besides the negative metabolic alterations that alcohol causes, it is also a diuretic

that can increase water loss. There is NO reason why serious athletes should drink alcoholic beverages at any time.

- *Engage in social activity or exercise after the flight.* This will help you get on the local schedule more quickly and will aid in reducing the stress associated with travel.

2. For a large phase shift:

- *Arrive at your destination at least one day early for each time zone crossed.* For flights crossing more than six time zones, give yourself one week to get back on a regular schedule and to feeling good. Cost and scheduling limitations may keep athletes from arriving as early as needed so get on the local schedule as quickly as possible, but with as much rest as possible, is important.

- *Exercise and get involved in social activities on your arrival in the new location.* It helps to get to know your new environment right away. The exercise and social activities will help reduce the stress of travel and will help you get on the local schedule more easily.

- *Maintain regular sleeping and eating times on arrival to your new destination.* The sooner you can eat and sleep on the schedule of your new destination, the more quickly your body will feel as if it can perform well. Eating and sleeping regularly and on schedule are keys to doing well when you travel.

- *Continue to eat and drink frequently before, during, and after travel.* Creating a snacking schedule at your new location maybe difficult, since you may not know where to buy good, high-carbohydrate snacks that you can have with you. However, maintaining a frequent eating and drinking schedule (eating something about every three hours) is an important strategy for helping you adjust to your new environment. Bring some snacks with you to get started, and then find a good source of snacks once you arrive. However, always avoid alcohol.

- *Have more protein than usual.* The stress associated with travel may slightly increase your protein requirement, so make a conscious effort to consume a little more protein each day. For instance, consuming a higher protein breakfast (add a boiled egg to your normal intake) could be useful in assuring that your protein requirement is met. However, the focus of your intake should continue to be carbohydrates.

Travel Location

If you're traveling most places in the United States and Western Europe, there's a high likelihood you'll be able to find foods you're familiar with. American-style breakfast cereals, for instance, can be found in virtually every grocery store, and there is bread everywhere you go. The preparation of many of the foods you'll find is different, however. If you're accustomed to having a cup of coffee in the morning, you may be surprised at the variety of ways different cultures treat the coffee bean.

All of this is to say that you should do whatever you can to keep your habits intact, because you're never sure of what the outcome will be if you suddenly change what you've been doing for years. One of the best little gadgets you can have with you is an in-cup electric water heater. You should make sure you've got the right power adapters with you so you can access the electric plugs in the

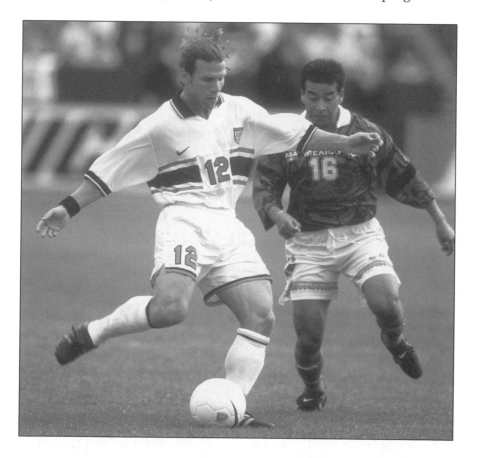

country you're traveling to. These little heaters allow you to enjoy familiar freeze-dried soups, and you can have your coffee the way you like it as well. This is one of the best little inventions ever made for a traveling athlete.

Some countries have reputations for unsafe water or food supplies. If you have any doubt at all, call your nearest American Consular office, or call your travel agency. They should be able to provide you with the information you need. If you've got the time, you should go to your local bookstore and pick up a good travel book for the location you're heading to. If it's a good one, it will describe the foods that will be available and will tell you about the water supply.

When traveling abroad, you should have the following items with you even if you feel the food and water supply are safe and familiar (you can adjust the quantities depending on your length of stay):

- Power cord adapters and converters to fit the power supply of the country you're traveling to
- An in-cup electric heater
- A water-filter pump
- A box of saltine crackers
- Powdered sports beverage packets to make 20 quarts of beverage
- 2 quarts of bottled water
- A medium-size box of raisins (or other favored dried fruit)
- 5 individually packaged low-fat granola bars
- 2 nonfat powdered milk packets
- 1 small box of your favorite cereal

Dealing With the Water Supply

It doesn't matter where you're going, you'll need water for one reason or another. Different water supplies can cause gastrointestinal (GI) difficulties, even if the water supply is perfectly safe. Different levels of bromide or fluoride in the water may, for instance, give someone severe gut pain. Of course, drinking bottled water or bottled sports drinks is a good solution if these are available. However, if bottled drinks are not easily available (I've been in populated places in the United States where it's virtually impossible to find a bottle of Gatorade), you need a way to deal with the situation. Obviously, you can't travel with cases of bottled drinks. However, you should travel with powdered packages of sports beverages and a water filter to purify the water. The best water filters (that take out parasites and bacteria) can be found at your local camping goods store. They don't take up much space, work extremely efficiently, and assure that you won't be scratched from a race because of a water-borne microbe. These water filters are also at the top of the list of excellent inventions for the traveling athlete. They work, and they can give you the peace of mind you need so you can deal with other more pressing matters.

Eating Locations

Travel inevitably keeps you from eating when and where you'd like to eat, so plan ahead for what you might select before you walk in. Seeing the dizzying array of foods and menu items can easily influence your order if you're not already committed to your selection.

Airports are filled with fast-food restaurants that typically offer high-fat and high-sugar foods. These are not easy places to make the right selection. In general, you will want to stick with foods that aren't fried. However, if you don't have a choice, minimize the fried food and maximize the carbohydrate. For instance, if you're really hungry, you might want to order a double-patty hamburger. However, it would be better to order two regular hamburgers because you get twice the bread (carbohydrate).

In restaurants, try to find pasta, baked potato, bread, vegetables, and salad. You might have to ask for a substitution (for instance, a baked potato instead of French fried potatoes) but don't be afraid to ask. Restaurants in airports or ports may be less likely to want to make you happy by satisfying your special needs because they know they'll probably never see you (or your business) again. Nevertheless, you should always ask for exactly what you want. Even when ordering baked potatoes, you should ask that they give you everything on the side rather than on the potato. You don't need that, and you shouldn't be afraid to tell them. See table 8.2 for key words to look for when looking over a menu.

Summary

The key to successful travel is advance planning. No assumptions should be made about the availability of foods or drinks that will satisfy your needs. Bring some limited items with you when traveling to be certain you have some key foods and drinks that will keep you happy and nourished. Don't try new foods until *after* the athletic event, and then only on the recommendation of your local hosts. Experimenting on your own can be dangerous. Find out as much as you can about where you're traveling to by going to a local bookstore, or learn about it through the Internet. Your travel agent and nearby American Consular office are also excellent sources of information. Give yourself plenty of time to get acclimated to the location you're traveling to. It takes about one day for each time zone you cross, so a trip from New York to Paris should have you arriving at least six days before the event. If that's not possible, do whatever you can to reduce stress by getting plenty of rest, relaxing with friends, and eating on the local schedule.

Table 8.2 Selecting Items Through a Careful Review of the Menu

Generally Avoid	Fried, crispy, breaded, scampi style, creamed, buttery, au gratin, gravy
Generally Seek	Marinara, steamed, boiled, broiled, tomato sauce, in its own juice, poached, charbroiled
Mexican: Avoid	Deep fat fried shells, fried flour tortillas, refried beans, corn chips, sour cream, guacamole
Mexican: Seek	Low-fat refried beans, chicken or lean beef and bean burritos, baked soft corn tortillas, salsa, rice, baked flour tortillas
Italian: Avoid	Cream sauces, high-fat dressings, rich desserts
Italian: Seek	Pasta with marinara sauce, cheese pizza or with vegetables, salad with dressing on the side, low-fat Italian ice, low-fat frozen yogurt
Chinese: Avoid	Deep fried egg rolls, deep fried wontons, sweet and sour pork, tempura
Chinese: Seek	Stir fry and steamed dishes, chicken and vegetables with rice, clear both soups
Burger places: Avoid	High-fat dressings in salad bars, mayonnaise, French fries, milkshakes
Burger places: Seek	Salad bars with low-fat dressings, baked potatoes, grilled items
Café: Avoid	Pre-buttered items, limit coffee intake
Café: Seek	Pancakes, toast, bagels, waffles, fruit, fruit juices, whole grain cereals, breads, muffins,

Adapted, by permission, from E.R. Burke and J.R. Berning, 1996, Training nutrition: The diet and nutrition guide for peak performance Carmel, IN: I.L. Copper, pp. 131-140.

PART III

Performance Nutrition Plans

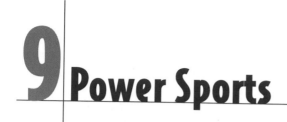

Power Sports

Hockey Night in Atlanta

Several years ago, Atlanta had a professional hockey team, a farm team for Tampa Bay, called The Atlanta Knights. I'm not sure if it's possible to have more fun working with a group of athletes than I had working with this group. Besides having the first professional female player, Ms. Manon Rheaume (her presence added a whole new dimension to hockey!), they also had an experienced coach who had done and seen everything in hockey, from the pros to the Olympic Games. When the coach asked me to work with the team to make certain they were doing the right things nutritionally, he invited me to join the team in practice and to go to the games to get a sense of what was going on. I also had all the team members in the lab to assess bone density, body composition, and nutrient intake. I learned from my data collection and observations was that these athletes worked hard day after day. When they weren't playing, they were either practicing or traveling somewhere to play. When they were on the ice, it was no-holds-barred all-out skating that was almost as exhausting to watch as it was to do. I also learned that when practice was over or when a game was finished, they didn't have any food in the locker room, so it was often more than two hours after this strenuous activity before they got something to eat. It was this point that I decided would be my first point of attack.

I spoke with the coach about getting some food into the locker room for the players to eat right after practice or a game. My main point was that the high-intensity activity of hockey was depleting their muscle energy stores (glycogen) and that a key to assuring its replacement for the next day of activity was to have 200 to 400 calories of carbohydrate *immediately* following practice. The coach agreed that it was a good idea, so he gave me a small budget, and I put one of my graduate students to work on getting some good-tasting carbohydrates in the locker room. To make it easier, the Gatorade Company donated some Gatorpro (high-carbohydrate meal replacement) and Gatorload (high-carbohydrate supplement) for the team. I explained the importance of having something to eat immediately after practice or the game. I said they should try to eat some food *before* they showered and dressed. After I spoke, the coach said it was a good strategy to follow, and that was that. For the rest of the year, the team ate and drank immediately after practice and games, and they also managed to win the league trophy at the end of the year.

A couple of years after the team moved to another city, I ran into one of the players at a restaurant. He told me he had been recruited to play for one of the major league teams and, at the end of his first week there, noticed he was beginning to feel run down. He remembered what I did with the Knights and requested that his new team also have food in the locker room for right after practice and games. He told me the whole team is now eating pasta and French bread in the locker room. There's just no stopping a good idea!

Different activities place different metabolic requirements on muscle systems, and these differences alter the nutritional requirements among athletes involved in various types of sports. This chapter focuses on sports that require a high level of power and speed over short distances and time. In the athletic world, these athletes are the true anaerobes among us. They're not interested in their ability to move efficiently over long distances, but want to be there first in short distances. When a baseball player steals a base, there is nothing about that four-to-five-second experience that requires aerobic efficiency. It is entirely dependent on anaerobic metabolism, which is dependent on phosphocreatine and glycogen as fuels. Bodybuilders need explosive power to train but almost never place continuous stress on the muscles for longer than 1.5 minutes, the anaerobic maximum.

There has been a clear evolution in the way athletes have eaten to support top athletic performance. Around the year 200 A.D., Diogenes Laertius wrote that Greek athletes of the time had a training diet that consisted of dried figs, moist cheeses, and wheat products.[1] American Olympians at the Berlin Games of 1936 had a daily intake that included beefsteak, lots of butter, three eggs, custard, 1.5 liters of milk, and as much as they could consume of white bread, dinner rolls, fresh vegetables, and salads. With each successive Olympic Games, athletes have consumed and avoided foods based on the knowledge of the time. Since the 1960s, however, there has been a purposeful scientific effort to learn what athletes need and why they need it. This scientific endeavor has led to a much-improved understanding of how muscles work for power and how they work for speed. The science of sports nutrition has also helped us understand the different nutritional demands associated with different types of activities. A failure to consider the nutritional implications of the activity will most certainly lead to problems in training and performance outcomes that are below the capabilities of the athlete.

Baseball

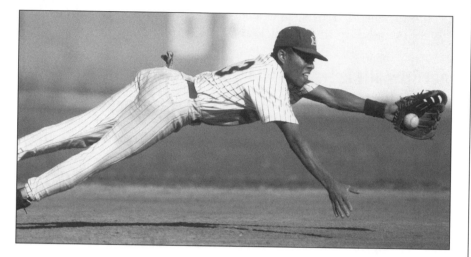

Baseball is a wonderful sport that requires an almost equal combination of teamwork *and* individual effort. It's also a highly mental game, requiring that the athlete stay constantly alert to make split-second judgments for the right play. It's safe to say that physically tired baseball players are also likely to be mentally tired (glucose is the fuel for both the brain and muscles) and prone to bad judgment and poor physical performance. David Halberstam, in his book *The Summer of '49* (New York: William Morrow, 1989), describes the pennant race between the Red Sox and Yankees. A theme in this book is how players would get worn out during the long baseball season, with the outcome of the pennant race determined, to a degree, by the number of players who remained relatively fresh by the end of the season. There are clearly many factors that contribute to players getting worn out during a long season, including frequent travel, hard-fought games, and constantly changing time zones.[2] But there are also nutritional factors, including what food and fluids are consumed over the long summer and fall season. When steak and beer are constantly on the menu, as was common for many baseball players in the past, you could have predicted that physical and mental fatigue would eventually take its toll. Alcohol interferes with B-vitamin metabolism (and therefore energy metabolism), and also increases the chance for dehydration. We have also learned that, while occasional red meat is a useful means of supplying good quality protein, iron, and zinc, it should not be the focus of an athlete's diet. What these baseball players really needed was plenty of bread, cereal, fruits, and vegetables to constantly replace the glycogen used up in the quick and powerful actions of the game.

Nutritionally Relevant Factors for Baseball

• *It's often played in a hot and humid environment.* Optimally hydrated muscles are composed of more than 70 percent water, and it should be the athlete's goal to maintain this optimal hydration state. A failure to do so will lead to a progressive reduction in total body water with a concomitant reduction in athletic performance. There is also good evidence to suggest that poor hydration makes the athlete more prone to injury, by reducing mental function (poor hydration is associated with higher core temperatures that can reduce coordination) and by making muscles less resilient (thus increasing the risk of muscle tears and pulls).

Baseball players (particularly pitchers) are known to experience a reduction in peak torque arm strength between pre- and postseason measurements.[3] It is likely that a good deal of this power reduction is due to overuse injury to the pitching arm. There is evidence that reduced throwing power could also be due to reduced strength in the legs, which are important in the throwing motion.[4] Weak legs, therefore, could exacerbate injury to the arm because of an altered throwing motion. It is also likely that the degree to which the progressive reduction in power occurs could be reduced with a regular program of optimal hydration and energy intake.

A study of baseball players strongly suggests that conditioning plays an important role in the ability of the athlete to maintain an optimal hydration state. This study found that, at fixed exercise intensities, the more-fit baseball players were able to maintain body temperature with a lower sweat rate than players who were less fit.[5] In another study, it was found that blood flow to the pitching arm (in pitchers) increased up to 40 pitches, but steadily declined after that. By the 100th pitch, blood flow to the pitching arm was 30 percent below baseline.[6] It is possible that the decrease in blood flow to the pitching arm matches a decrease in the general hydration state of the pitchers. Since it is well established that blood volume is a key factor in the maintenance of athletic performance, the performance of pitchers may be strongly influenced by their ability to stay hydrated.

Given the possibility for frequent exposure to hot and humid environments, baseball players should consider the following strategy for maintaining their hydration state:

1. Drink plenty of fluids prior to each game (a minimum of 16 ounces one hour prior to the game, followed by a constant sipping of fluids).

2. During the preseason, take weight before and after each game and practice to learn how much weight has been lost. Then determine how much fluid should be consumed during a typical game (1 pint of fluid = 1 pound of body weight). Your goal should be to drink enough fluids to maintain body weight (±1 pound) during the game. Different people have different sweat rates, so your drinking schedule is likely to be different from those of every one of your teammates.

3. Use each opportunity (between innings) to consume fluids. Since baseball involves multiple bouts of high-intensity movements, the drain on stored glycogen is high. Therefore, fluids consumed should be carbohydrate containing. Fluids containing a 6 to 7 percent carbohydrate solution are best both for replacing carbohydrate and for encouraging a fast absorption of water.

4. Immediately after the game, eat and drink enough carbohydrate to reconstitute your glycogen stores and body water.

5. Avoid or limit the consumption of alcohol and caffeinated beverages. Both alcohol and caffeine have a diuretic effect (cause you to urinate), placing you in a negative water balance.

• *It requires power and speed.* The greater the power and speed, the higher the reliance on phosphocreatine and carbohydrate (primarily glycogen) for muscular fuel. Phosphocreatine is synthesized from three amino acids (from protein), so an adequate intake of protein is necessary to assure that sufficient phosphocreatine can be manufactured. However, since we are an energy-first system, the protein consumption must be in the context of an adequate total intake of energy (calories). Since baseball players reach their peak at around age 28, they have the advantage of being fully grown.[7] Therefore, the provision of energy to support growth is not necessary, making it easier for developed players to obtain the needed energy. Inadequate energy intake causes the consumed protein to be burned as a fuel rather than used as a building block for other substances such as creatine. Creatine is a preformed component of meat. (Preformed creatine simply means that it is already made—we don't have to synthesize it from three amino acids—so it is readily available to the muscles.) Therefore, the occasional intake of meat is beneficial. While vegetarians may not get the benefit of this preformed creatine from meat, with enough protein intake vegetarians are fully capable of making their own creatine. In the context of an adequate energy intake, baseball players should consume a diet that derives 60 to 65 percent of its energy from carbohydrates, 20 to 25 percent of its energy from fat, and 15 percent of its energy from protein.

• *Many games are played during the season (several games/week).* Multiple games and practices each week can easily lead to overtraining with the associated problems of fatigue, weakness, and increased risk of illness. The key to limiting the impact of overtraining is the consumption of a high-carbohydrate diet to maintain muscle glycogen levels. It has been shown that daily practices or competitions will lead to a progressive reduction in muscle glycogen storage, with a related reduction in endurance and performance. Since baseball players are highly dependent on muscle glycogen as a fuel, this reduction would lead to a discernable lowering of performance with time. Studies have also shown that fatigue associated with daily training can be dramatically reduced in athletes who maintain a high-carbohydrate (more than 60 percent of calories) intake.

• *Games typically last for two to three hours.* Normal blood glucose flux is approximately three hours. That is, from the time you finish eating a meal, blood glucose stays in the normal range for about three hours. After this, blood glucose falls below the normal range (80–120 milligrams per deciliter), and people begin to feel hungry. In the exercising person, blood glucose is likely to go below the normal range earlier than three hours. Since blood glucose is an important factor in maintaining normal mental function and is also important in delivering fuel to muscles that have exhausted stored carbohydrate, athletes should take steps to maintain blood glucose for the entire competition. Therefore, baseball players should consume a carbohydrate-containing solution at every opportunity (between innings).

• *There's an opportunity to rest during the game.* Baseball players have a wonderful opportunity to maintain both fluid and carbohydrate status because of the inning structure of the game. When a team is on offense, every player should use this time to consume a carbohydrate solution.

• *Pitchers work harder when they're pitching than other players on the team (which is why they pitch every three to five games).* Pitchers are better able to maintain muscular power (both in the legs and arms) by maximizing glycogen storage and hydration state before and during each game. The principle of glycogen loading (a general tapering of activity coupled with a high-carbohydrate and fluid intake—refer to chapter 7 for more detailed information) can be followed with starting pitchers since they typically have several days between starts.

• *Catchers work hard and carry more equipment weight, so they are likely to need more breaks than other players.* The weight and insulating effect of the equipment worn by catchers add to their energy and fluid requirements. Since catchers are constantly in motion, working with the pitcher, and since they tend to play on a more frequent rotation than starting pitchers, it's safe to say that, pound for pound, catchers have the highest energy and fluid requirements of any of the baseball positions.

Bodybuilding

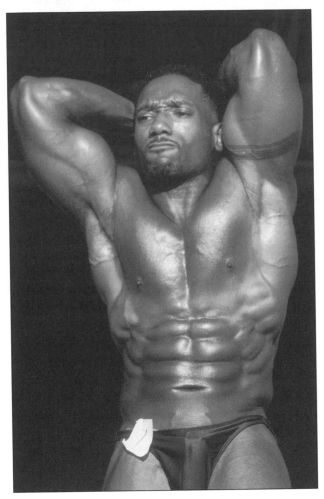

Bodybuilders strive for a physique that is high in muscle mass and extremely low in body fat. The low body fat is a necessary adjunct to performance, which requires a high level of muscular definition to achieve a high score. A high body fat level would serve to mask the underlying muscle formation. To achieve this high level of muscle mass, bodybuilders must place a high level of repetitive stress (typically via free weights and muscle-resistance equipment) on each muscle group. This is never done aerobically (i.e., low-level muscular force over long time periods). Instead, bodybuilders rely on high-intensity repetitions that rarely last longer than 30 seconds per muscle group, and never last longer than 1.5 minutes. In preparation for competition, bodybuilders couple this hard muscle training with the consumption of extra energy to enlarge the muscle mass. Typically, the diet is predominantly composed of high-protein foods and supplements.

Once the muscle mass is enlarged, bodybuilders go into a second training phase that involves a reduction in energy and a small aerobic component in the training.[8] This second phase is aimed at reducing body fat levels (particularly subcutaneous fat) to allow for a greater visual muscle definition. During the week prior to competition, bodybuilders typically decrease total energy intake and increase carbohydrate intake to glycogen load the muscles. There is also a great deal of fluid and sodium manipulation to aid in muscle definition. During this week, both fluids and sodium are typically restricted. There is evidence that fluid restriction is dangerous, particularly in younger bodybuilders, where both low blood potassium and phosphorus have been seen.[9] In addition, there is evidence that the energy (calorie) restriction common during the period immediately before the competition causes a loss of lean body (muscle) mass, suggesting that the energy restriction is too severe.[10]

Perhaps there is no sport that is so prone to nutritional *mis*information than bodybuilding. In a study evaluating advertisements in bodybuilding magazines, it was found that there was no scientific evidence for 42 percent of the products for which beneficial nutritional claims were made. Only 21 percent of the advertised products had appropriate documentation to support their claims, and 32 percent of the products that had some scientific documentation were marketed in a misleading manner.[11] In a study of male and female bodybuilders, it was found that multi drug abuse was prevalent (up to 40 percent of the subjects), and that a majority of bodybuilders reported following regimens that led to severe dehydration.[12] In this same study, it was found that women had calcium intakes that were extremely low, and that the general nutritional and dietary practices placed them, as a group, in a high-risk category for poor health.

Nutritionally Relevant Factors for Bodybuilding

• *Bodybuilders strive for a high level of muscle mass.* A higher level of muscle mass nutritionally translates into a higher need for energy. While the total amount of protein needed to maintain this larger mass is higher, the proportion of protein provided by foods actually remains the same. Ideally, bodybuilders should consume approximately 1.5 grams of protein per kilogram of body weight, but this should be consumed in the context of an adequate total energy consumption where most of the energy is derived from carbohydrates. Most of the studies of bodybuilders strongly suggest that protein consumption is significantly higher than the body's ability to use it anabolically (i.e., to use it to build tissue). Therefore, the excess protein is simply burned as a fuel or, in the case of excess total energy consumption, stored as fat. This has been confirmed by the finding in one study, which found that bodybuilders had significantly higher protein intakes than lean control subjects, and that they also relied more heavily on protein as a fuel to meet the energy requirements of the muscles.[13] It is very likely that bodybuilders believe excess protein assists in building body mass because they consume foods that do not, by themselves, provide sufficient energy to enlarge the lean mass. The extra protein consumed, therefore, serves to fill the energy gap, and meeting energy needs can clearly be done more effectively with carbohydrate than with protein. The nutritional key to building muscle mass is to consume enough energy to support the larger mass. For instance, if you now weigh 180 pounds and you wish to weigh 190 pounds, you should eat as if you already weigh 190 pounds.

• *Bodybuilders strive for an extremely low level of fat mass.* Body fat percentage is, to a great degree, determined by a person's genetic makeup. However, it is also clear that it can be influenced by dietary and exercise habits. From a dietary standpoint, it is clearly important to consume a low level of fat, since it takes very little energy to convert dietary fat to stored fat. Carbohydrate, on the other hand, is not as efficiently converted to stored fat. Since carbohydrates are more efficiently burned as a fuel for high-intensity muscular work and are not as efficiently converted to fat for storage, fat intake should be kept low (15 to 25 percent of total calories). This is slightly below the general population recommendation that no more than 30 percent of total calories be provided from fat. It also appears that eating small and frequent meals helps to prevent the manufacture of fat from the energy in foods. If you consume 1,500 calories in a single meal, the normal processing of so much energy at one time will inevitably lead to a percentage of this intake being stored as fat. However, if this 1,500-calorie meal is consumed in two meals that are three hours apart (750 calories per meal), the body is better at using this energy without storing it as fat. Therefore, eating a low-fat diet *and* eating small but frequent meals are both important strategies for obtaining a low body fat percentage.

Bodybuilders commonly go through repetitive patterns of weight gain and weight loss in an attempt to build muscle and then reduce body fat levels. The average reported weight loss experienced during the competitive season is 6.8 kilograms (15 pounds), and the average reported weight gain is 6.2 kilograms (14 pounds). This cyclic dieting leaves bodybuilders with a food preoccupation that leads to binge eating after competitions, as well as psychological stress.[14] A much more logical approach to building muscle safely is to consume an extra 300 to 500 calories (beyond current needs) from carbohydrate to support a larger muscle mass, and then do activities that sufficiently stress the muscles so they will enlarge.

• *Bodybuilders appear to be excessively dependent on nutritional and quasi-nutritional products and ergogenic aids to achieve the desired body composition.* Self-experimentation with ergogenic aids and nutritional products is common in many sports. (See chapter 4, "Training With Supplements.") However, bodybuilders appear to be especially targeted to marketing efforts for these products. It is easy to become convinced that these products actually work because the placebo effect is very real in nutrition. That is, if you *believe* something will help you, then it will probably lead to a benefit even if there is no physiological or biological basis for the improvement. The best scenario, however, is for athletes to consume products and foods that have a physiological and biological reason for improvement, and the athlete also believes they work. This will give twice the benefit to the athlete.

• *Bodybuilders commonly rely on excessive water loss to achieve the desired appearance.* Dehydration is dangerous (there are numerous deaths yearly from dehydration, both among athletes and non-athletes) and diminishes athletic performance. With bodybuilders, even though it is important to have a cut appearance, achieving this through dehydration is an unacceptable strategy since it can lead to organ failure and death. Bodybuilders should achieve their desired appearance through hard work and the development of a relatively low level of body fat (see section above).

• *Nutrient intake (i.e., vitamins and minerals) appears to be inadequate in this population.* The focus on nutritional products (protein powders and shakes, amino acid supplements, creatine monohydrate supplements, etc.) rather than food serves to place bodybuilders at nutritional risk. Consumption of a low-fat, high-carbohydrate, moderate-protein intake *that provides adequate energy (calories)* from a wide variety of foods will help to assure a good nutrient intake. Vitamin and mineral supplements are useful only when there is a known deficiency or risk of deficiency for a specific nutrient.

Football (U.S.)

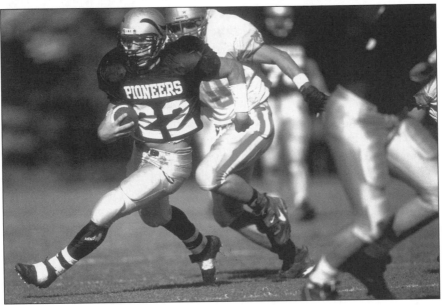

Football is the epitome of the anaerobic sport, with the length of plays almost never exceeding 15 seconds and a rest period between each play. However, when the ball is in play, the football players are giving 100 percent muscular effort to move the ball. In addition, football players carry the extra burden of heavy equipment, which adds to the energy requirement. Clearly, the fuels most used in this type of activity are phosphocreatine and muscle glycogen, so the traditional "steak and potatoes" pregame meal may not be the ideal meal to assure an optimal storage of muscle glycogen, since there is a relative overemphasis of protein (steak) and a relative underemphasis of carbohydrate (potato). In a recent study of college football players, it was found that supplementing with creatine monohydrate had a performance-enhancing effect (improved lifting volume and sprint performance).[15] However, findings from this and other studies should be reviewed carefully before embarking on a path of ergogenic aid supplementation. For instance, the total energy-intake adequacy of the subjects in this study was not evaluated, so it is unclear if the derived benefit is because of the increased creatine intake or from an improvement in the total energy intake of the subjects. In another study evaluating nutrient supplementation on athletic performance, football players who consumed chromium picolinate supplements

224

for nine weeks experienced no improvement in either body composition or strength relative to a group of football players who did not supplement.[16]

The stop-and-go nature of football, which vacillates between bouts of maximal effort and rest during a game, is also associated with a high level of body-water loss. This loss of body fluid impacts negatively on cooling ability, athletic performance, and the ability to concentrate.[17] In a study of the consumption of carbohydrate-containing beverages among football players, it was found that these beverages were better able to maintain plasma volume than water alone.[18] Since maintenance of plasma volume is strongly associated with athletic performance, football players should consider consuming a well-designed sports beverage to maintain endurance and performance. Adequate fluid consumption before, during, and after games and practices should be an important part of the training regimen.

Football players at every level have recently been getting bigger and stronger each year, and have a relatively positive body image when compared to other male athletes.[19] In a survey of High School All-American Football Teams from 1963 to 1971 and from 1972 to 1989, it was found that there have been significant increases in the ratio of weight to height (body mass index) in the 1970s and 1980s that did not exist earlier.[20] In other words, football players are getting heavier (relative to their heights) at a rate much higher than existed prior to 1963.

Increased weight by itself may not be a good thing for football players. In one study, it was found that football linemen with higher body fat percentages and higher body mass indexes had higher rates of lower-extremity injuries.[21] In another study, football players with a higher body fat level had a 2.5 times higher relative risk of injury than those with lower body fat levels.[22] In addition, it was found that there was an unexpectedly high rate of obesity among adolescent football players. Since body image is inversely related to body fat percentage in male athletes (i.e., higher body fats are associated with poor body image), it is important to help athletes understand how to increase weight properly if higher weight is desirable.[23] Taken together, these findings strongly suggest that increasing lean (muscle) mass rather than simply increasing weight should be a priority for football players.

Weight loss is often an issue for lightweight football players. These players, who must maintain weight below a given threshold to be eligible to play, often display eating patterns that are unhealthy. In one study, it was found that 20 percent felt their weight-control practices frequently interfered with their thinking and other activities, and 42 percent had a pattern of dysfunctional eating. Almost 10 percent of those surveyed were practicing binge-purge (bulimic) eating behaviors.[24]

Many have questioned whether the recent increases in football-player size are due to improved preselection in the sport (i.e., attracting bigger players to begin with), improved nutrition, or an increased reliance on anabolic steroid hormones. It is possible, of course, for all or any combination of these factors to contribute to the recent increases seen in the body mass index. Football players appear to be eating better than their non-football-playing counterparts. In a study of junior high school and high school football players, it was found that, in general, nutrient and energy intakes were better than those seen in the U.S. population of same-age boys.[25] Energy intakes, which are often below recommended levels in other sports, appear to be near at least 94 percent of the requirement in the assessed football players. Zinc was found to be one of the nutrients to be low in this study. In another study of football players, low zinc levels were found to have a negative impact on maximal workloads. Since zinc intake is strongly associated with the consumption of red meat, football players should consider a periodic, regular consumption of meat. However, this meat consumption should not interfere with or replace the consumption of carbohydrates, which are key to maintaining performance in stop-and-go activities. Vegetarians may be at risk for inadequate zinc intake, so they should be assessed by a qualified medical professional to determine if zinc supplements are warranted.

As with athletes in other professional sports, time-zone changes make a difference in performance outcomes. It has been found, for instance, that when games are played at night, West Coast teams have a clear advantage over eastern and central time-zone teams.[26] The West Coast teams feel as if they're playing earlier in the day relative to the other teams, so they do not suffer from end-of-day fatigue to the degree that other teams do. West Coast teams have a 75 percent and 68 percent winning percentage when playing Central and East Coast teams, respectively, and still maintain a high winning percentage even when playing in away games (approximately 68 percent). All of this strongly suggests that football players who travel across time zones to play should do whatever it takes to overcome normal circadian rhythms. Among the positive actions that players can take is to eat small amounts of foods frequently and to consume plenty of fluids during travel.

Nutritionally Relevant Factors for Football

• *Football requires a high level of strength and speed of short duration but high frequency.* Football players are involved in activities that require repeated bouts of high effort interspersed with periods of rest. This type of activity requires a high level of carbohydrate to properly fuel the muscles. Therefore, football players should enter the game with their muscle glycogen levels full. However, even with muscle glycogen storage at its peak, a player cannot play an entire game without depleting muscle glycogen in specific muscle groups. Therefore, football players should take every opportunity to consume a carbohydrate-containing beverage during breaks in the game. All of the pregame, during-game, and postgame hydration techniques reviewed earlier in chapter 2, "Staying Hydrated," should be followed to assure a constant availability of carbohydrate to the muscles.

• *Linemen require a high level of mass.* While high mass affords linemen a clear advantage, the ability to move the mass quickly is equally important. Therefore, linemen should strive for a high level of muscle mass not just higher weight. To achieve this, consumption of a diet that meets the energy requirements for the higher mass is needed and, in this context, a relatively low intake of fat (less than 25 percent of total calories) and a moderate intake of protein (12 to 15 percent of total calories or about 1.5 grams of protein per kilogram of body weight). This type of diet, coupled with exercise that places stress on the muscles, helps to enlarge the muscle mass. Increasing total energy intake through the consumption of a high level of fatty foods greatly enables an increase in fat storage (and therefore mass), but fat does not contribute to strength. Thus fatty foods negatively alter the strength-to-weight ratio and make it more difficult for a lineman to move quickly and powerfully off the line.

• *Backfield defensive positions and pass receivers require high agility, speed, and quick reaction time.* High speed and agility require a relatively low level of body fat. Therefore, these football players should consume foods that limit fat storage (i.e., a high-carbohydrate, low-fat intake). Since multiple 40 yard sprints down the field to catch (or defend against) long passes will quickly deplete muscle glycogen storage, consumption of a carbohydrate-containing beverage at natural breaks during the game is desirable. During hot and humid days, consuming this beverage will also enhance the ability to maintain a desirable hydration state.

• *Repeated high-intensity activity while carrying equipment (pads, helmet, etc.) translates into high sweat losses.* The fluid in sweat must be replaced to maintain optimal performance. To do this, consumption of sports beverages that contain a 6 to 7 percent carbohydrate solution are useful in maintaining the body's water level *and* replenishing carbohydrate fuel. When assessed, athletes typically place themselves in a state of voluntary underhydration, so there is every reason to set up a strategy that causes football players to consciously consume fluids during every possible break in the game.

Gymnastics

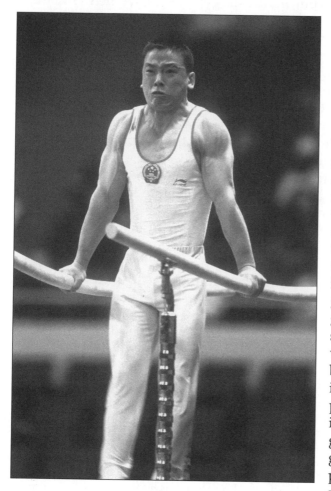

The number of young gymnastics competitors continues to increase, so it is especially important that growth, weight, bone health, eating behavior, and other developmentally important factors are carefully monitored. The tradition in gymnastics is to have small gymnasts, and gymnasts themselves commonly view this small body image as ideal. Weight is a prevailing theme in gymnastics, regardless of the gymnastics discipline. Even in men's gymnastics, it is suggested that controlling energy intake to achieve lower weight is an appropriate and desired approach if a gymnast is to achieve success.[27] But there is an expectation for growth in children, so there should be a concomitant expectation for increasing weight. Without accepting this fact, many young athletes, including gymnasts, may try to achieve a low weight through unhealthy means. While it is true that a lowering of excess body fat will reduce body mass and, perhaps, lower the risk of traumatic injuries to joints, trying to achieve this through inappropriate means may also place the gymnast at risk.[28]

Elite-level gymnastics has four separate disciplines, including men's gymnastics, women's artistic gymnastics, women's rhythmic gymnastics, and women's rhythmic group gymnastics. Although the total time spent in gymnastics practice is high for elite gymnasts (up to 30 hours of practice each week), the actual time spent in conditioning and skills training is considerably less. Gymnasts begin practice with a series of stretches and then initiate a series of basic skills on the floor mat as part of the warm-up routine. Following warm-up, each gymnast takes a turn practicing one of the events. The time performing a skill in practice never exceeds that of the competition maximum and is usually a small fraction of it. Because practice involves repeated bouts of highly intense, short-duration activity, gymnasts rest between each practice bout to regenerate strength. With the exception of the group competition in rhythmic gymnastics, none of the competition events within each of these disciplines has a duration longer than 90 seconds. This duration categorizes gymnastics as a high-intensity, anaerobic sport.

As anaerobes, gymnasts rely heavily on Type IIB (pure fast-twitch) and Type IIA (intermediate fast-twitch) muscle fibers (see chapter 5, "Eating for Anaerobic Power").[29] These fibers, while capable of producing a great deal of power, are generally regarded as incapable of functioning at high intensity for longer than 90 seconds. Type II fibers have a low oxidative capacity, which limits fat usage as an energy substrate during gymnastic activity, and a poor capillary supply, which deprives these fibers of nutrient, oxygen, and carbon dioxide exchange during intensive work. Because of these factors, gymnastics activity is heavily dependent on creatine phosphate and carbohydrate (both glucose and glycogen) as fuels for activity.

A number of studies have evaluated the nutrient intake of elite gymnasts. In general, these studies demonstrate an inadequacy in the intake of total energy, iron, and calcium.[30,31,32] Heavy gymnastic training and inadequate nutrient intake are implicated as causative factors in the primary amenorrhea experienced by many young gymnasts, and may also contribute to the secondary amenorrhea experienced by older gymnasts. A woman 18 years of age and older, who has never had a period (delayed menses), is considered to have primary amenorrhea. A female who has experienced menses in the past, but is not currently experiencing periods over a span of time (several months or even years) is considered to have secondary amenorrhea. While inadequate calcium intake is associated with poor bone development and increased risk of stress fracture, inadequate iron intake is associated with anemia, which is a risk factor in the development of amenorrhea.[33]

Nutritionally Relevant Factors for Gymnastics

• *Gymnasts are required to do difficult tumbling and acrobatic skills that are easier for smaller people to do.* Artistic gymnasts are commonly small (30th percentile for height-to-age ratio), but extremely muscular (90th percentile for arm muscle circumference).[34] It is possible that this tendency for small stature is due to a self-selection in the sport (i.e., only those who are small remain in the sport competitively because they tend to be more successful) or because of an inadequate nutrient intake. Both of these factors are possible, either together or separately. Gymnasts and gymnastics coaches know that the top gymnasts tend to be small, so many of them try to achieve this small size by reducing food intake. There are many problems with this strategy, not the least of which is the possibility of delayed growth with poor skeletal development. In the relatively few cases where this occurs because of an overzealous coach or a gymnast who has made severe cuts in food intake, the outcome may be grim, leading to life-threatening eating disorders. Luckily, however, the vast majority of gymnasts do very well in this sport, thrive as adults, and have healthy families.

The key thing to remember is that unhealthy athletes don't stay competitive for very long, so it's in everyone's interest to eat enough to sustain health and growth. Further, gymnasts should think more about optimizing body composition rather than maintaining or reducing weight. Clearly, one of the difficulties that arises from severe dieting is that weight goes down but so does muscle mass. In fact, muscle mass is likely to be reduced more than fat mass with dieting, making it *more difficult* for gymnasts to perform difficult skills. This relative increase in body fat (i.e., a greater proportion of remaining weight is fat) may cause gymnasts to further reduce food intake to a point that it is diagnosable as an eating disorder. If this occurs, the gymnast is in danger and requires serious and speedy intervention from a qualified health professional.

• *Gymnasts are sensitive to the strength-to-weight ratio both from appearance and performance standpoints.* It is called "artistic" gymnastics, so there's no getting around the fact that how a person looks in accomplishing the skills makes a difference in the score. Being strong makes it easier to achieve the required skill, so it looks better and more effortless when it is completed (i.e., it looks more artistic). Gymnasts are constantly being reminded to smile while in competition, and this just serves to give the appearance that the skills are easily done. The key is to be sufficiently conditioned and strong so that the skills can be completed with ease. In the United States, there is concern that gymnasts start learning skills too early, when they should be focusing on conditioning. After all, a well-conditioned athlete will learn the skill more quickly and with less risk of injury. However, there is tremendous pressure on coaches to demonstrate that the gymnasts are progressing nicely, and the best way to do that is to put them in junior competitions. Of course, a gymnast in competition needs to perform some skills. But a more balanced approach that focuses on conditioning early in the gymnast's career, and delays the introduction of specific gymnastics skills, may actually improve the skill-learning curve later on—when it really counts.

To improve conditioning, gymnasts *must* consume sufficient energy and nutrients to meet the combined demands of growth, maintenance, and improvement in musculature. The focus on gymnastics training should be on getting strong rather than on staying small (i.e., work on the *strength* part of the strength-to-weight ratio rather than on the weight part), and this can only be accomplished through a training program that satisfies nutritional needs. In fact, well-conditioned and strong gymnasts rarely have to worry about weight, because it takes care of itself quite nicely.

• *Gymnasts (and many other female athletes) have delayed menarche, which may play a role in bone health.* If a gymnast fails to achieve menses by age 16, she should see a physician to determine the cause and, if needed, a remedy. There are many possible causes for a delay or cessation of menses, including

- low body fat,
- poor iron status,
- high physical stress,
- high psychological stress,
- high cortisol level: (Cortisol is a hormone produced by the body to counteract the soreness created from activity. It is commonly high in athletes and interferes with estrogen production.)
- low energy intake.

It is conceivable that gymnasts may have *all* of these factors. Regardless of the cause(s), a delay in menstrual onset may negatively impact bone health and increase the later risk of early osteoporosis development. To reduce the risk of delayed menstrual onset, gymnasts should have periodic checks to determine iron status and should do whatever possible to eat normally.

• *Gymnasts commonly reach their competitive peak at around ages 16 to 18.* In hardly any other sport, except perhaps figure skating, does the athlete reach peak competitive form at such a young age. It's hard to be the best at anything without spending a tremendous amount of time practicing at it, and that's where the nutritional risk occurs. Adolescents in the middle of their growth spurt have an extremely high requirement for energy and nutrients. It's difficult to imagine how anyone can consume a sufficient amount of energy to support both the adolescent growth spurt and all the energy burned from the hours of activity needed to reach the peak of performance capabilities. However, with planning, it *is* possible. In fact, gymnasts who do it right by eating enough to support the combined energy needs of growth, physical activity, and tissue maintenance look better, do better, enjoy the sport more, and stay in the sport longer.

Hockey

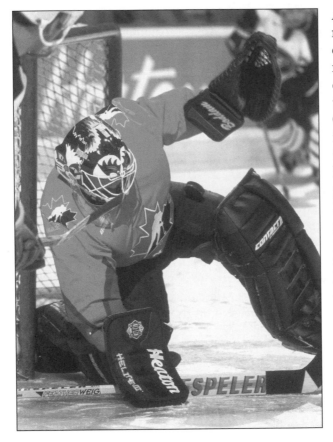

Although you may have thought of hockey as a male sport, anyone who watched the 1998 Winter Olympic Games in Nagano knows that women play hockey, too, and play it very well. Regardless of the gender of the player, hockey is a no-holds-barred, high-speed, full-effort sport. If you watch closely the way hockey players go in and out of play, they skate at full tilt while they're on the ice but almost never skate for more than 1.5 minutes continuously. This high-speed effort places a great deal of emphasis on anaerobic metabolism, which means the energy focus is on phosphocreatine and carbohydrate (glycogen and glucose). My own experiences with the Atlanta Knights hockey team, and the experiences of others who have worked on improving the nutritional practices of hockey players, strongly suggests that it is possible to make positive dietary changes in hockey players.[35] These changes can help them in making the right changes in hockey players can help them in weight maintenance during the season and during the off-season, and improvements in endurance have been seen with proper fluid and carbohydrate replacement.

In a study of elite hockey players from Sweden, it was determined that the distance skated, the number of shifts skated, the amount of time skated within shifts, and the skating speed all improved with carbohydrate loading.[36] The authors of this study concluded that individual differences in performance in hockey players are directly related to muscle glycogen metabolism. These findings are confirmed from a study of seven professional hockey players, which found that 60 percent of the muscle glycogen in the quadriceps muscle is burned during a single game.[37] Since hockey players frequently skate in practice or have successive game days, it is possible for muscle glycogen to become virtually depleted on an improper intake. Data from this study reveal that most players consume a diet high in protein and low in carbohydrate, a diet that is guaranteed to cause fuel-supply problems in working muscles.

Making a shift away from a high-fat, high-protein intake toward one that is higher in carbohydrates is not easy, however, and may increase the chance of consuming too little energy because carbohydrates are a less dense source of calories than fats. This was seen in one study where players from one hockey team were placed on a special dietary regimen that reduced fat and protein intake and increased carbohydrate intake.[38] This team was compared to another team that maintained the usual nutrient intake (i.e., high fat, high protein, low carbohydrate). In this study, the hockey players with the higher carbohydrate intake had some measurable changes in hormone balance that were best explained by inadequate total energy intake. Therefore, if a switch is made from a higher fat diet to one that is lower in fat and higher in carbohydrates, care must be taken that the total energy (i.e., calories) intake is sufficient to meet the athlete's needs.

Nutritionally Relevant Factors for Hockey

• *Frequent games place a high demand on muscle glycogen.* There is good evidence for muscle glycogen depletion in hockey players, strongly suggesting that those who play this sport must consume diets high in carbohydrates. However, it's not just the intake of carbohydrates that's important, but the strategies used in their consumption to optimize muscle glycogen storage. In general, a diet should provide 60 to 65 percent of the total energy intake from carbohydrate. The pregame meal should consist almost entirely of carbohydrates that are mainly starch based, such as pasta, potatoes, rice, breads, and cereals. Fruits, vegetables, and high-bran (i.e., high crude fiber) foods may increase gas production in the gut, so should be avoided or consumed sparingly in the pregame meal. (Of course, at other times, all of these foods are nourishing and good to eat.) Every opportunity should be taken during games to provide carbohydrate (carbohydrate-containing beverages during breaks in play; carbohydrate supplements (such as carbohydrate gels) and beverages between periods). Postgame carbohydrate consumption during the first hour following the game is critical to capitalize on the circulating glycogen synthetase (a hormone that helps to store muscle glycogen when carbohydrates are made available). Pregame and normal intake carbohydrates should focus on starch-based, complex carbohydrates, and during-game and immediately postgame carbohydrates should be sugar-based or simple carbohydrates (that is, carbohydrates that are more refined and have less fiber).

• *Changing food intake to provide more carbohydrates may result in an inadequate energy consumption.* Surveys of hockey players strongly suggest that normal energy intakes tend to be high in fat, high in protein, and low in carbohydrate. This is a diet that does not adequately support the type of muscular metabolism that takes place. However, because of the higher energy concentration in this type of intake, it is easier for hockey players to obtain the total energy they need. The simple reason for this is that for the same weight of food, fats provide more than twice the caloric content of carbohydrates (9 calories per gram vs. 4 calories per gram). Making a switch to foods that are lower in fat and higher in carbohydrate while maintaining the same eating frequency may serve to create a negative energy balance that could also be detrimental to performance.[39] Inadequate energy almost guarantees a catabolism (i.e., breakdown) of muscle that is used as a fuel, so the hockey player would eventually lose weight and become weaker. The solution (perhaps the *only* solution) is to make certain that hockey players increase their eating frequency to six times per day (breakfast, midmorning snack, lunch, midafternoon snack, dinner, evening snack) to assure that there is both an increase in carbohydrate and an adequate total energy intake.

• *High intensity activity causes body temperature to rise quickly, with a resultant high sweat rate.* It's hard to imagine anything more performance damaging than dehydration. Considering the amount of equipment, pads, and high-intensity work of hockey players, they are considered to be at risk for dehydration. Therefore follow a good hydration plan (see chapter 2, "Staying Hydrated"). Hockey players should consume plenty of fluids prior to the game and take every opportunity to consume fluids during and after the game. Given the need for carbohydrates and the need for fluids, a good strategy is to consume a carbohydrate-containing beverage whenever possible.

Track and Field

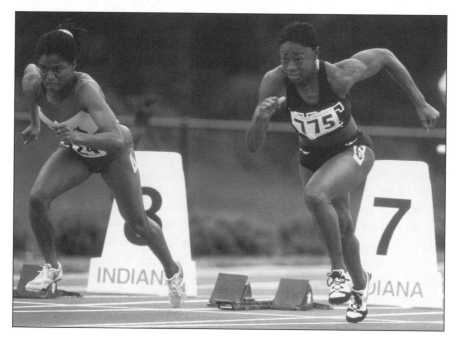

Track and field competition includes a number of events of short duration that rely on power through anaerobic energy. Sprints and hurdle events include races up to and including 400 meter. Field events include jumps and throws.

Have you ever seen an overweight sprinter? I haven't either, and that should be enough evidence that you don't have to do aerobic activity to lower body fat. In fact, a study performed by one of my students showed that high-intensity activity was as effective as low-intensity activity in lowering body fat.[40] Sprinting has been recommended as a normal component of interval training in many sports. Regardless of whether it's done for training, or represents the sport itself (as in the 100-meter dash), sprinting has specific energy requirements that must be accounted for and satisfied to perform at an optimal level. Sprints, which by their very nature rarely last longer than 10 seconds, primarily use the fuels phosphocreatine and carbohydrate. Since muscles with an adequate storage of phosphocreatine can support high-intensity exercise for up to 10 seconds, it is likely that many athletes use primarily phosphocreatine for the entire duration of the sprint. One study, in which creatine monohydrate

was supplemented to increase the muscular storage of phosphocreatine, found that it promoted gains in fat-free (i.e., muscle) mass as
well as sprint performance.[41] This indirectly supports the notion that
sprint performance is highly dependent on phosphocreatine. Carbohydrate intake also appears to make a difference in sprint performance. In a study evaluating the impact of high-, moderate-, and
low-carbohydrate intakes, the high-carbohydrate intakes produced
better initial sprint performance than lower intakes of carbohydrate.[42]

In some sports, the "sprint" may be the difference between winning or losing even when the majority of time is spent doing lower-
intensity exercise. For instance, 10K runners and marathoners run
almost the entire distance at a high pace, but at a pace that is within
the athlete's conditioned ability to provide oxygen to the muscles. At
the end of these races, however, the athlete goes into a sprint pace
(often described as the "kick") that exceeds oxidative capabilities. It
has been found that high-carbohydrate intakes, when compared to
moderate-carbohydrate intakes, are better able to maintain muscle
glycogen in athletes working at 75 percent peak $\dot{V}O_2$ for one hour
followed by five one-minute sprints on four consecutive days.[43]

Nutritionally Relevant Factors for Sprinting

• *There is a high demand for phosphocreatine and carbohydrate fuels in
sprints.* By its very definition, a sprint requires the fastest possible
movement over the prescribed distance. Metabolic limitations control the maximum distance humans can sprint, and sprints never last
longer than 1.5 minutes. On short sprints, there is a high dependence
on phosphocreatine as a fuel. It has been hypothesized that the
ingestion of extra creatine, typically as a supplement in the form of
creatine monohydrate, may improve phosphocreatine storage. (Please
refer to the chapter on supplements for more detailed information.)
This increased storage could theoretically increase the number of
short all-out sprints an athlete could do and might also improve the
time muscles can rely on phosphocreatine as a fuel. There is some
scientific evidence that supplementing with creatine monohydrate
does, in fact, improve both sprint frequency and sprint distance.
However, there are inherent design weaknesses in some of these
studies that should keep athletes from jumping on the creatine
supplement bandwagon. For instance, these studies have not evaluated the energy-intake adequacy of the athletes studied, so the

improvements seen in performance may be due to the energy (i.e., calories) supplied by the creatine (four calories per gram) that could more easily (and more cheaply!) be supplied by carbohydrate. Also, the issue of the safety of frequent and long-term creatine monohydrate ingestion has, to date, never been adequately addressed.

Creatine is a normal constituent of the diet and is highest in meats (beef, pork, poultry, fish, etc.). Therefore, in the context of a high-carbohydrate diet, it seems useful for sprinters to consider consuming small amounts of lean meats regularly. For nonmeat eaters, care should be taken to consume sufficient protein and calories so the synthesis of creatine can occur in the body. The *only* way for the body to synthesize phosphocreatine is for the athlete to consume sufficient energy, so it is also important that sprinters consume enough *total* energy.

• *Pure sprinters may be inhibited from carbohydrate supercompensation, while endurance athletes may require carbohydrate supercompensation to support the end-of-race "kick."* Pure sprinters must move a mass quickly over a relatively short distance. Clearly, the amount of mass that must be moved is a factor in how quickly it can be moved. Sprinters with high strength-to-weight ratios have an advantage over those with lower strength-to-weight ratios. One of the effects of carbohydrate loading (or supercompensation) is to force more carbohydrate (glycogen) into the muscles so it is available for muscular work. Glycogen is stored with water, however, in a 1:3 ratio: that is, for each gram of glycogen stored, the body stores three grams of water. At times, athletes who undergo a carbohydrate-loading regimen mention that they feel stiff and heavy. Clearly, this is not the way a sprinter should feel at the beginning of a race, but it is a perfectly acceptable feeling for long-distance runners. Therefore, pure sprinters should regularly consume a high-carbohydrate intake that provides sufficient total calories, but should avoid any carbohydrate loading regimen that might serve to force extra glycogen and water into the muscles.

Swimming (100- to 400-Meter)

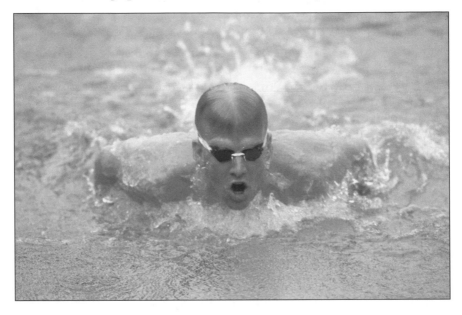

Perhaps there is no other sport where so much time must be spent practicing to gain such incrementally small levels of improvement. Swimmers spend a considerable amount of time in the water to perfect techniques that will better overcome drag and to improve their capacity to sustain both aerobic and anaerobic energy production. In the shorter (sprint) distances where races are typically less than two minutes in length, the majority of energy is predominantly derived anaerobically from phosphocreatine and glycogen (see table 9.1). While these sprint races don't last very long, the amount of energy needed to sustain a high level of power output is tremendously high, and the majority of it (over 55 percent) must come from glycogen and phosphocreatine.

All this time practicing has a high energy and nutrient cost that must be considered when developing a training plan. In a study of national developmental-training-camp swimmers it was found that the average energy (5,221 calories for males, 3,573 calories for females) and nutrient intakes were adequate, but that there was a large between-swimmer variation in intake.[44] This variation, coupled with a tendency for these swimmers to consume excessive amounts of fat and insufficient amounts of carbohydrate, suggests that a large proportion of swimmers may have dietary habits that do not optimally support training and compe-

Table 9.1   Relative Contribution of Aerobic and Anaerobic Energy Sources During Exercise of Different Lengths

Time	Anaerobic %	Aerobic %
0-30 seconds	80	20
30-60 seconds	60	40
60-90 seconds	42	58
90-120 seconds	36	64
120-180 seconds	30	70
Expressed Cumulatively		
0-60 seconds	70	30
0-90 seconds	61	39
0-120 seconds	55	45
0-180 seconds	45	55

Note: As the exercise time increases, power production decreases and a greater proportion of energy is derived aerobically. Aerobic metabolism is less reliant on glycogen and phosphocreatine because of an ability to metabolize fat for energy.

Adapted from Lamb 1995.

tition needs. The desire for higher fat foods from meats and dairy products has been tested in male swimmers, and it was found that they tend to like the sensory appeal of fat-containing animal products, even when undergoing a high level of exercise.[45]

High-level swimmers, who are often young high school students and college-age young adults, must spend a great deal of time in the pool to gain a speed improvement, which commonly translates into multiple training sessions each day. Typically, swimmers practice in the early morning and late afternoon (before and after school and classes). They generally accept the idea that they must get an hour or two of laps in *before* classes begin to have a chance of improving. This means that they must get up at 5:00 A.M. to get to the pool, then head for the pool again right after school or work. The problem, therefore, is trying to assure that swimmers consume sufficient energy *and* consume the energy in a form that is most supportive of the training plan. For swimmers, that means making the time between and during practices to eat lots of foods that are high in carbohydrates. However, swimmers must do this in a way that assures the stomach is empty before getting into the water. This means the focus, during practice and swim meets, should be on carbohydrate-containing fluids, such as sports beverages. Having large amounts of solid foods shortly before getting into the water causes a fluid shift away from the muscles and into the GI tract and may cause cramping.

Nutritionally Relevant Factors for Swimming

• *There are high training hours and an intensive training protocol.* Competitive swimmers work hard and long at getting better, and all that work translates into a tremendously high caloric need. Since swimmers often have a practice early in the morning, it's important to make plans for taking in some carbohydrates immediately upon awakening to assure that there's time for the food to leave the stomach before practice. A failure to consume some carbohydrate (even 100 to 200 calories is better than nothing) prior to practice will limit the benefits the athlete might derive from practice. Fluids (apple or grape juice, or a sports beverage) are good to sip on during the trip to the pool. Following the morning practice, swimmers should have some high-carbohydrate breakfast foods (cereal, toast, bagel, etc.) *immediately available* to eat to replenish the energy consumed during practice and to begin storing more energy for the afternoon practice. Also, because so much energy is needed, high school swimmers should seek approval from school administrators to consume a midmorning snack of 200 to 400 calories. Swimmers who practice *sprinting* in the pool should be aware that phosphocreatine (a major fuel for sprints) is likely to become depleted in muscle cells, and that it takes time to regenerate the phosphocreatine to get the cells ready for the next sprint. When total sprinting time meets or exceeds two minutes, there should be a recovery period of up to four minutes to allow cells time to replenish the depleted phosphocreatine. A failure to allow for this recovery period will force the swimmer to work at a lower intensity and for shorter periods on subsequent sprints. If that happens, the swimmer will be learning to sprint in a way that could adversely impact on competitive times.[46]

• *Body weight reduction may be necessary to improve bathing suit appearance and reduce drag.* The paper-thin material used for racing suits makes it impossible for swimmers to hide their physiques. Since everyone wants to look good, swimmers may be motivated to reduce body weight. However, many swimmers could easily experience a reduction in performance with weight loss if it resulted in a loss of muscle and a resultant loss of power. If weight were lost in such a way so as to reduce drag, there could be a performance benefit, but most weight-loss strategies backfire and hinder performance. Therefore, swimmers wishing to lose weight to either look better or go faster (or both) should only do so under the direct supervision of a qualified health professional. Also, the focus should be on fat reduction and muscle maintenance rather than weight reduction per se.

• *Swimmers rely heavily on glycogen and phosphocreatine.* Sprinting performance is very dependent on carbohydrate (to make stored glycogen) and phosphocreatine. With sufficient total energy intake that focuses on carbohydrates (at least 30 calories of carbohydrate per kilogram of body weight) and includes an adequate amount of protein (about 1.5 to 2.0 grams per kilogram of body weight), there is every reason to believe that athletes can store enough glycogen and make enough phosphocreatine to fuel their muscles properly. However, there is tremendous motivation for many athletes to consume creatine monohydrate supplements (a precursor to phosphocreatine) to gain a competitive edge. While creatine monohydrate supplements *may* improve the number of high-intensity sprints a swimmer is able to do, swimmers should be aware that regular creatine consumption is associated with an increase in weight. Since this weight increase is likely to be from water, it could reduce the swimmer's buoyancy and increase drag. It is likely that a greater benefit could be achieved by creating opportunities to eat in order to assure an optimal total energy intake.

• *Swimmers need to consume fluid.* It's hard to imagine that, with so much water around, a swimmer could get dehydrated! The fact that swimmers are working in a hypothermic environment (water is usually colder than air temperature) makes it easier for the excess heat generated from muscular work to be dissipated. However, there are other good reasons for swimmers to consider whether their hydration state is adequate. Poorly hydrated athletes may develop a lower blood volume that causes the heart to work harder to bring oxygen and nutrients to cells, and there is less volume in which to place metabolic by-products. Also, many competitions take place *outside*, where swimmers spend a great deal of time waiting for their event, and where they can easily become overheated. Excess water storage could clearly be a problem for swimmers by increasing weight and drag, but insufficient body water can impact on performance and concentration. Therefore, a good rule of thumb is to constantly sip small amounts of water or sports beverage, and also to avoid strategies (glycogen loading, glycerol, creatine) that could force excessive amounts of water to be stored (please refer to chapter 5 for more detailed information).

Wrestling

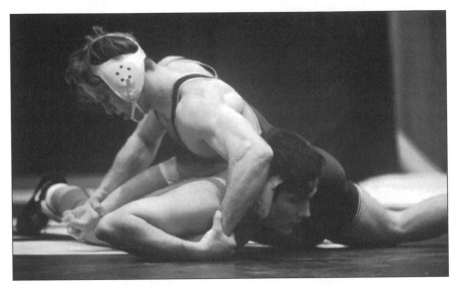

Wrestling has been around as a sport for thousands of years. Early sculpted artifacts and paintings from France, Egypt, and ancient Babylon show wrestlers involved in holds that are essentially the same as those used today. In the early Olympic Games in Greece, the wrestling competition was *the* important competition.[47] The basic strategy in all this time has not changed: wrestlers attempt to force the shoulders of their opponent onto the mat to win the match. If neither wrestler is able to score such a fall, the winner is determined by officials who use a point system, which involves providing points for near falls, holding an opponent close to his back, and controlling the opponent.

In 1997, there was news coverage of the tragic deaths of three collegiate wrestlers. Each death occurred during strenuous weight-loss workouts and initiated a badly needed discussion of the techniques used by wrestlers to achieve "weight." Jeff Reese, a University of Michigan junior, died of kidney and heart failure while working out in a rubber suit in a 92-degree room so that he could qualify for a lower weight class. Billy Saylor (19 years old and three-time Florida State champion) of Campbell University and Joseph LaRosa (22 years old) of the University of Wisconsin also died while trying to lose a large amount of weight to qualify for a lower weight class. The outrage resulting from these deaths has finally led to a serious discussion about the rules that encourage the manipulation of normal weight and the techniques used (supplements, dehydration, fasting) to achieve a weight well below the athlete's natural weight to allow qualification in a lower weight class. An important outcome of this discussion should be an improvement in the information wrestling coaches have about weight loss, sports nutrition, training diets, dehydration, and body composition. In surveys of wrestling coaches that evaluate knowledge in these areas, a high proportion of the coaches have a less-than-adequate knowledge base to be guiding young athletes in these areas.[48] The American College of Sports Medicine position on weight loss in wrestlers states:[49]

> Despite a growing body of evidence admonishing the behavior, weight cutting (rapid weight reduction) remains prevalent among wrestlers. Weight cutting has significant adverse consequences that may affect competitive performance, physical health, and normal growth and development. To enhance the education experience and reduce the health risks for the participants, the ACSM recommends measures to educate coaches and wrestlers toward sound nutrition and weight control behaviors, to curtail "weight cutting," and to enact rules that limit weight loss.

The general goal of this weight-loss strategy is to qualify for a weight class during a weigh-in on the night before a match, and to gain as much weight as possible between the weigh-in and the match on the next day. Sadly, there is evidence that wrestling at a weight below the predicted minimum wrestling weight appears to be associated with greater wrestling success.[50] There is also good evidence that successful weight gain during this short period is important for success. In one study evaluating the relative weight gains of wrestlers, the heavier wrestler was successful 57 percent of the time.[51]

There is concern on many levels about the weight-loss techniques commonly practiced by wrestlers. There is some evidence that undernutrition may lead to altered growth hormone production in wrestlers that, if present over several seasons, could lead to growth impairment.[52] In another study, it was determined that dietary restriction reduced protein nutrition and muscular performance.[53] These data are confirmed by findings indicating that weight loss by energy restriction significantly reduced anaerobic performance of wrestlers. Those on a high-carbohydrate refeeding diet tended to recover their performance while those with lower intakes of carbohydrate did not.[54] Besides the obvious physiological changes that occur from rapid weight loss, there is good evidence that rapid weight loss in collegiate wrestlers causes an impairment of short-term memory, a fact that could impact on scholastic achievement in these student athletes.[55]

Nutritionally Relevant Factors for Wrestling

• *"Making weight" is a hazard to both performance and health.* There is ample evidence to suggest that the weight cycling associated with making weight (i.e., weight loss to make weight followed by weight recovery for performance) is dangerous and can lead to glycogen depletion, a lower muscle mass, a lower resting energy expenditure, and an increase in body fat.[56] Should this occur with frequency, it is likely that the reduction in resting energy expenditure could make it more difficult for dietary restriction to achieve the desired weight, leading the wrestler to take more draconian (and more dangerous) measures to achieve the desired weight outcome. Wrestlers and coaches should follow a reasonable model for achieving desired weight, such as that offered by the Wisconsin Interscholastic Athletic Association, to avoid health and performance difficulties.[57] This program develops reasonable goals for weight, and provides nutrition education information to help wrestlers achieve desired weight reasonably and to understand the implications of improper weight-loss methods. The basic message of these weight-achievement guidelines is that a cap is placed on the maximum amount of weight change that can occur during the course of a season, and a monitoring system has been added to assure that sudden and dramatic weight change does not occur at any point in the season.

• *The anaerobic nature of wrestling implies a high need for carbohydrate.* While there is an aerobic component to Olympic wrestling (matches may continue for five minutes without a break), high school wrestling is primarily an anaerobic sport (three two-minute periods). The demand for carbohydrate in this type of activity is extremely high, and there is evidence that wrestlers perform better on high-carbohydrate intakes. In addition to supplying adequate carbohydrate, it is of great concern that wrestlers commonly resort to dehydration as a means of achieving desired weight. There is nothing that could be more dangerous or more performance reducing than entering competition in a dehydrated state. Wrestlers should resist going into a dehydrated state because of the clear dangers (including organ failure, heatstroke, and death) associated with this strategy, and should understand that well-hydrated athletes perform better than dehydrated ones.

• *Wrestlers and coaches should become better educated on the potential hazards of improper nutrition.* Sport should be health enhancing. No amount of argument can convince me that it is OK to place a young athlete in harm's way to achieve a falsely low weight goal, especially since the achieved weight has *nothing* to do with the weight at which the wrestler actually competes. Everyone involved in the sport should endorse the development of widely accepted weight-to-height norms that can be applied reasonably to wrestlers. Importantly, weight should be taken immediately before the competition, rather than at a time that permits drastic shifts in eating behaviors that *are* dangerous. Until the rules change, wrestlers and coaches should all be required to understand the hazards associated with the current "making weight" procedures.

Summary

In general, athletes involved in sports involving power and speed should focus on foods that provide enough total energy, primarily from carbohydrates, so that sufficient glycogen can be manufactured and stored for muscular work. Since phosphocreatine and glycogen are the primary fuels for high-intensity activites, there should also be enough protein (about 1.5 to 2.0 grams per kilogram of body weight) to assure that creatine can be synthesized. Fluid intake is also important, since inadequate fluid intake limits glycogen storage and also makes it difficult to maintain body temperature. Fluid intake also helps to maintain blood volume, which has been found to be a critically important factor in performance.

10 Endurance Sports

The Triathlete Who Wanted to Have the Perfect Food

Several years ago, I was staying at the Drake hotel in Chicago for an American Dietetic Association meeting. It just so happened that the meeting was scheduled at the same time as the famous Chicago Triathlon. Because the Drake hotel was on the lakefront, it was the center of triathlon activity. It was fantastic to see triathletes there of all ages, all enthusiastically preparing themselves for the race. The sports industry was in the hotel ballroom also, showing off the latest in handlebars, running suits, and quick-tie laces. Everywhere I looked there were folks eating bananas and Powerbars. This was a sports nutritionist's fantasyland, one that was so fascinating I could hardly pull myself away to go to my meetings.

The morning before the triathlon I was waiting in line to be seated for breakfast and found myself standing behind a wonderfully fit gentleman in running shorts and T-shirt. (I found out later that the Drake hotel had made attire exceptions during the period of the race to accommodate the athletes, so half of those waiting to eat were in suits, and the other half were wearing running gear. It made those of us in suits feel a bit silly.) When the runner in front of me was offered a table, he turned around and asked if I would like to join him. I didn't hesitate for a fraction of a second and said "Yes."

Sal was a 71-year-old triathlete from Oregon who was built like a rock. You'd be hard pressed to find anyone his age more trim and fit than he was. During our discussion, I asked why he did triathlons, and he said he used to do marathons but came to find them boring. He liked the variety, ebb, and flow of the triathlon, and he said it better suited his personality. He did mention that the marathon also had it's own ebb and flow, and that it was really several races in one: the beginning, where you establish your pace and position; the middle, where you try to hold your own and preserve some energy; and the end, where you strategize about the best place to make your move. The problem he had with marathons, with his increasing age, was that he would start to lose his concentration and think about women, or where he was going to go to have dinner. There just wasn't enough going on in the race to keep his mind on where he was and what he was supposed to do. With the triathlon, however, he didn't have a chance to lose his concentration. He said he was only sorry he hadn't found the triathlon before he was 65. If he had, he would have been much more competitive!

When he found out what I did for a living he started pumping me for answers about the best foods to eat to prepare for the triathlon. It was clear that he was willing to eat almost anything that he felt might give him a competitive edge, so I wanted to be clear and careful about what I said. The triathlon is clearly an endurance event, so carbohydrates are key. But it is also three events joined in one, with a swimming portion that's at least a quarter of a mile, a bicycle race that's at least 12 miles, and a run that's at least 3.1 miles. Then I remembered what one of my colleagues had said about eating for the triathlon. "The key," he said, "is beans." Beans are high in carbohydrates but are also a good source of protein and other nutrients. In addition, they have some beneficial "side effects" for the triathlon. Since they make you a bit bloated with gas, beans help you float and reduce drag for the swimming portion. For the biking portion, they help to "propel" you along the way, and for the running portion no one will run too closely behind you. Clearly, the perfect food for the triathlon! When I finished describing the perfect food, thinking that I had clearly done so in jest, Sal called the waitress over and asked for a serving of beans for breakfast. As a 71-year-old athlete, he said he'd try anything!

Endurance events such as road cycling, long-distance swimming, the marathon, triathlon, and 10-kilometer run all require a high level of endurance and place a relatively low premium on anaerobic power. These are events that force competitors to perform at the margin of their maximal aerobic capabilities over long distances. As training, nutrition, and improved selection of athletes in endurance sports improve, records continue to fall. This suggests that doing the right things can and will result in moving the known envelope of speed in endurance events.

The winner of the Marathon event at the Atlanta Olympic Games in 1996 won with an average running pace of slightly under a 5-minute mile. Despite this incredible speed, the athlete had to maintain this pace at a level that allowed a sufficient oxygen uptake and utilization to support primarily "aerobic" muscular metabolism. That is, the majority of all muscular work took place with fuel being burned in the presence of sufficient oxygen. This is an efficient way to burn muscular fuel, and allows the athlete to undergo muscular work for a long time.

Aerobic training does some wonderful things to the athlete's ability to use oxygen. The intermediary (Type IIA) fibers, which tend to behave more like fast-twitch (power) fibers than slow-twitch (endurance) fibers, develop a dramatic improvement in mitochondrial content and the enzymes involved in oxidative metabolism.

The training impact on oxygen usage is well known. In studies looking at blood lactate concentration, trained athletes are far more capable of tolerating high levels of blood lactate than untrained subjects doing the same intensity of work.

The conversion of the behavior of the intermediary fibers results in an improvement in the athlete's aerobic endurance. The increased ability to use oxygen results in an improvement in the ability to burn fat as a primary fuel, reducing the reliance on carbohydrates. As you can see in table 10.1, athletes in aerobic sports have a far better ability to use oxygen than athletes in power sports.

Since even the leanest athletes have a great deal of energy stored as fat, this increased ability to burn fat dramatically improves endurance. However, since carbohydrate is needed for the complete combustion of fat, carbohydrate is still the limiting energy source for endurance work, because athletes have a relatively low storage of carbohydrate. This is clearly demonstrated by findings that athletes

Table 10.1   Oxygen Uptake in Olympic-Level Athletes in Selected Sports

Sport	Maximal oxygen uptake (mL/kg per minute)
Cross-country skiing (male)	84
Cross-country skiing (female)	65
Runners (male)	80
Runners (female)	58
Speed skaters (male)	77
Speed skaters (female)	54
Cyclists (male)	73
Rowers (male)	62
Weight lifters (male)	55
Sedentary (male)	43
Sedentary (female)	40

Adapted from Katch, Katch, and McArdle 1993.

consuming a high-fat diet have a maximal endurance time of 57 minutes; on a normal mixed diet their endurance rises to 114 minutes; and on a high-carbohydrate diet, their maximal endurance rises to 167 minutes.[1]

Considerations for Endurance Sports

Endurance sports are those where the predominant form of energy metabolism is oxidative (it takes place in the presence of oxygen). This requires that the athlete have the ability to bring in and deliver enough oxygen to the muscles to support the level of physical work that is being done. Endurance (aerobic) work is at an intensity below a person's maximal work capacity, since working at a maximal capacity exceeds a person's ability to bring sufficient oxygen into the system. That's why sprinters, who are working at maximal capacity, can go very fast but only for relatively short distances. Endurance athletes can't go as fast as sprinters but can go much longer distances because they are metabolizing energy using a much more clean-burning and efficient oxidative system. In order to maintain the efficiency of their systems, endurance athletes need to keep in mind certain considerations, including overtraining, overuse injury, and dietary adequacy.

Overtraining

I recently received an email from a world-class runner who wrote:

> I've just come off three weeks of particularly intense training. I went "hard" four days a week. I have plateaued and am now resting to allow my body to absorb all the good work I did but am still feeling a little bit lethargic. I sleep well but don't feel rested. My coach is concerned that I may have become anemic. As you know, my nutritional analysis has always come up good. Should I get some blood tests? Take iron? Take something else? I'm worried.

These signs are typical of someone who "overtrained" and is now suffering the consequences. Overtraining has some well-established warning signs, including increased muscle soreness, delay of muscular recovery, inability to perform at the previous training load, poor quality sleep, decreased vigor, swelling of lymph nodes, high illness frequency, and loss of appetite. Many of these signs are a result of working at a level harder than the body's capacity to recover from it. Overtraining rarely leads to an improvement in performance, and, in fact, commonly reduces performance because it ultimately increases the likelihood that the athlete will become sick or injured.

Overtraining is a problem for many athletes (10 to 20 percent of those who train intensively) and appears to be a condition that is relatively common in endurance athletes. Among other factors that may increase the risk of developing overtraining syndrome, a poor intake of carbohydrates and fluids is known to be a problem.[2] Overtraining syndrome is an untreated excessive training overload with inadequate rest that results in chronic decreases in performance and the ability to train. Other problems may result and may require medical attention. Factors associated with the development of overtraining syndrome include

- frequent competition, particularly if it involves quality efforts;
- monotonous training with insufficient rest;
- preexisting medical conditions (e.g., colds or allergies);
- poor diet, particularly inadequate intake of carbohydrates, or dehydration;
- environmental stress (e.g., altitude, high temperatures, and humidity); and
- psychosocial stressors (e.g., work or school conflicts).

According to the American College of Sports Medicine, overtraining syndrome can be effectively eliminated through a logical training program that allows for adequate rest and recovery with proper nutrition and hydration.[3] Studies of marathon runners suggest that, after running a marathon, even athletes who consume a high-carbohydrate diet take seven days to return muscle glycogen to pre-race levels.[4] A continuation of regular training prior to full muscle glycogen resynthesis will inevitably lead to a degradation of performance. Athletes, therefore, need to understand that rest after a particularly hard and intensive session is best. For athletes who fear that a reduction in training may cause a diminution of competitiveness, getting sufficient rest may not be easy. Therefore, it is recommended that those working with athletes help them understand that overtraining is associated with a *reduction* in performance, so rest and recovery should be an integral part of the training plan.

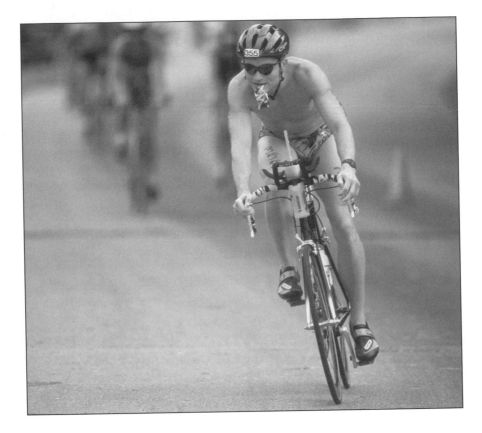

Overuse Injury

Overuse injuries occur when an athlete repeats the same physical task over and over again. In it's simplest and most benign form, you could consider a blister caused by the rubbing of a running shoe an overuse injury. In a more serious form, the constant pounding of legs on hard pavement causes bones to vibrate in specific areas, and, with enough vibrational stress, the bone can develop a painful crack called a stress fracture. This is analogous to taking a wire clothes hanger and bending it repeatedly in the same place. After a while, the hanger develops a crack and eventually breaks. Because endurance athletes spend so many hours training, overuse injury is a real concern.

In one study, triathletes developed skeletal injury early in the competition, which became worse as the competition progressed. These injuries to muscles appear to alter the use of energy substrates as the triathlon progresses and as the body heals the injuries following the competition.[5] However, while protein breakdown and muscular damage occur during a race, the well-trained athlete should experience no alteration in fitness provided nutritional status is maintained.[6] This is because adequately nourished athletes have a better capacity to heal the minor tissue damage that occurs during training and competition. In addition, athletes who can maintain carbohydrate and fluid levels during exercise are likely to have better brain function, and this translates into a smoother running style that is less prone to injury development. Loss of mental capacity, which can easily occur with either a carbohydrate or fluid storage, causes a breakdown in coordination that can increase structural stresses that lead to injury.

Dietary Adequacy

Since it is well established that low glycogen stores reduce the time an athlete is able to exercise, athletes should regularly consume carbohydrate to maintain or replace their limited glycogen stores.[7] This requires a carbohydrate intake of between 7 to 10 grams per kilogram of body weight per day. As you can see from table 10.2, even for 100-pound athletes, this represents a substantial amount of calories from carbohydrate.

The time that endurance athletes consume food is also important and may impact on glycogen storage and resynthesis. In a study of highly trained male cross-country runners, it was found that food intake was adequate and well timed except for the period following competition. While it is recommended that endurance athletes consume carbohydrates immediately following competition to encourage restoration of glycogen stores, these athletes delayed eating carbohydrate foods until, on average, 2.5 hours following competition.[8] This delay caused poor glycogen replacement, and subsequent days of exercise had the negative effect of reduced endurance. In another study of marathon runners, it was found that a significant

Table 10.2   Energy Intake for Endurance Athletes

Energy substrate	Per pound of body weight per day	Calories per day for 100-lb athlete	Calories per day for 200-lb athlete
Carbohydrate	3.2 to 4.5 grams	1,280–1,800	2,560–3,600
Protein	0.7 to 0.9 grams	280–360	560–720
Fat"	0.35 to 0.6 grams	312–540	623–864
Total calories per day	2,808–3,888	1,872–2,700	3,743–5,184

"Fat values based on 20 percent of total caloric intake.

proportion of total energy intake occurs after 4:00 P.M., rather than earlier in the day when it's needed the most.[9] This is clearly a missed opportunity, since trained endurance athletes have an improved ability—one that's been proven—to store muscle glycogen if carbohydrates are provided after exercise.[10,11]

There is no substitute for consuming sufficient energy and carbohydrates for endurance events. Supplements do not appear to work, and substances advertised as ergogenic aids do not appear to work. The key is to eat enough and to eat it on time. Further, there is some evidence that endurance athletes start to focus on nutrition several days to one week prior to a major competition.[12] This is clearly a strategy that inhibits development of optimal nutritional status, and may place the athlete at risk for nutritional weaknesses.

Endurance athletes, because of the time spent training and competing, may have to find strategies for providing energy and nutrients *during* the activity. This is not easy, since providing the wrong foods or the right foods at the wrong time may not be well tolerated. Add to this the nervous stomach many athletes get just before a race, and it makes taking in nutrients difficult. The point is that, if possible, endurance athletes should try sports beverages, carbohydrate gels, and any other source of energy and nutrients that might be well tolerated, because it is likely that they need the energy.

While each type of race alters slightly the proportion of carbohydrate and fat that is burned as fuel (more intensity = proportionately more carbohydrate; lower intensity = proportionately more fat), it's the carbohydrate level that will ultimately determine if the athlete will "hit the wall." That is, when the carbohydrate tank is empty, the athlete will stop. Since so much time is spent racing, every available opportunity must be capitalized on to assure that the athlete has enough food energy to continue the race and to store enough energy (glycogen) to do well during the next day of racing.

In general, athletes should consider doing whatever is necessary to take in sufficient energy and nutrients (bringing Baggies filled with food to meetings, eating while walking to class, snacking while going to the car), or all that good training will be wasted. Eating on a frequent schedule is important for another reason. Athletes who do not eat frequently become fatigued or injured more easily making them prone to products sold by "snake-oil" salesmen. There is no doubt whatsoever that much of the attention given to ergogenic aids and nutrient supplements by athletes, whether they're cyclists, runners, or swimmers, is to overcome a failure to have planned to eat enough and to eat on time.

Maintaining hydration status is important for operating at optimal physiological levels of efficiency. Endurance athletes should practice consuming fluids frequently, even in the absence of thirst, to reduce the chance of dehydration. Consumption of a carbohydrate-containing beverage with small amounts of sodium is useful in fluid absorption and in maintaining the drive to drink.

Nutrient Supplementation

There is ample evidence that athletes who do consume a high-carbohydrate diet that provides an adequate total energy level are also likely to obtain sufficient amounts of other nutrients, including vitamin C, thiamin, riboflavin, niacin, calcium, magnesium, and iron.[13] There is no reason, therefore, to believe that a diet high in complex carbohydrates will lead to nutrient deficiencies. These findings certainly place in doubt the necessity for supplement usage, which is common among endurance athletes. One study found that supplement usage (especially vitamins C and E, calcium, and zinc) was common in marathon runners. Forty-eight percent of the runners questioned reported using at least one supplement within the three-day period surrounding the Los Angeles Marathon.[14] Other studies confirm that nonsupplemented marathon runners, soccer players, wrestlers, and basketball players have adequate serum concentrations of vitamin C and vitamin B-6, so supplementation of these vitamins does not appear to be warranted.[15,16] In a study evaluating the effectiveness of magnesium supplementation on marathon runners, it was found that the supplementation did not improve resistance to muscle damage during the race, did not enhance muscle recovery following the race, and did not improve running performance.[17]

Male marathon runners were evaluated to determine if the consumption of a commercial ergogenic aid supplement containing vitamins, minerals, amino acids, and unsaturated fatty acids in a complex was useful in improving performance. The results indicate that the ergogenic aid had no effect on improvements in oxygen consumption or any other important metabolic or physiological parameter that might be useful to endurance athletes.[18]

Vitamin E may be an important exception regarding its provision as a supplement for endurance athletes. Since vitamin E is a fat-soluble vitamin and, therefore, delivered in fats (particularly vegetable oils), it is possible that the need for this important antioxidant may exceed its usual provision because the dietary focus of endurance athletes is carbohydrates. The endurance-sports combination of high oxidative work, which brings 10 to 15 times more oxygen into working muscle cells, and low-fat intake may limit the delivery of sufficient vitamin E to the cells and predispose these cells to oxidative damage. This exercise-induced increase in free radicals (caused by the oxidative damage of polyunsaturated fats in cells to produce peroxide) has been documented, suggesting that more antioxidants are needed.[19] While supplementing animals with vitamin E has shown a reduction in oxidative stress, there are no good studies to support the idea that this also happens in exercising humans.[20] In another study, on the other hand, there was no evidence of oxidative stress after a triathlon race in highly trained competitors.[21] However, since oxidative stress is involved in numerous disease states, it seems reasonable to suggest that endurance athletes should consider supplementing with 300 to 400 milligrams of vitamin E per day. This level has been tested with athletes and appears to be well tolerated with no undesirable side effects.[22] This strategy is meant as a security blanket only, since there is no apparent deficiency of vitamin E, but only a suggestion that oxidative stress may exist and may be mediated somewhat with more vitamin E in the system.

Concerns for Female Endurance Athletes

Female endurance athletes must consume sufficient energy and nutrients to avoid amenorrhea. There are many reasons for amenorrhea (cessation of regular menstrual periods), including high physical stress, high psychological stress, inadequate energy intake, poor iron status, high cortisol levels, and low body fat levels. It is conceivable that female endurance athletes have *all* of these factors working against them. While some of these factors are clearly out of a woman's control, food intake is not one of those. Female athletes should do whatever is within their means to consume sufficient total energy that is high in carbohydrates and provides all the nutrients needed for good health. Amenorrhea is strongly associated with a loss in bone density and an increase in stress fracture risk. In addition, this places the athlete at increased risk for early osteoporosis.

Distance Running

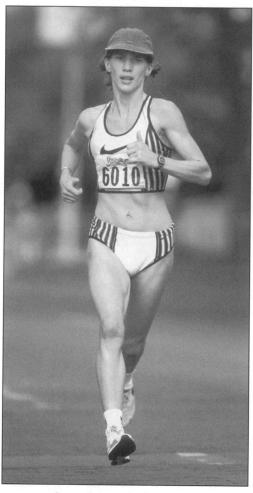

Distance running is commonly thought of as any distance that is 10,000 meters (6.2 miles) or longer. To go these distances, runners place a premium on staying in an aerobic metabolic pathway during the majority of the run. This means that fats contribute to a significant proportion of total energy used, limiting the dependence on carbohydrate. Since carbohydrate storage is limited but fat storage, from a practical standpoint, is limitless, fat storage enables long-distance runners to go very long distances provided they stay aerobic. This is confirmed by a recent study that found that only 2 to 7 percent of the total energy burned in aerobic activity was derived anaerobically.[23] However, carbohydrate storage is still the key to performance because when the carbohydrate runs out, the fats are no longer efficiently burned as a fuel.

Nutritionally Relevant Factors for Distance Runners

• *Amenorrhea, low bone density, and stress fractures are risks.* The distances that long-distance runners run weekly to train may predispose them to stress fractures, despite encouraging an increased bone mass from the stresses placed on the skeleton.[24] While stress fractures occur more frequently in women runners than in men (reduced estrogen in female athletes negatively impacts on bone density), all runners should assure that their calcium intake is adequate to reduce the risk of fracture. There is a clear relationship between amenorrhea and lower bone density, so amenorrheic runners should seek the advice of a physician to determine if there are other reasonable steps that can be taken to reduce the risk of stress fractures.[25]

Long-distance runners appear to hit their peak at an age that is considerably older than athletes in other sports. For women, this may be a real concern if the running is accompanied with amenorrhea (and associated with low estrogen levels), which could lead to a long-lasting bone disease that has lifelong implications. Care should be taken to reduce the risk of osteoporosis, especially if there is long-lasting amenorrhea. To reduce the risk, female athletes should do the following:

- Consume calcium (1,500 mg/day) from food, or a combination of food and supplements.
- Avoid overconsumption of protein as excess protein consumption is associated with higher urinary calcium losses.
- Control the production of stress hormones (particularly cortisol), by maintaining hydration and blood sugar during exercise.
- Avoid overtraining, which is associated with amenorrhea.

Inadequate energy intake is a red flag that nutrient intake may also be low. In a study comparing the nutrient intakes of trained female runners who either were not menstruating or not menstruating normally, it was found that there were clear nutritional differences between these groups, despite being matched on height, weight, training distance, and body fat percent.[26] The runners who were not menstruating had zinc intakes well below the recommended level of intake and lower than those found in the runners who had normal menses. In addition, the runners who had normal menses had higher intakes of fat. It appears that higher fat intakes were associated with more adequate total energy consumption. This suggests that high carbohydrate diets, which are preferred for optimal performance, make it more difficult to consume the needed level of energy because carbohydrates have a lower caloric density than high-fat foods. Therefore, athletes need to concentrate on consuming more food when carbohydrates constitute the main energy source. Since failure to menstruate normally is a strong risk factor in the development of weaker bones and resulting stress fractures, female runners have good cause to be fully aware of the adequacy of their energy and nutrient intakes. There is almost no injury that is more frustrating or career ending than the development of frequent stress fractures.

• *Enormous amounts of energy are needed.* It may be hard to imagine that people who are so "thin" need so much energy. In fact, long-distance runners burn so much energy that they find it difficult to replace all they need. Consuming lots of snacks between meals, eating before, during, and after practice (and competitions), and having good meals that are high in carbohydrates, moderate in protein, and low in fat is important.

Tapering activity prior to a competition works in improving competition performance.[27] It does so by improving glycogen stores, but it also helps to make the runner calmer, which gives the runner an improved economy of running motion that improves endurance. The importance of tapering exercise and carbohydrate loading prior to an important event cannot be overemphasized.

Most surveys of distance runners confirm that total energy and carbohydrate intake are below the recommended levels, suggesting that runners must make a concerted effort to consume the recommended amounts before, during, and after exercise.[28,29] In a case study assessing the nutrient intake of an ultra-endurance runner during a race, it was found that if the pre-event and during-event guidelines for food and beverage are followed, then athletes will have sufficient energy and fluids to successfully complete the event.[30]

• *Fluids are crucial.* Fluid consumption should be on a fixed time schedule (every 10 to 15 minutes) to avoid underhydration and thirst. There may be no single thing that is more important for assuring a long-distance runner's success. Drink now, drink again in 15 minutes, and when you think you've had enough, drink some more.

Sufficient fluid intake is critical in endurance running since a great deal of body heat is generated over a long period of time, and this heat is liberated through sweat evaporation. Many studies strongly suggest that 7-percent-carbohydrate solutions with electrolytes are effective as both water replacement and energy replacement beverages.[31] Long-distance runners should develop the habit of frequent fluid consumption to maintain water status, whether they are thirsty or not. It has been found that a fluid intake of 0.5 to 1 liter per hour is sufficient to prevent significant dehydration in most athletes in mild environmental conditions, but a greater intake of fluids is needed for athletes running at higher intensities or in more severe environmental conditions in order to avoid heat stress.[32]

• *Distance runners typically carry very low body fat.* Successful long-distance runners commonly look "thin," and this body profile may be advantageous to them in dissipating heat during long runs.[33] Maintaining a relatively low body fat percentage may thus be desirable in long-distance running, since that would contribute to a smaller body mass and also, by itself, improve heat dissipation. However, since very low body fat levels are associated with amenorrhea, female athletes should seek a balance between low body fat levels and normal hormone function.

Triathlon

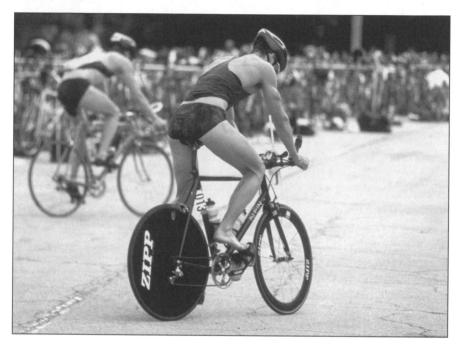

Muscular balance in the upper and lower body is important to successful triathletes, because the three events each have a different muscular focus. Since *all* the major muscles are put to the test in triathlons, these athletes must consume enough total energy to assure that the fuel capacity for each working muscle starts out full. Swimmers, for instance, have a much higher upper-body strength requirement than cyclists.[34] Triathletes, however, need strength in all the muscles. Interestingly enough, it may be this general requirement for use of all the muscles that makes the triathlon a sport with no preference for a unique body type or shape.[35] It looks like anyone who's willing to train really hard can do it.

Triathlons have different lengths, depending on the location and sponsor. An Olympic Distance Triathlon consists of a 1.5-kilometer swim, a 40-kilometer cycle, and a 10-kilometer run. The most well-known Ironman competition in Hawaii includes a 2.4-mile swim, a 112-mile bike run, and a 26-mile, 385-yard run. A recent survey of *lower-level* triathletes indicated that even they have average weekly training loads that would make most mere mortals want to cry. This survey demonstrated that the average swimming distance per week for these triathletes was 8.8 kilometers, the cycling distance was 270 kilometers, and the running distance was 58.2 kilometers.[36] All this training makes you wonder if these athletes ever take time to rest. In fact, studies have shown that triathletes would do well to taper down their activity prior to a competition. One study showed a statistically significant improvement in performance values that were well above their pretaper training level when triathletes reduced the total time spent training prior to a competition.[37]

Different sports apparently induce athletes to consume different foods and, therefore, take in different levels of nutrients. Calcium intake appears to be lower in triathletes than in athletes participating in team sports such as volleyball and basketball. Of all the athletes surveyed in a large French study with 10,373 subjects, calcium intakes were below the recommended level for the triathletes, and females had lower calcium intakes than males.[38] This is bad news for athletes who place so much repetitive stress on the skeleton, and it may place them at increased risk for stress fractures.

Nutritionally Relevant Factors for Triathletes

• *Maintenance of normal hydration.* There may be no more important performance-related factor for triathletes than to create a strategy for maintaining hydration state during this grueling event. Triathletes need to find a sports beverage that is well tolerated and develop a drinking schedule that, at the end of the competition, results in the smallest possible weight loss. Drinking enough (typically between .25 to .5 liters every 15 minutes) to avoid any level of underhydration is probably the best ergogenic thing a triathlete can do.

There has been some concern that triathletes, who wear a wet suit during the swimming phase of the triathlon, when the water temperature is relatively warm, may predispose themselves to heat stress during the cycling and running portions of the race. In a study evaluating this issue, wearing a wet suit did not adversely impact on the athlete's subsequent body temperature during the cycling and running states, provided that the athlete maintained a good hydration state.[39] The importance of good hydration as it relates to triathlon performance is the theme of numerous studies, all of which state that it is one of two keys to a successful race (the other being maintenance of carbohydrate stores). It also appears that triathletes are typically unsuccessful at maintaining good hydration during a competition, with a water-related body weight loss that commonly exceeds 4 percent.[40] It also appears that triathletes may be predisposed to hyponatremia (low blood-sodium level), which is a result of using replacement fluids that contain no electrolytes.[41,42] The levels of the water loss and the hyponatremia are both factors that can clearly impact on performance, which underlines the importance that triathletes should give to proper fluid replacement during training and during an event. The focus on *proper* fluid replacement is important, since there are published cases of GI distress in triathletes who consumed fluids that were too concentrated with carbohydrate and/or electrolytes.[43]

• *Consumption of sufficient energy.* The energy requirement for carbohydrate in the triathlete exceeds the body's ability to store it. Therefore, triathletes should develop a strategy for adequate consumption of carbohydrate energy during a race (typically 1 to 1.5 grams of carbohydrate per kilogram of body weight per hour).[44] To do this, the athlete should find sports beverages that contain carbohydrate in a form and concentration that are well tolerated. Some triathletes have found that the consumption of carbohydrate gels, bananas, or crackers can be consumed during the cycle portion of the race (taken with a water chaser). If this is tolerated, it is an excellent way to boost the carbohydrate-fuel level in the body before the beginning of the running portion of the race.

It is clear that nutrition interventions that provide more fluids and carbohydrates to triathletes work. Following such an intervention, triathletes were able to consume a level of energy and nutrients that was closer to their requirement than before the intervention, and this improvement led to an improvement in endurance performance.[45]

• *Risk of overtraining.* Getting sufficient rest and tapering exercise prior to a race have been shown to be two of the best training strategies a triathlete can follow. By contrast, triathletes who increase the training frequency prior to an important race are not likely to do their best. Sufficient rest is just as important as sufficient training to do well.

• *Planning a meal schedule.* The triathlon includes different distances, depending on whether it's a sprint, the Olympic distance, a long course, or the ironman. The sprint can take as little as 45 minutes to complete, and the ironman often takes longer than eight hours. Regardless of the competition distance, triathletes train hard—and they find themselves juggling their training with work or school. Eating and drinking often takes a back seat to all the other demands of life, yet they are critically important to the success an athlete can realize. The only solution is to sit down and make a schedule that includes working, training, eating, resting, and drinking. Treat them all as having equal importance.

Many (if not most) triathletes have more than one workout each day, and some race weekly or bimonthly. This places a tremendous energy requirement on the athlete that is commonly not met. The more time an athlete takes to train, the less time there is to eat, so there is a natural conflict between the increased requirement for energy and the reduced time to supply what is needed. This problem makes a clear case for *planning* time for eating as much as *planning* time for training. If an athlete's training has a fixed schedule (it usually does) but the eating doesn't, the athlete will suffer.

Long-Distance Swimming

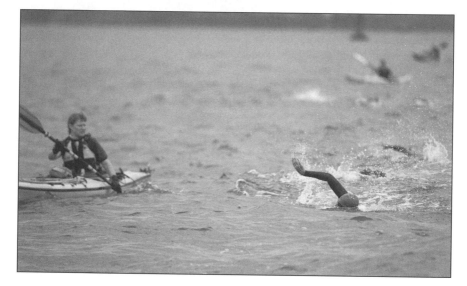

Distance swimmers are unique folks, because they must spend so much time in the water to realize incrementally miniscule improvements in time. A key to performance appears to be the swimmer's capacity to go faster without increasing blood lactate levels, or to go faster while utilizing a lower percentage of their maximal aerobic capacity.[46] This means the swimmer is working harder but still able to maintain a predominantly aerobic (oxidative) metabolic pathway. This translates into terrific aerobic fitness and the ability to maintain enough glycogen and oxygen in the system to assure and efficient energy burn. Maintaining lower blood lactate concentrations may also be a function of maintaining a sufficient blood volume (lactate in a larger volume = lower lactate concentration). This is, of course, largely dependent on adequate hydration and a good electrolyte status (sodium helps maintain blood volume).

Nutritionally Relevant Factors for Distance Swimmers

• *Lower bone densities.* Swimmers, when compared to other athletes, appear to have lower bone densities.[47] The reason for this is easy to understand, since the impact stress of being in water is less than that of thumping your legs on hard ground. However, it may also be related to spending many hours doing laps in an indoor pool while other athletes are running outside, where they can increase their exposure to sunlight and manufacture more vitamin D. The vitamin D difference may be enough to influence bone development. Of course, for those long-distance swimmers lucky enough to live in areas warm enough for outdoor pools, this is not an issue. However, there is one study suggesting that swimmers, particularly female swimmers, may not consume sufficient calcium, a factor that could clearly contribute to lower bone mineral density.[48] Clearly, having sufficient calcium (1,500 milligrams/day) is critical to maintaining strong bones, but swimmers should also make an effort to spend some time outside to assure an adequate vitamin-D synthesis.

• *Replacement of fluids.* The main focus for swimmers involved in an all-day meet (which it usually is!) is the replacement of adequate fluids to maintain blood volume and to provide a constant source of carbohydrate. It's hard to imagine that being in all that water could lead to dehydration, but failure to drink sufficient fluids can be a serious performance detriment.

• *Consumption of carbohydrates during long competitions.* Have a snacking plan for competitions so you don't get hungry. These competitions can last a long time, and they may make you seriously hungry by the time you're ready to get in the water. In an endurance event, you don't want to start by being hungry! Sip on sports beverages and snack on crackers and other simple carbohydrate (mainly starchy) foods to get a constant trickle of carbohydrates into the system. That way you'll start the event being fully energized.

• *Eat enough to support the activity.* Swimming long distances uses a tremendous amount of energy, so make certain enough food is consumed to maintain weight or to increase weight if you're trying to build muscle. Swimmers often complain that they can't keep their weights up during the long swim-competition season, and that means they're burning muscle to meet their needs.

Cycling

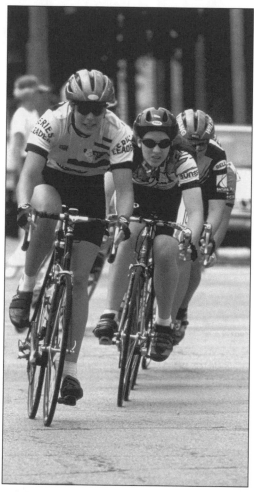

There are a number of endurance events that take place over several days of competition. The Tour de France cycle race is notable for its extreme endurance demands on participating athletes, and each stage of the race places different physiological demands on the cyclist. They pedal approximately 4,000 kilometers over three weeks with only a single day of rest allowed! The energy expenditure ranges are the highest values that have ever been reported for athletes over a period longer than seven days.[49] They consume approximately 62 percent of their energy from carbohydrates, 15 percent from protein, and 23 percent from fat. Over 49 percent of total energy consumption takes place *between* meals. Some days have long hard hills, while other days have roads that are more level. Studies of Tour de France cyclists indicate that they consume approximately 30 percent of their total daily energy intake in the form of a liquid carbohydrate-enriched beverage.[50] Since so much time during the day is spent on the bike, there may be no other way to adequately consume sufficient energy.

In studies of athletes at the 1996 Olympic Games in Atlanta, U.S. athletes participating in cycling and mountain biking had the highest prevalence (45 percent) of having been told that they had asthma.[51] By contrast, 20 percent of the total U.S. athletes reported they actually had asthma. This suggests that asthma may be a contributing factor in determining the sport an athlete selects to participate in. It is possible, for some athletes, that asthma might be triggered by an allergic response, and this could be an allergic response to food. Cyclists with asthma should be extremely careful about avoiding foods or other substances that could trigger an asthmatic response.

Nutritionally Relevant Factors for Cyclists

• *Recovering from multiday events.* The energy cost of multiday cycling events is enormous, and it may be the meal planning of the athlete's team that makes the difference between winning and losing. There is a clear requirement for carbohydrate, and this conflicts with the huge requirement for energy because carbohydrate foods have a low-energy density. (By contrast, fats have a high-energy density but are not needed to the degree that carbohydrates are.) Therefore, carbohydrates should be consumed in large quantities and frequently, and the focus should be on starchy carbohydrates (pasta, bread, rice, potatoes, etc.)

• *Consumption of food and fluid during long rides.* Cyclists have an advantage over other endurance athletes in that they can easily carry fluids and foods on the bike frame or in jersey pockets. Since there is less bouncing while riding than while running, cyclists can usually consume some solid foods without experiencing GI distress. Cyclists should take advantage of this on long rides by bringing along sport beverages to drink and some crackers, bananas, carbohydrate gel, or bread to eat. These high carbohydrate foods should be well tolerated and can significantly boost the carbohydrate delivery to working muscles.

• *Training is very time and energy consuming.* The longer athletes train, the more energy they need, but the less time they have to consume it. Therefore, cyclists should consider the training period as a time to take in a proportion of their daily caloric requirements. To do this, cyclists should find foods that are well tolerated, such as bananas and crackers, and bring them along during the ride. Sports beverages are also an important source of energy, so these should be consumed instead of plain water as a rehydration beverage. A failure to eat during training will inevitably lead to an inadequate total energy consumption and a decrease in performance.

Summary

Endurance athletes spend many hours training and have enormous energy needs. However, these training times make it difficult to consume the needed foods. Athletes should plan multiple eating breaks throughout the day (something high in carbohydrate to consume every three hours) to assure an adequate total energy consumption. Fluid intake is also critically important, and endurance athletes should develop the habit of drinking frequently (every 10 to 15 minutes) regardless of thirst. There is a large body of evidence that suggests lower levels of either carbohydrates or fluids inhibit endurance.

11 Combined Power and Endurance Sports

Tradition Doesn't Always Win

Several years ago, the university I worked at hired a top-notch, experienced coach for our basketball team. He did wonders in recruitment, and his practices were, from what I heard, character-building experiences. The team went well beyond its expectations during the first year, chalking up the best season in the history of the university. All this was accomplished despite a team that was, essentially, inherited from earlier recruitment efforts. At the beginning of the next season, disaster loomed ahead. Several of the players were ineligible because of academic difficulties, a couple of recruits were transfers who couldn't play right away because of NCAA rules, and the star guard broke his foot during the first game of the season. Put simply, due to factors well out of the coach's control, the bench was thin—very thin.

There is no easy game in NCAA Division I basketball, and I've yet to see a game between Division I teams where one team has truly coasted. It doesn't matter if it's a preseason game, an out-of-division game, or a "Holiday Classic," these teams play to win. From a physiological standpoint, it's difficult to imagine anyone who could stand the rigors of an entire game played at the pace these athletes play. Basketball is a sport that combines power and endurance, and it's all-out, be-faster-than-your-opponent-or-you-lose game. When a bench is thin, it forces those who do play into a position where they need all the nutritional and training help they can get.

When I observed one of the games, I noticed that the players weren't following an optimal hydration strategy during the game. This was happening despite the good efforts of the athletic training staff, which was obviously trying to do everything within their means to get the players to drink on schedule. Besides, these trainers were busy trying to keep the players they had physically functional (I've never seen so much tape). After observing this, I thought I'd send off a memo to the coach and athletic training staff to remind them of the importance of what they already knew, that game-time hydration (with carbohydrate) is critical to performance—salting the memo with science as my crutch. The most important response to this memo was that the coach wanted to talk with me. (This, by the way, is a characteristic of all successful coaches. They want all the information they can get, and they want it *now*.) After numerous attempts at schedule juggling, we talked and it all boiled down to this: the university had a contract with a beverage company to supply the sports beverage, and the athletes didn't like it. As a result, the athletes were provided with plain water during the games. Plain water during games has problems, not the least of which is that it doesn't provide the all-important carbohydrate. In addition, because it contains no sodium, it doesn't drive the desire to drink. Therefore, athletes tend to drink less than they need.

After some experimentation, we found a beverage the athletes liked and it was "hidden" in the containers of the contract company. (This is known as a win-win solution!) The result was, to say the least, *very* good. The experience helped to solidify my belief that if you have parties willing to listen to the facts, good things will happen.

This chapter provides nutrition information for sports where athletes intermittently perform at high intensity. That is, the high-intensity efforts are interspersed throughout a competition that has periods of lower physical effort. This is characteristic of team sports such as basketball, volleyball, and soccer, and is also typical of figure skating. This is different than other sports, where the focus is either mainly power or mainly endurance. For instance, there is nothing in gymnastics training or competition that requires a great deal of aerobic endurance, and marathon runners spend all their time trying to have a better aerobic endurance. In many team sports, the premium is on both. Soccer players must run the field back and forth at a controlled pace until an opportunity presents itself where players must run at peak speed to take advantage of an offensive opportunity to quickly get back in an appropriate defensive position. Basketball players may jog back and forth in a steady aerobic pace, but a player has to have some clear jumping *power* to grab a rebound or some quick-move sprinting ability to split the defense.

In 1995, Mark Davis at the University of South Carolina found that repeated sprint work is enhanced with consumption of a carbohydrate-electrolyte beverage.[1] While it has been well established for years that carbohydrate-electrolyte beverages enhance submaximal (below maximal aerobic capacity) endurance performance, this was the first finding to clearly show the benefits of such a beverage during high-intensity, short-duration efforts such as those found in football or basketball. Compared to a trial when a placebo (water) was consumed, subjects performed seven additional one-minute sprints of cycling at 120 to 130 percent of peak $\dot{V}O_2$ when they consumed a 6 percent carbohydrate-electrolyte beverage. This is equivalent to making a dramatic improvement in sprint capability during the last 5 to 10 minutes of a basketball game.

In a similar study, also in 1995, Nicholas et al. found that sports drinks (i.e., carbohydrate-electrolyte beverages) can help maintain high-intensity efforts during high-intensity activities that consist of intermittent sprinting, running, and jogging.[2] Again, these findings have strong implications for improved maintenance of high-intensity activity over the course of a typical basketball and soccer game.

The effects of the intake of the individual components of a sports beverage (electrolytes, water, or carbohydrate) and the combination of all components on exercise performance have also been studied. Compared to the electrolyte-only trial, performance during the water-only and carbohydrate-only trials were approximately 6 percent faster. However, the combination of carbohydrate and fluid caused a performance enhancement that was approximately 12 percent faster than the electrolyte trial, and 5 to 6 percent faster than when water only or carbohydrate only were consumed.[3] These findings support the thesis that carbohydrate enhances water absorption, and that carbohydrate has the most limited storage of any energy substrate in the system. The high demands on carbohydrate during high-intensity work require a constant vigilance to assure proper and speedy replacement. This study was based on earlier work, which found that exercise performance improved significantly with carbohydrate feedings.[4] It has also been found that the optimal level of carbohydrate concentration *during exercise* is 6 percent. This concentration was best for fluid absorption and also helped to efficiently deliver carbohydrate. A level greater than this (about 8 percent) caused fluid absorption to be reduced or, depending on the source of carbohydrate, to stop totally.[5]

When basketball players jump (leap!) for the ball, or soccer players sprint toward the ball and jump high to kick it, these activities can be compared to certain forms of strength training. In a study of resistance-trained athletes, it was found that athletes tended to perform more repetitions for the same weight when carbohydrate was consumed versus a water placebo. Blood glucose and lactate concentrations were higher with the carbohydrate trial, suggesting that more carbohydrate was available and used to sustain the high-intensity exercise.[6] In a study recently published, head-to-head comparisons of Gatorade, Powerade, and AllSport were made.[7] It was found that Gatorade stimulates fluid absorption faster than either Powerade or AllSport. This difference can be attributed to both the type of carbohydrate and the concentration of carbohydrate in the beverages. Gatorade has a carbohydrate-concentration level that is consistent with the positive findings in virtually all the studies (6 percent) and contains an equal mixture of sucrose and glucose. Powerade and AllSport have higher carbohydrate concentrations and include a large quantity of fructose. Fructose has been shown to cause gastrointestinal (GI) distress; it is also less efficient in raising blood glucose because it requires a secondary conversion in the liver following absorption.

A 1998 study has found that athletes who do repeated or sustained high-power efforts experience a reduction in performance when they are dehydrated.[8] Given the importance of carbohydrate beverages in effective rehydration during exercise, it seems clear that this might be a strategy that would help maintain the power and endurance of the athletes on the basketball team. The fluid consumption guidelines established by the American College of Sports Medicine are summarized in table 11.1.[9]

There are several general nutrition guidelines—involving what to do before, during, and after exercise and competition—that are good for virtually all athletes involved in sports that include periods of maximal intensity. See table 11.2 for these guidelines.

The two keys to these guidelines are fluids and carbohydrates in the context of a generally varied diet. Athletes should find ways to consume both fluids and carbohydrates at, literally, every opportunity. Recent findings tend to contradict the traditional and commonly followed belief that carbohydrate-containing beverages are useful only for endurance (aerobic) activities that last longer than 60 minutes. The best predictors of athletic performance are maintenance of blood volume and maintenance of glycogen/glucose. What follows are some strategies that might be useful for achieving both enhanced hydration and improved maintenance of system carbohydrate in different sports.

Table 11.1 ACSM Fluid Intake Guidelines

Timing	Amount	Adaptation
Before exercise (2 hours prior)	Drink 500 milliliters (17 ounces)	None
During exercise	Drink 600-1,200 milliliters (20–40 ounces) per hour	Drink 150-300 milliliters (5-10 ounces) every 15-20 minutes
After exercise	Based on pre- and postexercise body weight, drink enough fluid to restore body weight (16 ounces fluid = 1 pound body weight*).	Drink 50 percent over and above the volume ingested to restore preexercise body weight. This compensates for urine losses, which may induce hypo-hydration when only 100 percent of fluid is consumed.

*1.5 times loss in body weight should be consumed as fluid.

Table 11.2 General Guidelines for Athletes Involved in Sports That Include Intermittent Periods of High-Intensity Work

General nutrition	Maintain a diet high in complex carbohydrates, moderate in protein, and relatively low in fat. Strive for a varied consumption of foods to assure exposure to all the nutrients that the body's cells need. Varying your intake also helps to assure that you don't overexpose your cells to substances in foods that may be, with frequent exposure, harmful to general health.
The preexercise or precompetition meal	Consume starchy, easy-to-digest, high-carbohydrate foods. Consume plenty of fluids with meals and during the period between the meal and the exercise session or competition. When possible, consume the high-carbohydrate meal about 3 hours before exercise.
During-exercise replenishment	Consume a sports drink that is approximately a 6 to 7 percent carbohydrate solution. The drink should also contain a small amount of salt to encourage drinking during the competition. Drink 20 to 40 ounces of fluid per hour, depending on the environmental temperature and humidity and your predisposition to sweating. In some sports, there are no natural breaks in the action, which makes it difficult to consume fluids at this rate. In such cases, athletes and coaches should develop a clear strategy for fluid consumption that can take place during "time-outs" in the game. A good strategy will assure that there are adequate personnel available to provide fluids quickly and efficiently to every player on the field whenever a break in the action occurs.
Postexercise or postcompetition replenishment	Drink a sports drink to ensure quick rehydration and replenishment of depleted glycogen stores. Consume approximately 24 ounces per pound of body weight (1.5 liters per kilogram of body weight) lost during the activity. Muscle glycogen stores are efficiently replaced if the athlete consumes carbohydrate immediately following the activity. For the two hours immediately following activity, consume high-glycemic index foods (i.e., foods high in natural sugars or foods that are quickly and easily digested into sugars). The goal is to consume at least 50 grams (200 calories) of carbohydrate every hour until the next meal time. In general, strive to consume approximately 4 grams of carbohydrate per pound of body weight during the 24 hours following exercise or competition.

Adapted from Williams and Nicholas 1998.

Basketball

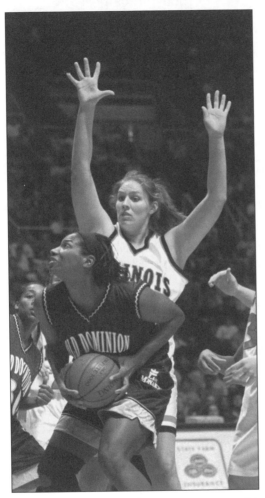

Basketball combines many of the best aspects of team cooperation and individual effort, with two guards, two forwards, and one center who *all* play both defense and offense during the 32 (high school) to 48 (professional) minutes of the game. Basketball is a game played around the world by both men's and women's teams and has been a highly visible part of the Olympic Games since the 1936 Olympics in Berlin. Among the most impressive winning streaks in basketball was the 10 national championships (7 won consecutively) by the John Wooden–coached UCLA men's teams. In a conversation many years later, one of John Wooden's players said that Wooden was brilliant at making sure his team was the best conditioned on the floor, and part of that conditioning regimen was making certain the players worked harder during practice than would be needed during any game against any opponent. But he also made certain all of the players ate and rested well enough to be ready to give a 100 percent effort.

It is clear from studies in intermittent high-intensity sports, that basketball players can gain an advantage by focusing on the consumption of the right foods and fluids during the pre-, during-, and postgame periods. In a study that surveyed the nutrition knowledge of college basketball coaches and coaches in other sports, it was found that only 33 percent of the coaches were confident that they responded correctly to questions related to nutrition.[10] In addition, this survey noted that coaches felt college athletes had problems with the consumption of junk food, had generally poor eating habits, and generally consumed unbalanced diets. In a survey of male and female basketball players, it was found that the diet of the female players was lacking in a number of nutrients, and that there was an excessive reliance on nutrient supplements.[11] None of this, of course, is consistent with what basketball players need to do to compete effectively.

Nutritionally Relevant Factors for Basketball

• *Basketball players have a halftime that can be used to replenish fluids and carbohydrates.* Basketball games have the advantage of having a 10 to 20 minute half-time break. This is an excellent opportunity for players to sip on a sports beverage to replace lost fluids and carbohydrates. Some players may also find they do well by eating some plain crackers and drinking water. However, this is not a good time to consume candy bars and other foods that, while they contain some sugar, are also high in fat. What basketball players really need at this time is carbohydrate and water, and eating anything else detracts from what they should have.

• *Time spent on the bench should be used to maintain hydration state.* Natural breaks in the game from official time-outs or substitutions should be taken advantage of by sipping on sports beverages, *whether the players feel they need it or not.* Sipping on beverages should become part of the game plan, just as important as making the right team defensive or offensive plays. A player may not want to do it, but it's the "team" thing to do.

• *Frequent practices and games can wear a player out.* Basketball players typically practice six days each week, and often have two practices in a single day. Add to that a match schedule that has them playing a least one game during the week, and it's easy to see why a typical basketball season can wear a player out. In general, players should eat enough carbohydrate to support both glycogen storage (critical to basketball performance) and also consume sufficient energy to maintain muscle mass. A common complaint of coaches is that they find it difficult to keep the weight of many players as high as they would like to, and this is a sure sign that the players are not eating enough to support the intense activity of practice and games. Teams that can make it through the season with weight maintained generally are stronger and have better endurance than those who don't.

• *Playing as well in the second half as in the first half wins games.* Teams that can manage to keep their strength and endurance up during the second half of the game tend to do better on the scoreboard than teams that don't. To do this, players should establish a pattern of frequent sipping on a carbohydrate-containing beverage, whether they think they need it or not. Studies show that this frequent sipping pattern helps players keep their strength and endurance longer than if they drink water alone or fail to drink at all.

Figure Skating

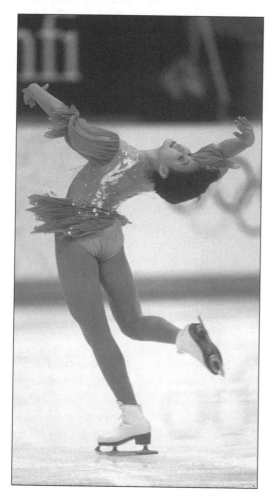

Figure skating took its name from the "figures" that competitors were required to complete. These figures were literally outlined on the ice as two- or three-lobed figure eights that "figure" skaters had to skate over and match as closely as possible to receive a top score. In 1991, however, the "figures" in competitive skating were removed and replaced with a short and long program, but the name "figure skating" has remained. Competitive figure skaters aim to produce performances that are smooth, graceful, artistic, and appear to be effortless. The short, curved blades and toe picks used by figure skaters permit these athletes to create movements with sharp turns and high jumps with spins. Figure skaters have three separate events, and training is specialized for each of these: individual figure skating, pairs skating, and ice dancing. Figure skating is a single-gender competition (i.e., males compete against males, and females compete against females), and pairs skating and ice dancing are mixed-gender events.

In individual figure skating, there is an expectation of grace and effortlessness in the performance, but there is also a competitive premium placed on achieving difficult spins and jumps that favor strong but smaller athletes. Since the density of air and the resistance of ice do not change for each athlete, large athletes have a greater ice resistance and are confronted with greater relative air resistance than smaller competitors. Therefore, larger skaters require significantly greater strength to do the same skills as smaller skaters. The top successful figure skaters have recently been smaller than in previous years.

In pairs skating, it is common to see the male partner considerably larger and stronger than the female. For anyone who has seen a pairs competition, the reason is obvious: the male must lift and throw his female partner frequently during the competition, and this is easier if he's lifting someone smaller. Finding the right physical match is difficult, and poorly matched pairs skaters have difficulty performing at the top level even if they are superb individual skaters.

In ice dancing, there is a much smaller premium on a large male and smaller female since there are no throws or overhead lifts in the competition. Given the intricacy of foot movement and grace found in ice dancing, the sport is well named. The constant movement coupled with a lower power requirement makes this the most "aerobic" of the three skating disciplines.

In studies of figure skaters, it has been found that they possess an average aerobic capacity but have the ability to produce high power peaks.[12] That is, when they need to, they can call upon their muscles to produce a tremendous amount of power all at once. It has also been found that young female skaters consume diets that are relatively high in fat and protein and relatively low in carbohydrate, calcium, and iron.[13] Although there has been a traditional concern that competitive figure skaters may not consume sufficient total energy, a recent study suggests that this concern may be unfounded for most skaters.[14] However, there appears to be a portion of these skaters who may be at risk for certain disordered eating patterns and, when this occurs, nutrient intake is likely to be low.

As with any elite sport, injuries occur. There is particular concern about the rate of injuries among pairs skaters. In one study, the female senior pairs skaters reported an average of 1.4 serious injuries over a nine-month period, while other skaters had injury rates that were averaging 0.5 serious injuries per skater over this same time period.[15] Most of these injuries are lower-extremity injuries that might be related to boot design, but other researchers suggest that injuries might be related to poor conditioning.[16]

Nutritionally Relevant Factors for Figure Skating

• *Skaters are extremely concerned about their weight, since appearance on the ice is important in this sport.* Achievement of optimal weight is best achieved through the consumption of a low-fat, moderate-protein, high complex-carbohydrate intake plus a good exercise and conditioning program. Although dieting is counterproductive, there is good evidence that this is the weight-management strategy of choice among skaters. The consumption of adequate energy from carbohydrate is important for both performance and achievement of a desirable body composition. Inadequate energy intake may predispose the skater to nutrient deficiencies, low energy expenditure, and high body fat levels that can increase the risk of injury, create ill-health, and reduce athletic performance.

• *The high jumps in figure skating place a great deal of reliance on phosphocreatine and muscle glycogen.* Adequate energy intake from carbohydrate, interspersed with a regular intake of meats (to provide creatine or sufficient protein to *make* creatine) is important for skaters. For vegetarian skaters, assuring an adequate total protein and total energy consumption is critical to maintaining muscle mass and synthesizing creatine. The quick burst of muscular activity associated with the high jumps required in competitive figure skating is not possible without sufficient storage of phosphocreatine and muscle glycogen. For dance skating competitions, the fuel requirement involves more muscle glycogen than phosphocreatine, so these athletes are likely to do better with slightly less protein (or meat), but still require an adequate total energy intake to perform adequately.

• *Practices are considerably longer than performances.* Although skating performances may only last several minutes, practices may last for an hour or longer, they may occur more than once each day, and they may be very early in the morning or very late at night (ice time is hard to find). This means that skaters must alter eating patterns to satisfy their practice needs. For very early-morning practices, skaters should eat and drink something before taking the ice, to be certain that muscles are well fueled. For late-night practices, a small dinner two hours before practice followed by another small dinner immediately after practice will help assure that muscles are well fueled. Skating while the muscles are on "empty" will not help them become more conditioned and may actually be counterproductive in inducing a training benefit.

Soccer

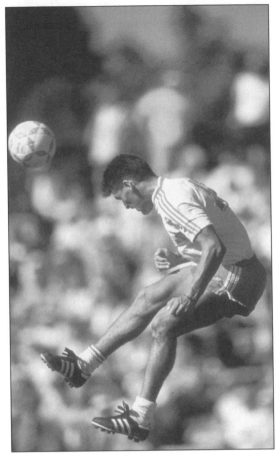

The popularity of soccer worldwide is enormous, and is increasing in popularity in the United States. This is a wonderful sport from a fitness standpoint, as the average distance covered by a typical soccer player during a match is approximately 10 kilometers.[17] In addition, soccer players appear to have significantly greater bone mineral densities (likely to be due from all the running stresses placed on the bones) than age- and weight-matched controls.[18,19] While much of this activity is aerobic, a good deal of it is anaerobic as players sprint to go for the ball. It appears as if there is less activity in the second half of the game when compared to the first, and that lower muscle glycogen levels may be the cause of this reduction in activity. It was suggested long ago that the ingestion of carbohydrates immediately before, during, and after a game may play an important role in reducing player fatigue during a game.[20]

In studies of professional soccer players' nutrient consumption, it was found that energy and nutrient intake was similar to that of the general population, despite having a far higher energy and nutrient requirement.[21,22] While the recommended training diet for soccer players should be comprised of 55 to 65 percent carbohydrate, 12 to 15 percent protein, and less than 30 percent fat,[23] the athletes in this and other surveys had diets that were considerably lower in carbohydrate and higher in fat.[24] It is generally believed that playing soccer places a high demand on glycogen stores, so glycogen depletion could cause premature fatigue and reduced performance during a match.[25] Of course, adequate energy intake, estimated to be approximately 4,000 calories for males and 3,200 calories for females, is also important. Without sufficient energy intake, glycogen will become depleted regardless of the makeup of the diet.

Nutritionally Relevant Factors for Soccer

• *Play in soccer is expected to be continuous, making it difficult for players to consume fluids.* Since soccer players may not have an opportunity to regularly consume fluids during a game, pregame hydration status is particularly important. When possible (between periods and during official breaks), players should do whatever is reasonably possible to consume some sports beverage to rehydrate and to replace carbohydrates.

• *Surveys suggest the consumption of carbohydrates is less than optimal for soccer players.* Carbohydrate consumption is critical for the achievement of optimal soccer performance. Since surveys suggest that soccer players typically consume diets that match those of the general public, with a carbohydrate intake of around 50 percent of total calories, players should make a conscious effort to improve carbohydrate intake.

• *Pregame glycogen storage is critical.* Soccer players spend a lot of time running up and down the field, and this places a tremendous drain on muscle glycogen. Players who begin the game with more stored glycogen will experience an endurance advantage. To achieve a higher glycogen storage, players should consistently consume plenty of carbohydrates and fluids and also focus mainly on carbohydrates during the pregame meal.

Tennis

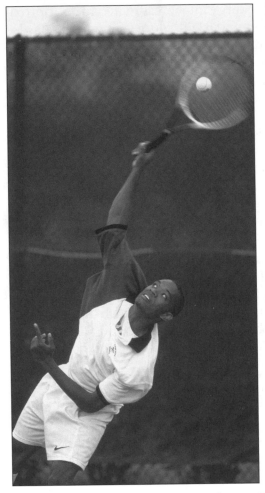

It is generally agreed that tennis has both aerobic and anaerobic components, but the majority of energy supply appears to come from anaerobic systems.[26,27] It is this heavy reliance on the anaerobic metabolic system that is likely to be the reason why it has been found that carbohydrate supplementation improves the stroke quality during the final stages of a tennis match.[28] Since long-lasting, high-intensity exercise is highly dependent on carbohydrate as a fuel, it makes perfect sense that tennis players should assure that carbohydrate is available to the muscles as a fuel.

While carbohydrate consumption may be of concern, it appears that collegiate tennis players (Division I) have been well coached to consume sufficient fluids in hot environments. In a study evaluating fluid and electrolyte balance during multiday match play in a hot environment, it was found that the athletes successfully maintained overall balance, resulting in no occurrence of heat illness.[29]

It also appears, from data on young tennis players, that the adequacy of energy intake is better than that seen in other sports (gymnastics and swimming). It is well established that menstrual onset is, to a great degree, dependent on the adequacy of energy intake. In general, females experience the first menses at age 13. Females who have energy deficits, however, may have up to a two-year delay in the age of menarche. Tennis players, however, appear to have only a slight delay (13.2 years) in the age of menarche, suggesting that energy consumption is good.[30] Typically, there is less concern in tennis on "making weight." The focus is on conditioning, regardless of where the weight ends up.

Nutritionally Relevant Factors for Tennis

• *Tennis is commonly played outside on courts where the reflective temperature off the court is higher than the environmental temperature.* The heat at courtside can quickly cause heat illness if tennis players fail to take steps to adequately hydrate themselves. Players should be aware of the signs of heat disorders (thirst, fatigue, vision problems, inability to speak normally) and take quick action if they, a partner, or an opponent appears to have any heat-related symptoms (see table 11.3).

• *Tennis has natural breaks after each odd game, when the opponents change sides.* These natural breaks in a tennis match are, perhaps, why it has been found that tennis players are in relatively good hydration state during and following a match. However, since carbohydrate supplementation has been found to improve end-of-game strokes, players should make certain that the beverage consumed contains

Table 11.3   Heat Disorder Symptoms

Heat cramps	Muscle spasms that occur involuntarily during or after exercise, typically with the muscles that did most of the work during the exercise.
Heat exhaustion	Weak and rapid heart rate with low blood pressure, headache, dizziness, and severe weakness. Body temperature is not elevated to dangerous levels, but sweat rate may be reduced, increasing the risk of high body temperature. Blood volume is typically low. At this stage, the athlete should stop exercising, go to a shady area or cool building, and consume fluids to rehydrate.
Heatstroke	A failure of the body's ability to maintain temperature. Characterized by a failure to sweat. Circulatory system collapse may lead to death. Immediate steps should be taken to cool the body by applying ice, placing the person in cold water, and/or applying alcohol rubs. This is an emergency condition, so medical assistance should be called immediately.

Reprinted by permission from M.H. Williams, 1997, *Nutrition for fitness and sport,* 5th ed. (New York: McGraw-Hill), 208-209. Reproduced with the permission of The McGraw-Hill Companies.

carbohydrate. These sports beverages, if sipped during a match, will help to assure that high-intensity activity can be maintained for a longer period of time.

Summary

Sports that require a combination of power and endurance have only recently received the same kind of scientific attention that endurance sports have enjoyed for many years. Interestingly, studies on these sports indicate that carbohydrate consumption is useful in enhancing performance *even if the activity lasts less than one hour*. This is an important finding, since the traditional thought has been that water is an appropriate hydration beverage for activities lasting less than one hour, but that carbohydrate-containing sports beverages are important to consume for activities lasting longer than one hour. We now know that even in these shorter activites, carbohydrate consumption is performance enhancing. Since many of these sports (basketball, soccer, tennis) place an enormous caloric drain on the system, athletes should develop eating strategies (i.e., eating enough) that encourage maintenance of muscle mass during long and arduous seasons.

Appendix A

Following are six sample meal plans to assist athletes and coaches in planning meals that meet needed energy and nutrient requirements. Energy requirements are calculated as 30 to 50 calories per kilogram of body weight, although energy requirements vary by duration and intensity of activity and by growth phase. These meal plans meet carbohydrate requirements calculated as 8 grams per kilogram of body weight, and also provide a minimum of 1.5 grams of protein per kilogram of body weight. Data for these meal plans are derived from USDA nutrient database for standard reference (release SR11, 1996).

2,500 CALORIES

	Food	Cal	Carb	Prot	Fat
Breakfast	1 cup orange juice	112	25.8	1.7	0.5
	1 cup whole-wheat cereal	166	37.7	5.1	0.6
	1 cup skim milk	86	11.9	8.4	0.4
	1 banana	105	26.7	1.2	0.6
	Subtotals (19% of total calories)	**470**	**102.1**	**16.4**	**2.1**
Mid-AM snack	5 saltine crackers	63	10.2	1.3	17
	1 cup apple juice	117	29.0	0.2	0.3
	Subtotals (7% of total calories)	**180**	**39.2**	**1.5**	**2.0**
Lunch	1/2 chicken breast (broiled)	142	0.0	26.7	3.1
	2 slices bread, cracked wheat	132	26.0	4.4	1.1
	3/4 cup salad (lettuce and vegetables)	17	3.4	1.3	0.1
	1 tbsp lemon juice (for dressing)	4	1.3	0.1	0.0
	1 cup fruit cocktail (juice pack)	114	29.4	1.1	0.0
	Subtotals (17% of total calories)	**409**	**60.1**	**33.6**	**4.3**
Mid-PM snack	2 ounces cheese, cheddar	225	0.7	13.9	18.6
	1 apple (raw)	81	21.1	0.3	0.5
	Subtotals (13% of total calories)	**306**	**21.8**	**14.2**	**19.1**
Dinner	2.5 cups spaghetti and meat balls	720	83.8	40.3	25.2
	1 roll	119	19.6	2.9	3.0
	1 cup Caesar salad	9	1.3	0.9	0.1
	1 tbsp Caesar salad dressing	57	3.5	0.1	4.9
	1 orange	72	15.4	1.2	0.2
	Subtotals (40% of total calories)	**977**	**123.6**	**45.4**	**33.5**
Evening snack	1 cup popcorn (air popped)	35	6.9	1.1	0.5
	8 ounces Gatorade	75	21.1	0.0	0.2
	Subtotals (5% of total calories)	**110**	**28.0**	**1.1**	**0.5**
	Daily totals (grams)	**2,452**	**375**	**112**	**61**
	Percent of total calories		**60**	**18**	**22**

Other key nutrients provided by this food intake

Nutrient	Amount	Nutrient	Amount
Calcium	1,242 mg	Thiamin	1.8 mg
Iron	18 mg	Riboflavin	2.2 mg
Vitamin C	417 mg		

Note: This level of food intake is appropriate for an athlete weighing about 125 lbs.

2,500 CALORIES (LACTOVEGETARIAN)

	Food	Cal	Carb	Prot	Fat
Breakfast	1 cup orange juice	112	25.8	1.7	0.5
	1 cup whole-wheat cereal	166	37.7	5.1	0.6
	1 cup skim milk	86	11.9	8.4	0.4
	1 banana	105	26.7	1.2	0.6
	Subtotals (19% of total calories)	**470**	**102.1**	**16.4**	**2.1**
Mid-AM snack	5 saltine crackers	63	10.2	1.3	1.7
	1 cup apple juice	117	29.0	0.2	0.3
	Subtotals (7% of total calories)	**180**	**39.2**	**1.5**	**2.0**
Lunch	2 cups soba noodles	226	48.9	11.5	0.2
	4 pieces tofu, fried	141	5.5	8.9	10.5
	2 slices cracked wheat bread	132	26.0	4.4	1.1
	3/4 cup salad	17	3.4	1.3	0.1
	1 tbsp lemon juice (for dressing)	4	1.3	0.1	0.0
	1 cup fruit cocktail	114	29.4	1.1	0.0
	Subtotals (26% of total calories)	**632**	**114.5**	**27.4**	**11.9**
Mid-PM snack	2 ounces cheese, cheddar	225	0.7	13.9	18.6
	1 apple	81	21.1	0.3	0.5
	Subtotals (13% of total calories)	**306**	**21.8**	**14.2**	**19.1**
Dinner	8 ounces pasta (made without egg)	283	57.3	10.0	2.2
	1 cup marinara sauce	170	25.5	4.0	8.4
	2 tbsp parmesan cheese	46	0.4	4.2	3.0
	1 roll	119	19.6	2.9	3.0
	1 cup caesar salad	9	1.3	0.9	0.1
	1 tbsp caesar salad dressing	57	3.5	0.1	4.9
	Subtotals (31% of total calories)	**977**	**123.6**	**45.4**	**33.5**
Evening snack	1 cup popcorn (air popped)	35	6.9	1.1	0.5
	8 ounces Gatorade	75	21.1	0.0	0.2
	Subtotals (5% of total calories)	**110**	**28.0**	**1.1**	**0.5**
	Daily totals (grams)	**2,440**	**428.3**	**83.8**	**57.3**
	Percent of total calories		**67**	**13**	**20**

Other key nutrients provided by this food intake

Nutrient	Amount	Nutrient	Amount
Calcium	1,359 mg	Thiamin	2.0 mg
Iron	18 mg	Riboflavin	2.1 mg
Vitamin C	401 mg		

Note: This level of food intake is appropriate for an athlete weighing about 125 lbs.

3,000 CALORIES

	Food	Cal	Carb	Prot	Fat
Breakfast	1 cup orange juice	111.6	25.8	1.7	0.5
	1 cup strawberries	44.7	10.5	0.9	0.6
	1 cup whole-wheat cereal	116.2	26.0	3.3	0.7
	1 cup 1% milk	102.2	11.7	8.0	2.6
	1 roll	75.0	13.4	2.0	1.3
	1 tsp margarine	33.8	0.0	0.0	3.8
	1 tbsp strawberry jam	54.4	14.0	0.1	0.0
	Subtotals (18% of total calories)	**537.4**	**101.4**	**16.2**	**9.4**
Mid-AM snack	1 plain bagel	199.9	38.0	7.0	2.0
	1 tsp margarine	33.8	0.0	0.0	3.8
	1 tbsp jam or preserves	54.4	14.0	0.1	0.0
	16 ounces Gatorade	100.2	28.1	0.0	0.0
	Subtotals (11% of total calories)	**388.4**	**80.1**	**7.2**	**5.8**
Lunch	2 slices turkey (for sandwich)	46.8	0.0	9.6	0.7
	2 slices bread (for sandwich)	131	26.1	4.4	1.1
	Lettuce (for sandwich)	2.6	0.4	0.2	0.0
	1 tbsp mayonnaise (for sandwich)	49.5	0.2	0.1	5.5
	1 cup cranberry juice	216.3	54.7	0.0	0.4
	1 medium apple	81.4	21.1	0.3	0.5
	1/3 cup potato salad	216.6	25.7	2.9	11.5
	Subtotals (25% of total calories)	**744.6**	**128.1**	**17.4**	**19.6**
Mid-PM snack	3 Dutch-type pretzels	187.2	36.4	4.7	2.2
	16 ounces Gatorade	100.2	28.1	0.0	0.0
	1/2 cup grapes	29.0	8.0	0.3	0.2
	Subtotals (13% of total calories)	**316.4**	**72.4**	**5.0**	**2.3**
Dinner	1 1/2 cups chicken chow mein	382.5	15.0	46.5	15.0
	1 cup rice	199.5	43.3	4.0	0.5
	6 ounces tea	1.7	0.5	0.0	0.0
	1 orange	61.6	15.4	1.2	0.2
	Subtotals (21% of total calories)	**645.4**	**74.2**	**51.7**	**15.6**
Evening snack	1 banana	104.9	26.7	1.2	0.6
	2 ounces cheddar cheese	112.7	0.4	7.0	9.3
	2 squares graham crackers	109.1	20.8	2.3	2.7
	8 ounces Gatorade	50.0	14.0	0.0	0.0
	Subtotals (13% of total calories)	**376.8**	**61.9**	**10.4**	**12.5**
	Daily totals (grams)	**3,009**	**518**	**108**	**65**
	Percent of total calories		**67.1**	**14.0**	**18.9**

Other key nutrients provided by this food intake

Nutrient	Amount	Nutrient	Amount
Calcium	1,200 mg	Thiamin	3.7 mg
Iron	37.3 mg	Riboflavin	4.2 mg
Vitamin C	528.8 mg		

Note: This level of food intake is appropriate for an athlete weighing about 170 lbs.

3,500 CALORIES

	Food	Cal	Carb	Prot	Fat
Breakfast	1.5 cups orange juice	167.4	38.7	2.6	0.8
	1 cup strawberries	44.7	10.5	0.9	0.6
	1.5 cups whole-wheat Total	174.2	39.0	5.0	1.0
	1 cup 1% milk	102.2	11.7	8.0	2.6
	1 roll	75.0	13.4	2.0	1.3
	1 tsp margarine	33.8	0.0	0.0	3.8
	1 tbsp strawberry jam	54.4	14.0	0.1	0.0
	Subtotals (19% of total calories)	**651.3**	**127.3**	**18.7**	**10.0**
Mid-AM snack	1 plain bagel	199.9	38.0	7.0	2.0
	1 tsp margarine	33.8	0.0	0.0	3.8
	1 tbsp jam or preserves	54.4	14.0	0.1	0.0
	16 ounces Gatorade	100.2	28.1	0.0	0.0
	Subtotals (11% of total calories)	**388.4**	**80.1**	**7.2**	**5.8**
Lunch	1 roast beef sandwich	346.1	33.4	21.5	13.8
	1 cup cranberry juice	216.3	54.7	0.0	0.4
	1 medium apple	81.4	21.1	0.3	0.5
	2/3 cup potato salad	216.6	25.7	2.9	11.5
	1 peach	37.4	9.7	0.6	0.1
	Subtotals (25% of total calories)	**897.9**	**144.5**	**25.3**	**26.2**
Mid-PM snack	3 Dutch-type pretzels	187.2	36.4	4.7	2.2
	16 ounces Gatorade	100.2	28.1	0.0	0.0
	1 cup grapes	57.9	15.8	0.6	0.3
	Subtotals (10% of total calories)	**345.4**	**80.3**	**5.3**	**2.5**
Dinner	1.5 cups chicken chow mein	382.5	15.0	46.5	15.0
	1 cup rice	199.5	43.3	4.0	0.5
	6 ounces tea	1.7	0.5	0.0	0.0
	1 orange	61.6	15.4	1.2	0.2
	1 cup 1% milk	102.2	11.7	8.0	2.6
	1 tsp sugar (for tea)	15.4	34.0	0.0	0.0
	Subtotals (21% of total calories)	**762.9**	**89.8**	**59.8**	**18.2**
Evening snack	1 banana	104.9	26.7	1.2	0.6
	1 cup 1% milk	102.1	11.7	8.0	2.6
	3 graham crackers	163.6	31.2	3.4	4.0
	16 ounces Gatorade	100.3	28.1	0.0	0.0
	Subtotals (13% of total calories)	**470.9**	**97.7**	**12.6**	**7.2**
	Daily totals (grams)	**3,517**	**620**	**129**	**70**
	Percent of total calories		**68.4**	**14.2**	**17.4**

Other key nutrients provided by this food intake

Nutrient	Amount	Nutrient	Amount
Calcium	1,760 mg	**Thiamin**	5.1 mg
Iron	51.3 mg	**Riboflavin**	6.2 mg
Vitamin C	639.4 mg		

Note: This level of food intake is appropriate for an athlete weighing about 190 lbs.

4,000 CALORIES

	Food	Cal	Carb	Prot	Fat
Breakfast	1.5 cups orange juice	167.4	38.7	2.6	0.8
	1 cup strawberries	44.7	10.5	0.9	0.6
	2 cups whole-wheat Total	232.3	52.0	6.6	1.4
	2 cups 1% milk	204.3	23.3	16.1	5.2
	1 roll	75.0	13.4	2.0	1.3
	1 tsp margarine	33.8	0.0	0.0	3.8
	1 tbsp jam	54.4	14.0	0.1	0.0
	Subtotals (21% of total calories)	**811.5**	**152.0**	**28.4**	**13.0**
Mid-AM snack	1 plain bagel	199.9	38.0	7.0	2.0
	1 tsp margarine	33.8	0.0	0.0	3.8
	1 tbsp jam	54.4	14.0	0.1	0.0
	16 ounces Gatorade	100.2	28.1	0.0	0.0
	Subtotals (11% of total calories)	**388.4**	**80.1**	**7.2**	**5.8**
Lunch	1 roast beef sandwich	346.1	33.4	21.5	13.8
	1 medium baked potato	145.1	33.6	3.1	0.2
	1 tbsp sour cream (for potato)	25.7	0.5	0.4	2.5
	1.5 cups tossed salad	33.1	6.7	2.6	0.1
	1 tbsp Italian dressing for salad	68.7	1.5	0.1	7.1
	1.5 cups cranberry juice	216.3	54.7	0.0	0.4
	1 apple	81.4	21.1	0.3	0.5
	1 peach	37.4	9.7	0.6	0.1
	Subtotals (24% of total calories)	**953.9**	**161.1**	**28.5**	**24.6**
Mid-PM snack	3 Dutch-type pretzels	187.2	36.4	4.7	2.2
	16 ounces Gatorade	100.2	28.1	0.0	0.0
	1 cup grapes	57.9	15.8	0.6	0.3
	Subtotals (10% of total calories)	**345.4**	**80.3**	**5.3**	**2.5**
Dinner	2 cups chicken chow mein	510.0	20.0	62.0	20.0
	2 cups rice	399.5	86.6	8.0	1.0
	6 ounces tea	1.8	0.5	0.0	0.0
	1 orange	61.6	15.4	1.2	0.2
	1 cup 1% milk	102.2	11.7	8.0	2.6
	1 tsp sugar (for tea)	15.4	34.0	0.0	0.0
	Subtotals (28% of total calories)	**1089.9**	**138.1**	**79.3**	**23.7**
Evening snack	1 cup 1% milk	102.1	11.7	8.0	2.6
	3 graham crackers	163.6	31.2	3.4	4.0
	16 ounces Gatorade	100.3	28.1	0.0	0.0
	Subtotals (13% of total calories)	**470.9**	**97.7**	**12.6**	**7.2**
	Daily totals (grams)	**3,958**	**697**	**153**	**74**
	Percent of total calories		**68.6**	**15.1**	**16.4**

Other key nutrients provided by this food intake

Nutrient	Amount	Nutrient	Amount
Calcium	1,986 mg	Thiamin	6.5 mg
Iron	65.5 mg	Riboflavin	7.3 mg
Vitamin C	745.4 mg		

Note: This level of food intake is appropriate for an athlete weighing about 220 lbs.

	Food	Cal	Carb	Prot	Fat
Breakfast	1.5 cups orange juice	167.4	38.7	2.6	0.8
	1 cup strawberries	44.7	10.5	0.9	0.6
	2 cups whole-wheat Total	232.3	52.0	6.6	1.4
	2 cups 2% milk	242.4	23.3	16.3	9.4
	1 roll	75.0	13.4	2.0	1.3
	1 tsp margarine	33.8	0.0	0.0	3.8
	1 tbsp jam	54.4	14.0	0.1	0.0
	Subtotals (17% of total calories)	**849.6**	**152.1**	**28.6**	**17.2**
Mid-AM snack	1 plain bagel	199.9	38.0	7.0	2.0
	2 tbsp cream cheese	195.5	1.5	4.2	19.5
	1 banana	104.9	26.7	1.2	0.6
	16 ounces Gatorade	100.2	28.1	0.0	0.0
	Subtotals (12% of total calories)	**600.5**	**94.3**	**12.4**	**22.1**
Lunch	1 hamburger with roll	401.4	54.7	22.6	22.9
	1 medium baked potato	145.1	33.6	3.1	0.2
	1 tbsp sour cream (for potato)	25.7	0.5	0.4	2.5
	1.5 cups tossed salad	33.1	6.7	2.6	0.1
	1 tbsp Italian dressing (for salad)	68.7	1.5	0.1	7.1
	1.5 cups cranberry juice	216.3	54.7	0.0	0.4
	1 medium apple	81.4	21.1	0.3	0.5
	1 serving coffee cake	150.7	24.5	2.95	4.5
	Subtotals (22% of total calories)	**1122.5**	**168.0**	**32.0**	**38.2**
Mid-PM snack	3 slices whole-wheat toast	182.1	35.7	7.9	2.3
	1 tbsp jam	54.4	14.0	0.1	0.0
	16 ounces Gatorade	100.2	28.1	0.0	0.0
	1 banana	104.9	26.7	1.2	0.6
	Subtotals (11% of total calories)	**542.9**	**104.6**	**9.3**	**14.2**
Dinner	2 cups chicken chow mein	510.0	20.0	62.0	20.0
	2 cups rice	399.5	86.6	8.0	1.0
	6 ounces tea	1.8	0.5	0.0	0.0
	1 tsp sugar (for tea)	15.4	34.0	0.0	0.0
	1 orange	61.6	15.4	1.2	0.2
	1 cup 2% milk	121.2	11.7	8.1	4.7
	1 slice chocolate cake	162.4	24.6	2.0	7.2
	Subtotals (25% of total calories)	**1271.3**	**162.7**	**81.4**	**33.0**
Evening snack	1 cup ice cream	269.2	31.7	4.8	14.3
	3 graham crackers	163.6	31.2	3.4	4.0
	16 ounces Gatorade	100.3	28.1	0.0	0.0
	Subtotals (13% of total calories)	**637.9**	**117.7**	**9.4**	**18.9**
	Daily totals (grams)	**5,025**	**799**	**173**	**144**
	Percent of total calories		**61.7**	**13.4**	**24.9**

Other key nutrients provided by this food intake

Nutrient	Amount	Nutrient	Amount
Calcium	2,338 mg	**Thiamin**	6.8 mg
Iron	69.0 mg	**Riboflavin**	8.1 mg
Vitamin C	755.4 mg		

Note: This level of food intake is appropriate for an athlete weighing about 240 lbs.

Appendix B

Iron Content of Selected Foods in Descending Iron Amount

Food description and common serving amount	Iron (mg)
Product 19 cereal (1 oz)	18.00
Total cereal (1 oz)	18.00
Oysters, raw (1 cup)	15.60
Enchilada (1 enchilada)	11.00
Cream of Wheat (1 cup)	10.90
Malt-O-Meal (1 cup)	9.60
Cashew nuts, dry roasted (1 cup)	8.20
40% Bran Flakes, Kellogg (1 oz)	8.10
Seaweed, spirulina, dried (1 oz)	8.10
Cap'n Crunch cereal (1 oz)	7.50
Oatmeal, cooked from instant (1 pkt)	6.70
Peaches, dried (1 cup)	6.50
Spinach, cooked (1 cup)	6.40
Apricots, dried, uncooked (1 cup)	6.10
Duck, roasted, flesh only (1/2 duck)	6.00
Lima beans, dry, cooked (1 cup)	5.90
Beef liver, fried (3 oz)	5.30
Chickpeas, cooked, drained (1 cup)	4.90
Hamburger, 4 oz patty and roll (1 sandwich)	4.80
Red kidney beans, dry, canned (1 cup)	4.60
Cereal, most popular brands (1 oz)	4.50
Cheeseburger, 4 oz patty and roll (1 sandwich)	4.50
Chili con carne w/ beans (1 cup)	4.30
Figs, dried (10 figs)	4.20
Roast beef sandwich (1 sandwich)	4.00

Calcium Content of Selected Foods in Descending Calcium Amount

Food description and common serving amount	Calcium (mg)
Yogurt, w/low-fat milk, plain (8 oz)	415.00
Macaroni and cheese (1 cup)	362.00
Enchilada (1 enchilada)	322.00
Milk, low fat, 1% fat (1 cup)	313.00
Milk, skim, no fat (1 cup)	302.00
Orange juice, calcium fortified (1 cup)	300.00
Milk, low fat, 2% fat (1 cup)	297.00
Milk, whole, 3.3% fat (1 cup)	291.00
Figs, dried (10 figs)	269.00
Spinach, cooked (1 cup)	245.00
Cheeseburger, 4 oz patty and roll (1 sandwich)	236.00
Oysters, raw (1 cup)	226.00
Turnip greens, cooked (1 cup)	200.00
Oatmeal, cooked from instant (1 pkt)	168.00
Pasteurized processed cheese food, American (1 oz)	163.00
Bok choy, cooked (1 cup)	160.00
Feta cheese (1 oz)	140.00
Spaghetti w/meatballs and tomato sauce (1 cup)	124.00
Tofu (1 piece)	108.00
Kale, cooked (1 cup)	90.00
Chili con carne w/ beans (1 cup)	82.00
Chickpeas, cooked, drained (1 cup)	80.00
Hamburger, 4 oz patty and roll (1 sandwich)	75.00
Red kidney beans, dry, canned (1 cup)	74.00
Raisins (1 cup)	71.00
Broccoli (1 cup)	70.00

B-Vitamin Content of Selected Foods in Descending B-Vitamin Amount

Food description and common serving amount	B-1 (mg)	B-2 (mg)	Niacin (mg)
Product 19 cereal (1 oz)	1.50	1.70	20.00
Total cereal (1 oz)	1.50	1.70	20.00
Seaweed, spirulina, dried (1 oz)	0.67	1.40	3.60
Duck, roasted, flesh only (1/2 duck)	0.57	1.40	11.30
Oatmeal, cooked from instant (1 pkt)	0.53	0.38	5.90
Cap'n Crunch cereal (1 oz)	0.50	0.55	6.60
Malt-O-Meal (1 cup)	0.48	0.24	5.80
Roast beef sandwich (1 sandwich)	0.40	0.33	6.00
Hamburger, 4 oz patty and roll (1 sandwich)	0.38	0.38	7.80
40% Bran Flakes, Kellogg (1 oz)	0.37	0.43	5.00
Cereal, most popular brands (1 oz)	0.37	0.43	5.00
Cornflakes, Kellogg (1 oz)	0.37	0.43	5.00
Rice Krispies cereal (1 oz)	0.37	0.43	5.00
Oysters, raw (1 cup)	0.34	0.43	6.00
Cheeseburger, 4 oz patty and roll (1 sandwich)	0.33	0.48	7.40
Chicken potpie, home recipe (1 piece)	0.32	0.32	4.90
Cashew nuts, dry roasted (1 cup)	0.27	0.27	1.90
Bagels, plain (1 bagel)	0.26	0.20	2.40
Lima beans, dry, cooked (1 cup)	0.25	0.11	1.30
Spaghetti with meatballs and tomato sauce (1 cup)	0.25	0.30	4.00
Cream of Wheat (1 cup)	0.24	0.00	1.50
Raisins (1 cup)	0.23	0.13	1.20
Rice, white, cooked (1 cup)	0.23	0.02	2.10
Macaroni and cheese (1 cup)	0.20	0.40	1.80
Enchilada (1 enchilada)	0.18	0.26	0.00
Beef liver, fried (3 oz)	0.18	3.52	12.30
Chickpeas, cooked, drained (1 cup)	0.18	0.09	0.90
Spinach, cooked (1 cup)	0.17	0.42	0.90
Red kidney beans, dry, canned (1 cup)	0.13	0.10	1.50
Figs, dried (10 figs)	0.13	0.16	1.30
Yogurt, w/low-fat milk, plain (8 oz)	0.10	0.49	0.30
Milk, low fat, 2% fat (1 cup)	0.10	0.40	0.20
Milk, low fat, 1% fat (1 cup)	0.10	0.42	0.20
Turkey, roasted, light + dark (1 cup)	0.09	0.25	7.60
Milk, whole, 3.3% fat (1 cup)	0.09	0.40	0.20
Milk, skim, no fat (1 cup)	0.09	0.34	0.20
Chili con carne w/beans (1 cup)	0.08	0.18	3.30
Raisin bread (1 slice)	0.08	0.15	1.00
Tofu (1 piece)	0.07	0.04	0.10
Beef steak (3 oz)	0.06	0.21	3.30
Tuna salad (1 cup)	0.06	0.14	13.30
Chicken, roasted, breast (3 oz)	0.06	0.10	11.80
Feta cheese (1 oz)	0.04	0.24	0.30
Beef, corned (3 oz)	0.02	0.20	2.90
Apricots, dried, uncooked (1 cup)	0.01	0.20	3.90
Pasteurized processed cheese food, American (1 oz)	0.01	0.13	0.00
Peaches, dried (1 cup)	0.00	0.34	7.00

[B-1=Thiamin; B-2=Riboflavin]

(Source: USDA Home and Garden Bulletin #72)

Energy Distribution of Foods Commonly Consumed, in Alphabetical Order

Food description and common serving amount	Carb %	Prot %	Fat %	Calories
100% Natural Cereal (1 Oz)	52	9	39	138
1000 Island, salad drsng, reglr (1 Tablespoon)	13	0	87	62
40% Bran Flakes, Kellogg (1 Oz)	78	14	8	113
40% Bran Flakes, Post (1 Oz)	88	12	0	100
Alfalfa Seeds, Sprouted, Raw (1 Cup)	50	50	0	8
All-Bran Cereal (1 Oz)	77	15	8	109
Almonds, Whole (1 Oz)	13	13	74	183
Angelfood Cake, From Mix (1 Piece)	91	9	0	128
Apple Juice, Canned (1 Cup)	100	0	0	116
Apple Pie (1 Piece)	58	3	39	414
Apples, Raw, Unpeeled (1 Medium Apple)	100	0	0	84
Applesauce, Canned, Sweetened (1 Cup)	100	0	0	204
Applesauce, Canned, Unsweetened (1 Cup)	100	0	0	112
Apricot Nectar (1 Cup)	97	3	0	148
Apricots, Canned, Juice Pack (1 Cup)	94	6	0	132
Apricots, Canned, Juice Pack (3 Halves)	91	9	0	44
Apricots, Dried, Uncooked (1 Cup)	92	6	3	349
Apricots, Raw (3 Apricots)	92	8	0	52
Artichokes, Globe, Cooked (1 Artichoke)	80	20	0	60
Asparagus, Cooked Frm Raw (4 Spears)	60	40	0	20
Avocados, Florida (1 Avocado)	29	5	65	371
Bagels, Egg (1 Bagel)	77	14	9	198
Bagels, Plain (1 Bagel)	77	14	9	198
Baking Pwdr Biscuits, Home Recipe (1 Biscuit)	50	8	43	105
Bananas (1 Banana)	89	3	7	121
Barbecue Sauce (1 Tablespoon)	100	0	0	8
Bean Sprouts, Mung, Cooked (1 Cup)	63	38	0	36
Bean Sprouts, Mung, Raw (1 Cup)	67	33	0	36
Bean With Bacon Soup, Canned (1 Cup)	52	18	30	178
Beef And Vegetable Stew (1 Cup)	27	29	44	223
Beef Gravy, Canned (1 Cup)	35	29	36	125
Beef Noodle Soup, Canned (1 Cup)	43	24	33	83
Beef Potpie, Home Recipe (1 Piece)	31	16	53	510
Beef Roast, Rib, Lean Only (2.2 Oz)	0	46	54	149
Beef Steak, Sirloin, Broil, Lean (2.5 Oz)	0	62	38	142
Beet Greens, Cooked (1 Cup)	67	33	0	48

(continued)

Energy Distribution of Foods Commonly Consumed, in Alphabetical Order *(continued)*

Food description and common serving amount	Carb %	Prot %	Fat %	Calories
Beets, Cooked, Drained, Diced (1 Cup)	85	15	0	52
Beets, Cooked, Drained, Whole (2 Beets)	00	13	0	32
Black Beans, Dry, Cooked (1 Cup)	70	26	4	233
Black-Eyed Peas, Dry, Cooked (1 Cup)	70	26	4	201
Blackberries, Raw (1 Cup)	85	5	11	85
Blue Cheese (1 Oz)	4	24	72	100
Blue Cheese Salad Dressing (1 Tablespoon)	5	5	90	80
Blueberries, Raw (1 Cup)	86	4	10	93
Blueberry Muffins, From Mix (1 Muffin)	61	8	31	145
Blueberry Muffins, Home Recipe (1 Muffin)	58	9	33	137
Blueberry Pie (1 Piece)	57	4	39	389
Bologna (2 Slices)	4	16	80	180
Boston Brown Bread (1 Slice)	83	8	9	101
Bran Muffins, From Mix (1 Muffin)	67	8	25	144
Bran Muffins, Home Recipe (1 Muffin)	54	8	38	142
Brazil Nuts (1 Oz)	8	8	84	203
Broccoli, Frozen, Cooked (1 Piece)	67	33	0	12
Broccoli, Raw, Cooked (1 Spear)	58	29	13	69
Brown And Serve Sausage (1 Link)	0	15	85	53
Brown Gravy From Dry Mix (1 Cup)	65	14	21	86
Brownies w/Nuts (1 Brownie)	43	4	53	102
Brussels Sprouts, Raw, Cooked (1 Cup)	68	21	12	77
Butter, Salted (1 Tablespoon)	0	0	100	99
Buttermilk, Fluid (1 Cup)	49	33	18	98
Cabbage, Common, Cooked (1 Cup)	88	13	0	32
Cabbage, Common, Raw (1 Cup)	80	20	0	20
Cabbage, Red, Raw (1 Cup)	80	20	0	20
Camembert Cheese (1 Wedge)	0	28	72	113
Cantaloupe, Raw (1/2s Melon)	84	8	9	105
Cap 'n Crunch Cereal (1 Oz)	75	3	22	123
Caramels, Plain Or Chocolate (1 Oz)	74	3	23	119
Carrots, Raw, Whole (1 Carrot)	88	13	0	32
Cashew Nuts, Dry Roasted, Salted (1 Cup)	22	10	68	831
Catsup (1 Tablespoon)	100	0	0	16
Cauliflower, Cooked From Raw (1 Cup)	75	25	0	32
Cauliflower, Raw (1 Cup)	71	29	0	28

Food description and common serving amount	Carb %	Prot %	Fat %	Calories
Celery, Raw (1 Stalk)	100	0	0	4
Cheddar Cheese (1 Oz)	0	26	74	109
Cheerios Cereal (1 Oz)	70	14	16	114
Cheese Crackers, Plain (10 Crackers)	44	7	49	55
Cheese Crackers, Sandwich (1 Sandwich)	48	10	43	42
Cheese Sauce w/Milk (1 Cup)	30	21	50	309
Cheeseburger, Regular (1 Sandwich)	36	20	44	307
Cheesecake (1 Piece)	36	7	57	286
Cherries, Sweet, Raw (10 Cherries)	77	7	16	57
Cherry Pie (1 Piece)	58	4	38	422
Chicken à la King, Home Recipe (1 Cup)	10	23	66	462
Chicken And Noodles, Home Recipe (1 Cup)	29	25	46	354
Chicken Chow Mein, Canned (1 Cup)	72	28	0	100
Chicken Chow Mein, Home Recipe (1 Cup)	16	49	35	254
Chicken Gravy, Canned (1 Cup)	26	10	64	198
Chicken Noodle Soup, Canned (1 Cup)	51	23	26	70
Chicken Potpie, Home Recipe (1 Piece)	31	17	52	539
Chicken Rice Soup, Canned (1 Cup)	45	26	29	62
Chicken, Fried, Batter, Breast (4.9 Oz)	15	40	46	354
Chicken, Fried, Batter, Drumstick (2.5 Oz)	13	34	53	187
Chicken, Fried, Drumstick (1.7 Oz)	3	44	53	119
Chicken, Fried, Flour, Breast (3.5 Oz)	4	58	38	213
Chicken, Roasted, Breast (3.0 Oz)	0	80	20	135
Chicken, Roasted, Drumstick (1.6 Oz)	0	73	27	66
Chicken, Stewed, Light + Dark (1 Cup)	0	65	35	233
Chickpeas, Cooked, Drained (1 Cup)	65	22	13	276
Chili Con Carne w/Beans, Cnnd (1 Cup)	36	22	42	344
Chocolate Chip Cookies (4 Cookies)	49	4	47	211
Chocolate Milk, Low fat 1% (1 Cup)	64	20	17	163
Chocolate Milk, Regular (1 Cup)	50	15	35	208
Chop Suey w/Beef + Pork (1 Cup)	17	34	50	309
Clam Chowder, Manhattan, Canned (1 Cup)	59	20	22	82
Clam Chowder, New Eng, w/Milk (1 Cup)	41	22	38	167
Clams, Raw (3 Oz)	13	72	15	61
Coconut, Raw, Shredded (1 Cup)	16	4	80	303
Coffeecake, Crumb, From Mix (1 Piece)	65	9	27	235
Cola, Regular (12 Fl Oz)	100	0	0	164

(continued)

Energy Distribution of Foods Commonly Consumed, in Alphabetical Order (continued)

Food description and common serving amount	Carb %	Prot %	Fat %	Calories
Collards, Cooked From Raw (1 Cup)	71	29	0	28
Corn Chips (1 Oz)	42	5	53	153
CornFlakes, Kellogg (1 Oz)	92	8	0	104
CornFlakes, Toasties (1 Oz)	92	8	0	104
Corn Grits, Cooked With Salt (1 Cup)	91	9	0	136
Corn Muffins, From Mix (1 Muffin)	57	8	35	154
Corn Muffins, Home Recipe (1 Muffin)	60	9	32	141
Corn Oil (1 Tablespoon)	0	0	100	126
Corn, Canned, Cream Style (1 Cup)	88	8	4	209
Corn, Canned, Whole Kernel (1 Cup)	85	10	5	193
Corn, Cooked From Raw, Yellow (1 Ear)	78	12	9	97
Cottage Cheese, Creamed, Large Curd (1 Cup)	11	50	40	226
Cottage Cheese, Creamed, Small Curd (1 Cup)	11	50	39	209
Crabmeat, Canned (1 Cup)	3	75	22	123
Cracked-Wheat Bread (1 Slice)	74	12	14	65
Cranberry Juice Cocktail w/Vit C (1 Cup)	100	0	0	152
Cranberry Sauce, Canned, Sweetened (1 Cup)	99	1	0	436
Cream Cheese (1 Oz)	4	8	88	102
Cream Of Chicken Soup w/Milk, Canned (1 Cup)	32	15	53	187
Cream Of Mushroom Soup w/H_2O, Canned (1 Cup)	29	6	65	125
Cream Of Mushroom Soup w/Milk (1 Cup)	29	11	60	210
Cream Of Wheat, Cooked, Instant (1 Cup)	88	12	0	132
Creame Pie (1 Piece)	52	3	45	455
Croissants (1 Croissant)	46	8	46	236
Cucumber, w/Peel (6 Slices)	100	0	0	4
Custard Pie (1 Piece)	43	11	46	333
Custard, Baked (1 Cup)	38	18	44	307
Danish Pastry, Fruit (1 Pastry)	46	7	48	245
Danish Pastry, Plain, No Nuts (1 Ring)	46	6	48	1,331
Dates (10 Dates)	97	3	0	252
Devils Food Cake With Choc Frosting (1 Piece)	66	5	30	244
Doughnuts, Cake Type, Plain (1 Doughnut)	44	6	50	216
Doughnuts, Yeast Leavened, Glazed (1 Doughnut)	44	7	49	237
Eggnog (1 Cup)	39	12	49	347
Eggplant, Cooked, Steamed (1 Cup)	86	14	0	28
Eggs, Cooked, Fried (1 Egg)	4	26	69	91

Food description and common serving amount	Carb %	Prot %	Fat %	Calories
Eggs, Cooked, Hard Cooked (1 Egg)	5	29	66	82
Eggs, Cooked, Poached (1 Egg)	5	29	66	82
Eggs, Cooked, Scrambled/Omelet (1 Egg)	7	26	67	108
Enchilada (1 Enchilada)	30	25	45	320
English Muffin, Egg, Cheese, Bacon (1 Sandwich)	35	20	45	358
English Muffins, Plain (1 Muffin)	79	15	7	137
Evaporated Milk, Skim, Canned (1 Cup)	58	38	4	201
Evaporated Milk, Whole, Canned (1 Cup)	29	20	50	339
Fats, Cooking/Vegetbl Shorteng (1 Tablespoon)	0	0	100	117
Feta Cheese (1 Oz)	5	22	73	74
Fig Bars (4 Cookies)	79	4	17	212
Figs, Dried (10 Figs)	92	5	3	530
Filberts, (Hazelnuts) Chopped (1 Cup)	9	8	83	780
Filberts, (Hazelnuts) Chopped (1 Oz)	8	8	84	194
Fish Sandwich, Reg, w/Cheese (1 Sandwich)	37	15	48	427
Flounder Or Sole, Baked With Margarine (3 Oz)	0	54	46	118
Frankfurter, Cooked (1 Frank)	3	14	83	141
French Bread (1 Slice)	77	13	10	93
French Salad Dressing, Regular (1 Tablespoon)	5	0	95	85
French Toast, Home Recipe (1 Slice)	44	15	41	155
Froot Loops Cereal (1 Oz)	85	7	8	117
Fruit Cocktail, Canned, Juice Pack (1 Cup)	97	3	0	120
Fruit Punch Drink, Canned (6 Fl Oz)	100	0	0	88
Fruitcake, Dark (1 Piece)	58	5	37	171
Fudge, Chocolate, Plain (1 Oz)	73	3	23	115
Gelatin Dessert, Prepared (1/2 Cup)	89	11	0	76
Ginger Ale (12 Fl Oz)	100	0	0	128
Gingerbread Cake, From Mix (1 Piece)	74	5	21	172
Golden Grahams Cereal (1 Oz)	85	7	8	113
Graham Cracker, Plain (2 Crackers)	77	7	16	57
Grape Drink, Canned (6 Fl Oz)	100	0	0	104
Grape Juice, Canned (1 Cup)	97	3	0	156
Grape Soda (12 Fl Oz)	100	0	0	184
Grape-Nuts Cereal (1 Oz)	88	12	0	104
Grapefruit Juice, Raw (1 Cup)	96	4	0	96
Grapefruit, Raw, Pink (1/2 Fruit)	91	9	0	44
Grapes, Raw (10 Grapes)	100	0	0	40

(continued)

Energy Distribution of Foods Commonly Consumed, in Alphabetical Order *(continued)*

Food description and common serving amount	Carb %	Prot %	Fat %	Calories
Great Northern Beans, Dry, Cooked (1 Cup)	70	26	4	217
Ground Beef, Broiled, Regular (3 Oz)	0	33	67	242
Haddock, Breaded, Fried (3 Oz)	16	38	46	177
Half And Half, Cream (1 Tablespoon)	18	0	82	22
Halibut, Broiled, Butter, Lemon Juice (3 Oz)	0	60	40	134
Hamburger, Regular With Roll (1 Sandwich)	43	19	38	259
Hard Candy (1 Oz)	100	0	0	112
Herring, Pickled (3 Oz)	0	37	63	185
Hollandaise Sce, w/H$_2$O, Frm Mx (1 Cup)	22	8	70	256
Honey (1 Tablespoon)	100	0	0	68
Honey Nut Cheerios Cereal (1 Oz)	81	11	8	113
Honeydew Melon, Raw (1/10 Melon)	92	8	0	52
Ice Cream, Vanilla, Regular (1 Cup)	47	7	46	274
Ice Cream, Vanilla, Soft Serve (1 Cup)	39	7	53	387
Ice Milk, Vanilla, 4% Fat (1 Cup)	61	11	28	190
Ice Milk, Vanilla, Soft Serve 3% (1 Cup)	66	14	20	229
Italian Bread (1 Slice)	85	15	0	80
Italian Salad Dressing, Regular (1 Tablespoon)	5	0	95	85
Jams And Preserves (1 Tablespoon)	100	0	0	56
Jellies (1 Tablespoon)	100	0	0	52
Jelly Beans (1 Oz)	100	0	0	104
Kale, Cooked From Raw (1 Cup)	62	18	20	45
Kiwifruit, Raw (1 Kiwi)	92	8	0	48
Lamb, Chops, Arm, Braised, Lean (1.7 Oz)	0	52	48	131
Lamb, Chops, Loin, Broil, Lean (2.3 Oz)	0	58	42	130
Lamb, Leg, Roasted, Lean Only (2.6 Oz)	0	60	40	134
Lard (1 Tablespoon)	0	0	100	117
Lemon Juice, Canned (1 Cup)	83	5	12	77
Lemon Meringue Pie (1 Piece)	59	6	35	358
Lemon-Lime Soda (12 Fl Oz)	100	0	0	156
Lemons, Raw (1 Lemon)	83	17	0	24
Lentils, Dry, Cooked (1 Cup)	68	28	4	225
Lettuce, Crisphead, Raw, Wedge (1 Wedge)	75	25	0	16
Lettuce, Looseleaf (1 Cup)	67	33	0	12
Light, Coffee Or Table Cream (1 Tablespoon)	13	0	87	31
Lima Beans, Dry, Cooked (1 Cup)	73	24	3	269

Food description and common serving amount	Carb %	Prot %	Fat %	Calories
Lima Beans, Frozen, Cooked (1 Cup)	72	23	5	177
Lime Juice, Raw (1 Cup)	96	4	0	92
Lime Juice, Canned (1 Cup)	83	5	12	77
Limeade, Concen, Frozen, Diluted (6 Fl Oz)	100	0	0	80
Lucky Charms Cereal (1 Oz)	81	11	8	113
Macadamia Nuts, Oil Roasted, Salted (1 Cup)	7	4	90	1035
Macaroni And Cheese, Canned (1 Cup)	45	16	39	230
Macaroni And Cheese, Home Recipe (1 Cup)	38	16	46	426
Macaroni, Cooked, Firm (1 Cup)	81	15	5	193
Malt-O-Meal, With Salt (1 Cup)	87	13	0	120
Mangos, Raw (1 Mango)	92	3	6	153
Margarine, Regulr, Hard, 80% Fat (1 Tablespoon)	0	0	100	99
Margarine, Regulr, Soft, 80% Fat (1 Tablespoon)	0	0	100	99
Margarine, Spread, Hard, 60% Fat (1 Tablespoon)	0	0	100	81
Margarine, Spread, Soft, 60% Fat (1 Tablespoon)	0	0	100	81
Marshmallows (1 Oz)	96	4	0	96
Mayonnaise-Type Salad Dressing (1 Tablespoon)	26	0	74	61
Mayonnaise, Regular (1 Tablespoon)	0	0	100	99
Melba Toast, Plain (1 Piece)	80	20	0	20
Milk Chocolate Candy, Plain (1 Oz)	42	5	53	153
Milk Chocolate Candy, With Rice Crispies (1 Oz)	50	6	44	143
Milk Chocolate Candy, w/Almonds (1 Oz)	37	7	56	162
Milk Chocolate Candy, w/Peanuts (1 Oz)	31	10	59	167
Milk, Whole, 3.3% Fat (1 Cup)	30	22	49	148
Milk, Low Fat, 1% Fat (1 Cup)	45	30	25	107
Milk, Low Fat, 2%, No Added Solid (1 Cup)	38	26	36	125
Milk, Skim (1 Cup)	60	40	0	80
Minestrone Soup, Canned (1 Cup)	51	18	31	87
Mixed-Grain Bread (1 Slice)	74	12	14	65
Mixed Nuts w/Peanuts, Dry, Salted (1 Oz)	15	11	74	183
Mozzarella Cheese, Skim, Low Moisture (1 Oz)	5	40	56	81
Muenster Cheese (1 Oz)	0	26	74	109
Mushroom Gravy, Canned (1 Cup)	44	10	46	118
Mushrooms, Raw (1 Cup)	75	25	0	16
Nature Valley Granola Cereal (1 Oz)	57	9	34	133
Nectarines, Raw (1 Nectarine)	83	5	12	77
Noodles, Egg, Cooked (1 Cup)	76	14	9	194

(continued)

Energy Distribution of Foods Commonly Consumed, in Alphabetical Order (continued)

Food description and common serving amount	Carb %	Prot %	Fat %	Calories
Oatmeal Bread (1 Slice)	74	12	14	65
Oatmeal w/Raisins Cookies (4 Cookies)	59	5	37	246
Oatmeal, Cooked, Instant (1 Cup)	70	17	13	142
Ocean Perch, Breaded, Fried (1 Fillet)	15	34	52	191
Okra Pods, Cooked (8 Pods)	75	25	0	32
Olive Oil (1 Tablespoon)	0	0	100	126
Olives, Canned, Green (4 Medium)	0	0	100	18
Onion Rings, Breaded (2 Rings)	40	5	56	81
Onions, Raw, Chopped (1 Cup)	86	14	0	56
Orange Juice, Raw (1 Cup)	93	7	0	112
Orange Soda (12 Fl Oz)	100	0	0	184
Oranges, Raw (1 Orange)	94	6	0	64
Oysters, Breaded, Fried (1 Oyster)	24	24	53	85
Oysters, Raw (1 Cup)	22	54	24	148
Pancakes, Buckwheat (1 Pancake)	48	16	36	50
Pancakes, Plain, Home Recipe (1 Pancake)	58	13	29	62
Parmesan Cheese, Grated (1 Oz)	3	36	61	133
Parsley, Raw (10 Sprigs)	100	0	0	4
Parsnips, Cooked, Drained (1 Cup)	94	6	0	128
Pasteurized Processed Cheese, Swiss (1 Oz)	4	29	66	95
Pasteurized Processed Cheese, American (1 Oz)	0	23	77	105
Pea Beans, Dry, Cooked (1 Cup)	70	26	4	229
Pea, Green, Soup, Canned (1 Cup)	63	21	16	171
Peach Pie (1 Piece)	59	4	37	409
Peaches, Frozen, Sweetened (1 Cup)	97	3	0	248
Peaches, Canned, Juice Pack (1 Cup)	94	6	0	124
Peaches, Dried (1 Cup)	92	6	2	425
Peaches, Raw (1 Peach)	91	9	0	44
Peanut Butter (1 Tablespoon)	12	19	69	104
Peanut Butter Cookies (4 Cookies)	44	6	50	254
Peanut Oil (1 Tablespoon)	0	0	100	126
Peanuts, Oil Roasted, Salted (1 Cup)	12	17	71	903
Pears, Raw, D Anjou (1 Pear)	90	3	7	133
Pears, Canned, Juice Pack (1 Cup)	97	3	0	132
Pears, Raw, Bartlett (1 Pear)	88	4	8	113
Peas, Edible Pod, Cooked, Drained (1 Cup)	69	31	0	64

Food description and common serving amount	Carb %	Prot %	Fat %	Calories
Peas, Green, Frozen Cooked (1 Cup)	74	26	0	124
Pecan Pie (1 Piece)	47	5	48	600
Pecans, Halves (1 Cup)	10	4	85	769
Pepper-Type Soda (12 Fl Oz)	100	0	0	164
Peppers, Hot Chili, Raw, Green (1 Pepper)	80	20	0	20
Peppers, Sweet, Cooked, Green (1 Pepper)	100	0	0	12
Peppers, Sweet, Raw, Green (1 Pepper)	80	20	0	20
Pickles, Cucumber, Dill (1 Pickle)	100	0	0	4
Pine Nuts (1 Oz)	11	6	83	185
Pineapple Juice, Canned, Unsweetened (1 Cup)	97	3	0	140
Pineapple, Canned, Juice Pack (1 Cup)	98	3	0	160
Pineapple, Raw, Diced (1 Cup)	85	4	10	89
Pineapple-Grapefruit Juice Drink (6 Fl Oz)	100	0	0	92
Pinto Beans, Dry, Cooked (1 Cup)	74	23	3	265
Pistachio Nuts (1 Oz)	16	13	71	178
Pita Bread (1 Pita)	80	15	5	165
Pizza, Cheese (1 Slice)	53	20	27	297
Plums, Canned, Juice Pack (1 Cup)	97	3	0	156
Plums, Raw (1 Medium Plum)	100	0	0	16
Popcorn, Air Popped (1 Cup)	86	14	0	28
Popsicle (1 Popsicle)	100	0	0	72
Pork Chop, Loin, Broiled, Lean (2.5 Oz)	0	56	44	164
Pork Fresh Ham, Roasted, Lean (2.5 Oz)	0	53	47	152
Pork, Cured, Bacon, Regular, Cooked (3 Slices)	0	23	77	105
Pork, Cured, Canadian Bacon (2 Slices)	5	52	43	84
Pork, Link, Cooked (1 Link)	0	25	75	48
Pork, Luncheon Meat, Cooked Ham, Lean (2 Slices)	5	59	36	75
Potato Chips (10 Chips)	37	4	59	107
Potato Salad Made w/Mayonnaise (1 Cup)	34	9	57	329
Potatoes, Au Gratin (1 Cup)	34	15	52	331
Potatoes, Baked With Skin (1 Potato)	91	9	0	224
Potatoes, Boiled And Peeled (1 Potato)	90	10	0	120
Potatoes, Mashed With Milk (1 Cup)	86	9	5	173
Potatoes, Scalloped (1 Cup)	49	13	38	213
Potatoes, French Fried, Frozen, Oven Cooked (10 Strips)	61	7	32	112
Pound Cake, From Home Recipe (1 Slice)	53	7	40	113
Pretzels, Stick (10 Pretzels)	100	0	0	8

(continued)

Energy Distribution of Foods Commonly Consumed, in Alphabetical Order *(continued)*

Food description and common serving amount	Carb %	Prot %	Fat %	Calories
Pretzels, Twisted, Dutch (1 Pretzel)	75	12	13	69
Product 19 Cereal (1 Oz)	89	11	0	108
Provolone Cheese (1 Oz)	4	27	69	104
Prune Juice, Canned (1 Cup)	96	4	0	188
Prunes, Dried (5 Large)	97	3	0	128
Pudding, Choc, Cooked From Mix (1/2 Cup)	66	11	24	152
Pudding, Chocolate, Canned (5 Oz)	52	5	43	231
Pudding, Rice, From Mix (1/2 Cup)	68	10	23	160
Pudding, Tapioca, From Mix (1/2 Cup)	66	11	24	152
Pudding, Vanilla, Canned (5 Oz)	57	3	39	230
Pudding, Vanilla, From Mix (1/2 Cup)	66	11	24	152
Pudding, Vanilla, Instant From Mix (1/2 Cup)	68	10	23	160
Pumpernickel Bread (1 Slice)	75	14	11	85
Pumpkin And Squash Kernels (1 Oz)	12	17	71	165
Pumpkin Pie (1 Piece)	46	7	47	325
Quiche Lorraine (1 Slice)	19	9	72	600
Radishes, Raw (4 Radishes)	100	0	0	4
Raisin Bran, Kellogg (1 Oz)	80	11	9	105
Raisin Bran, Post (1 Oz)	80	11	9	105
Raisin Bread (1 Slice)	75	12	13	69
Raisins (1 Cup)	94	4	2	489
Raspberries, Raw (1 Cup)	81	6	13	69
Red Kidney Beans, Dry, Canned (1 Cup)	71	25	4	237
Refried Beans, Canned (1 Cup)	67	24	9	303
Relish, Sweet (1 Tablespoon)	100	0	0	20
Rice Krispies Cereal (1 Oz)	93	7	0	108
Rice, Brown, Cooked (1 Cup)	87	9	4	229
Rice, White, Cooked (1 Cup)	93	7	0	216
Ricotta Cheese, Part Skim Milk (1 Cup)	16	33	51	335
Roast Beef Sandwich (1 Sandwich)	40	26	34	341
Rolls, Dinner, Commercial (1 Roll)	68	10	22	82
Rolls, Dinner, Home Recipe (1 Roll)	67	10	23	119
Rolls, Frankfurter + Hamburger (1 Roll)	73	11	16	110
Rolls, Hard (1 Roll)	76	13	11	158
Rolls, Hoagie Or Submarine (1 Roll)	71	11	18	404
Root Beer (12 Fl Oz)	100	0	0	168

Food description and common serving amount	Carb %	Prot %	Fat %	Calories
Rye Bread, Light (1 Slice)	74	12	14	65
Rye Wafers, Whole Grain (2 Wafers)	75	8	17	53
Safflower Oil (1 Tablespoon)	0	0	100	126
Salami, Cooked Type (2 Slices)	3	24	73	135
Salmon, Baked, Red (3 Oz)	0	65	35	129
Salmon, Canned, Pink, w/Bones (3 Oz)	0	60	40	113
Salmon, Smoked (3 Oz)	0	50	50	144
Saltines (4 Crackers)	73	8	18	49
Sandwich Spread, Pork, Beef (1 Tablespoon)	21	10	69	39
Sandwich-Type Cookie (4 Cookies)	59	4	37	196
Sardines, Canned In Oil (3 Oz)	0	50	50	161
Sauerkraut, Canned (1 Cup)	83	17	0	48
Scallops, Breaded, Frozen, Reheat (6 Scallops)	21	32	47	190
Semisweet Chocolate (1 Cup)	40	3	57	965
Sesame Seeds (1 Tablespoon)	8	17	75	48
Shakes, Thick, Chocolate (10 Oz)	69	10	21	348
Shakes, Thick, Vanilla (10 Oz)	62	14	25	325
Sheetcake, With Frosting (1 Piece)	68	4	28	450
Sherbet, 2% Fat (1 Cup)	84	3	13	280
Shortbread Cookies (2 Cookies)	46	5	49	148
Shredded-Wheat Cereal (1 Oz)	81	11	8	113
Shrimp, Canned, Drained (3 Oz)	4	87	9	97
Shrimp, French Fried (3 Oz)	22	32	45	198
Snack Cakes, Devils Food, Creame Filled (Small Cake)	63	4	33	108
Snack-Type Crackers (1 Cracker)	47	0	53	17
Snap Bean, Cooked, Green (1 Cup)	83	17	0	48
Sour Cream (1 Tablespoon)	13	0	87	31
Soy Sauce (1 Tablespoon)	50	50	0	16
Soybeans, Dry, Cooked (1 Cup)	31	33	37	246
Spaghetti With Meatballs And Tomato Sauce (1 Cup)	46	22	32	340
Spaghetti, Cooked, Firm (1 Cup)	81	15	5	193
Spaghetti, Cooked, Tender (1 Cup)	82	13	6	157
Special K Cereal (1 Oz)	78	22	0	108
Spinach Souffle (1 Cup)	6	20	74	218
Spinach, Cooked From Raw (1 Cup)	58	42	0	48
Spinach, Raw (1 Cup)	50	50	0	16
Squash, Summer, Cooked, Drained (1 Cup)	65	16	18	49

(continued)

Energy Distribution of Foods Commonly Consumed, in Alphabetical Order *(continued)*

Food description and common serving amount	Carb %	Prot %	Fat %	Calories
Strawberries, Raw (1 Cup)	75	8	17	53
Sugar Cookies (4 Cookies)	52	3	45	240
Sugar Frosted Flakes, Kellogg (1 Oz)	96	4	0	108
Sugar Smacks Cereal (1 Oz)	85	7	8	117
Sugar, White, Granulated (1 Tablespoon)	100	0	0	48
Sunflower Oil (1 Tablespoon)	0	0	100	126
Sunflower Seeds (1 Oz)	12	14	74	170
Super Sugar Crisp Cereal (1 Oz)	93	7	0	112
Sweet (Dark) Chocolate (1 Oz)	41	3	57	158
Sweetened Condensed Milk (1 Cup)	66	10	24	1003
Sweet Potatoes, Baked, Peeled (1 Potato)	93	7	0	120
Swiss Cheese (1 Oz)	4	30	67	108
Syrup, Chocolate Flavored, Fudge (2 Tablespoons)	61	6	33	137
Table Syrup (Corn And Maple) (2 Tablespoons)	100	0	0	128
Taco (1 Taco)	31	18	51	195
Tahini (1 Tablespoon)	13	13	75	96
Tangerines, Raw (1 Fruit)	90	10	0	40
Tartar Sauce (1 Tablespoon)	5	0	95	76
Tea, Instant, Prepared, Unsweetened (8 Fl Oz)	100	0	0	4
Tea, Instant, Prepared, Sweetened (8 Fl Oz)	100	0	0	88
Tofu (1 Piece)	13	39	48	93
Tomato Juice, Canned With Salt (1 Cup)	83	17	0	48
Tomato Sauce, Canned With Salt (1 Cup)	86	14	0	84
Tomato Soup w/Water, Canned (1 Cup)	72	9	19	94
Tomato Soup With Milk, Canned (1 Cup)	53	14	33	166
Tomatoes, Raw (1 Tomato)	83	17	0	24
Tortillas, Corn (1 Tortilla)	75	12	13	69
Total Cereal (1 Oz)	81	11	8	109
Trix Cereal (1 Oz)	93	7	0	108
Trout, Broiled, w/Butter And Lemon Juice (3 Oz)	0	51	49	165
Tuna Salad (1 Cup)	20	35	45	379
Tuna, Canned In Oil, (3 Oz)	0	60	40	159
Tuna, Canned In Water (3 Oz)	0	93	7	129
Turkey, Roasted, Dark Meat (4 Pieces)	0	64	36	150
Turkey, Roasted, Light Meat (2 Pieces)	0	79	21	127
Turnip Greens, Cooked From Raw (1 Cup)	75	25	0	32

Food description and common serving amount	Carb %	Prot %	Fat %	Calories
Vanilla Wafers (10 Cookies)	62	4	34	187
Veal Cutlet, Med Fat, Braised, Broiled (3 Oz)	0	53	47	173
Vegetable Beef Soup, Canned (1 Cup)	49	29	22	82
Vegetable Juice Cocktail, Canned (1 Cup)	85	15	0	52
Vegetarian Soup, Canned (1 Cup)	65	11	24	74
Vienna Bread (1 Slice)	75	12	13	69
Vienna Sausage (1 Sausage)	0	18	82	44
Vinegar And Oil Salad Dressing (1 Tablespoon)	0	0	100	72
Waffles (1 Waffle)	52	13	35	208
Walnuts, Black, Chopped (1 Cup)	7	15	78	819
Watermelon, Raw (1 Piece)	82	7	11	170
Wheat Bread (1 Slice)	74	12	14	65
Wheat Bread, Toasted (1 Slice)	70	17	13	69
Wheat Thin Crackers (4 Crackers)	61	12	27	33
Wheaties Cereal (1 Oz)	88	12	0	104
Whipped Topping, Pressurized (1 Tablespoon)	0	0	100	9
Whipping Cream, Unwhipped, Heavy (1 Tablespoon)	0	0	100	54
Whipping Cream, Unwhipped, Light (1 Tablespoon)	0	0	100	45
White Bread (1 Slice)	74	12	14	65
White Cake With White Frosting (1 Piece)	64	5	31	261
White Sauce w/Milk From Mix (1 Cup)	35	17	49	241
White Sauce, Medium, Home Recipe (1 Cup)	24	10	67	406
Whole-Wheat Bread (1 Slice)	71	16	12	73
Whole-Wheat Wafers, Crackers (2 Crackers)	48	10	43	42
Yellow Cake With Chocolate Frosting (1 Piece)	66	5	30	244
Yellow Cake With Chocolate Frosting (1 Piece)	59	3	38	263
Yogurt, w/Low-Fat Milk, Plain (8 Oz)	43	32	24	148
Yogurt, w/Nonfat Milk (8 Oz)	57	43	0	120
Yogurt, With Low-Fat Milk, Fruit Flavored (8 Oz)	75	17	8	230

(Source: USDA Home and Garden Bulletin #72)

Endnotes

Chapter 1

1   Willett, W.C. 1994. Diet and health: What should we eat? *Science* 264:532-537.
2   Meredith, C.N., Zackin, M.J., Frontera, W.R., and Evans, W.J. 1989. Dietary protein requirements and body protein metabolism in endurance-trained men. *J. Appl. Phys.* 66(6):2850-2856.
3   Butterfield, G.E., and Calloway, D.H. 1984. Physical activity improves protein utilization in young men. *Br. J. Nutr.* 51:171-184.
4   Butterfield, G., Cady, C., and Moynihan, S. 1992. Effect of increasing protein intake on nitrogen balance in recreational weight lifters. *Med. Sci. Sport Exer.* 24:S71 (abstr).
5   Tarnopolsky, M.A., MacDougall, J.D., and Atkinson, S.A. 1988. Influence of protein intake and training status on nitrogen balance and lean body mass. *J. Appl. Phys.* 64(1):187-193.
6   Kaufmann, D.A. 1990. Protein as an energy substrate during intense exercise. *Ann. Sports Med.* 5:142.
7   Bach, A.S., and Babayan, V.K. 1982. Medium-chain triglycerides: An update. *Am. J. Clin. Nutr.* 36:950.
8   Seaton, T.B., Welle, S.L., Warenko, M.K., and Campbell, R.G. 1986. Thermic effect of medium-chain and long-chain triglycerides in man. *Am. J. Clin. Nutr.* 44:630.
9   Geliebter, A., Torbay, N., Bracco, E.F., Hashim, S.A., and van Itallie, T.B. 1983. Overfeeding with medium-chain triglyceride diet results in diminished deposition of fat. *Am. J. Clin. Nutr.* 37:1.
10   Scalfi, L., Coltorti, A., and Contaldo, F. 1991. Postprandial thermogenesis in lean and obese subjects after meals supplemented with medium-chain and long-chain triglycerides. *Am. J. Clin. Nutr.* 53:1130.
11   Katan, M.B. 1995. Fish and heart disease: What is the real story? *Nutr. Revs.* 53:228-230.
12   Bucci, L. 1993. *Nutrients as ergogenic aids for sports and exercise.* Boca Raton, FL: CRC Press, 20.
13   Simopoulos, A.P. 1991. Omega-3 fatty acids in health and disease and in growth and development. *Am. J. Clin. Nutr.* 54:438.
14   Brilla, L.R., and Landerholm, T.E. 1990. Effect of fish oil supplementation and exercise on serum lipids and aerobic fitness. *J. Sports Med.* 30 (2):173.
15   Bucci, L. 1993. *Nutrients as ergogenic aids for sports and exercise.* Boca Raton, FL: CRC Press, 19-20.
16   Williams, M.H. 1985. Drug foods: Alcohol and caffeine. In *Nutritional Aspects of Human Physical and Athletic Performance,* 2nd ed., Springfield, IL: Charles C Thomas, 272.
16a   Robinson, C.H., Lawler, M.R., Chenoweth, W.L., and Garwick, A.E. 1986. *Normal and therapeutic nutrition,* 17th ed. New York, NY: MacMillan Publishing Company, 152-153; 169; 198-199.
17   Belko, A.Z., Obarzanek, E., Kalkwarf, J.H., Rotter, M.A., Bogusz, S., Miller, D., Haas, J.D., and Roe, D.A. 1983. Effects of exercise on riboflavin requirements of young women. *Am. J. Clin. Nutr.* 37:509-517.
18   Belko, A.Z., Obarzanek, M.P., Rotter, B.S., Urgan, G., Weinberg, S., and Roe, D.A. 1984. Effects of aerobic exercise and weight loss on riboflavin requirements of moderately obese, marginally deficient young women. *Am. J. Clin. Nutr.* 40:553.
19   Belko, A.Z., Meredith, M.P., Kalkwarf, H.J., Obarzanek, E., Weinberg, S., Roach, R., McKeon, G., and Roe, D.A. 1985. Effects of exercise on riboflavin requirements: Biological validation in weight-reducing young women. *Am. J. Clin. Nutr.* 41:270.

20 Tremblay, A., Boiland, F., Breton, M., Bessette, H., and Roberge, A.G. 1984. The effects of a riboflavin supplementation on the nutritional status and performance of elite swimmers. *Nutr. Res.* 4:201.

21 Carlson, L.A., Havel, R.J., Ekelund, L.G., and Holmgren, A. 1963. Effect of nicotinic acid on the turnover rate and oxidation of the free fatty acids of plasma in man during exercise. *Metab. Clin. Exp.* 12:837.

22 Bergstrom, J., Hultman, E., Jorfeldt, L., Pernow, B., and Wahnen, J. 1969. Effect of nicotinic acid on physical working capacity and on metabolism of muscle. *J. Appl. Physiol.* 26:170.

23 Hilsendager, D., and Karpovich, P.V. 1964. Ergogenic effect of glycine and niacin separately and in combination. *Res. Q.* 35:389.

24 National Research Council. 1989. *Recommended Dietary Allowances*, 10th ed. Washington, DC: National Academy of Sciences.

25 Dalton, K., and Dalton, M.J.T. 1987. Characteristics of pyridoxine overdose neuropathy syndrome. *Acta. Neurol. Scand.* 76:8-11.

26 Schaumberg, H., Kaplan, J., Windebank, A., Vick, N., Ragmus, S., Pleasure, D., and Brown, M.J. 1983. Sensory neuropathy from pyridoxine abuse. *New Engl. J. Med.* 309:445-448.

27 Manore, M.M. 1994. Vitamin B-6 and exercise. *Int. J. Sport Nutr.* 4:89-103.

28 Fogelholm, M., Ruokonen I., Laakso, J.T., Vuorimaa, T., and Himberg, J.J. 1993. Lack of association between indices of vitamin B-1, B-2, and B-6 status and exercise-induced blood lactate in young adults. *Int. J. Sport Nutr.* 3:165-176.

29 Guilland, J.C., Penarand, T., Gallet, C., Boggio, V., Fuchs, F., and Klepping, J. 1989. Vitamin status of young athletes including the effects of supplementation. *Med. Sci. Sports Exerc.* 21:441-449.

30 Telford, R.D., Catchpole, E.A., Deakin, V., McLeay, A.C., and Plank, A.W. 1992. The effect of 7 to 8 months of vitamin/mineral supplementation on the vitamin and mineral status of athletes. *Int. J. Sport Nutr.* 2:123-134.

31 Suboticanec, K., Stavljenic, A., Schalch, W., and Buzina, R. 1990. Effects of pyridoxine and riboflavin supplementation of physical fitness in young adolescents. *Int. J. Vit. Nutr. Res.* 60:81-88.

32 Delitala, G., Masala, A., Alagna, S., and Devilla, L. 1976. Effect of pyridoxine on human hypophyseal trophic hormone release: A possible stimulation of hypthalamic dopaminergic pathway. *J. Clin. Endocr. Metab.* 42:603-606.

33 Dunton, N., Virk, R., Young, J., Leklem, J. 1992. Effect of vitamin B-6 supplementation and exhaustive exercise on vitamin B-6 metabolism and growth hormone. [Abstract]. *FASEB Journal* 6:A1374.

34 Moretti, C., Fabbri, A., Gnessi, L., Bonifacio, V., Fraioli, F., and Isidori, A. 1982. Pyridoxine (B6) suppresses the rise in prolactin and increases the rise in growth hormone induced by exercise. *New Engl. J. Med.* 307 (7):444-445.

35 Manore, M.M. 1994. Vitamin B-6 and exercise. *Int. J. Sport Nutr.* 4:89-103.

36 Dreon, D.M., and Butterfield, G.E. 1986. Vitamin B-6 utilization in active and inactive young men. *Am. J. Clin. Nutr.* 43:816-824.

37 Rokitzki, L., Sagredos, A.N., F., Büchner, M., and Keul, J. 1994. Acute changes in vitamin B-6 status in endurance athletes before and after a marathon. *Int. J. Sport Nutr.* 4:154-165.

38 Albert, M.J., Mathan, V.I., and Baker, S.J. 1980. Vitamin B-12 synthesis by human small intestinal bacteria. *Nature* 283:781-782.

39 Ryan, A. 1977. Nutritional practices in athletics abroad. *Physician Sports Med.* 5:33.

40 U.S. Senate. 1973. *Proper and improper use of drugs by athletes*. June 18 and July 12-13. Hearing Washington, DC: U.S. Government Printing Office.

41 Montoye, H.J., Spata, P.J., Pincney, V., and Barron, L. 1955. Effects of vitamin B-12 supplementation on physical fitness and growth of young boys. *J. Appl. Physiol.* 7:589.

42 Tin-May Than Ma-Win-May, Khin-Sann-Aung, and Mya-Tu, M. 1978. The effect of vitamin B-12 on physical performance capacity. *Br. J. Nutr.* 40:269.

43 Read, M., and McGuffin, S. 1983. The effect of B-complex supplementation on endurance performance. *J. Sports Med. Phys. Fitness* 23:178.

44   National Research Council. 1989. *Recommended Dietary Allowances*, 10th ed. Washington, DC: National Academy of Sciences.

45   McNulty, H. 1995. Folate requirements for health in different population groups. *Br. J. Biomed. Sci.* 52:110-112.

46   Baily, L.B. 1995. Folate requirements and dietary recommendations. *Folate in health and disease*, ed. Baily, L.B. New York: Marcel Dekker, 123.

47   Matter, M., Stittfall, T., Graves, J., Myburgh, K., Adams, B., Jacobs, P., and Noakes, T.D. 1987. The effect of iron and folate therapy on maximal exercise performance in female marathon runners with iron and folate deficiency. *Clin. Sci.* 72Z:415-420.

48   Weight, L.M., Noakes, T.D., Labadarios, D., Graves, J., Jacobs, P., and Berman, P.A. 1988. Vitamin and mineral status of trained athletes including the effects of supplementation. *Am. J. Clin. Nutr.* 47:186-192.

49   National Research Council. 1989. *Recommended Dietary Allowances*, 10th ed. Washington, DC: National Academy of Sciences.

50   Shock, N.W., and Sebrell, W.H. 1944. The effects of changes in concentration of pantothenate on the work output of perfused frog muscles. *Am. J. Physiol.* 142: 274.

51   Bialecki, M. and Nijakowski, F. 1967. Behavior of pantothenic acid in tissues and blood of white rats following short and prolonged physical strain. *Acta. Physiol. Pol.* 18:25.

52   Nice, C., Reeves, A.G., Brinck-Hohnsen, T., and Noll, W. 1984. The effects of pantothenic acid on human exercise capacity. *J. Sports Med.* 24:26.

53   Litoff, D., Scherzer, H., and Harrison, J. 1985. Effects of pantothenic acid on human exercise. *Med. Sci. Sports Exerc.* 17:287.

54   National Research Council. 1989. *Recommended Dietary Allowances*, 10th ed. Washington, DC: National Academy of Sciences.

55   National Research Council. 1989. *Recommended Dietary Allowances*, 10th ed. Washington, DC: National Academy of Sciences.

56   Hickson, J.F., and Wolinsky, I., eds. 1989. *Nutrition in exercise and sport*. Boca Raton, FL: CRC Press, 121.

57   Bramich, K., and McNaughton, L. 1987. The effects of two levels of ascorbic acid on muscular endurance, muscular strength, and on $\dot{V}O_2$max. *Int. Clin. Nutr. Rev.* 7:5.

58   Schwartz, P.L. 1970. Ascorbic acid in wound healing: A review. *J. Am. Diet. Assoc.* 56:497.

59   Kanter, M.M. 1994. Free radicals, exercise, and antioxidant supplementation. *Int. J. Sport Nutr.* 4:205-220.

60   Herbert, V. 1993. Does mega-C do more good than harm, or more harm than good? *Nutr. Today* Jan/Feb:28-32.

61   Wald, G., Brouha, L., and Johnson, R. 1942. Experimental human vitamin A deficiency and ability to perform muscular exercise. *Am. J. Physiol.* 137:551.

61a   Murray, R., and Horsun II, C.A. 1998. Nutrient requirements for competitive sports. In *Nutrition in Exercise and Sport*, 3rd ed., ed. Ira Wolinsky. Boca Raton, FL: CRC Press, 550.

62   Barr, S.I., Prior, J.C., and Vigna, Y.M. 1994. Restrained eating and ovulatory disturbances: Possible implications for bone health. *Am. J. Clin. Nutr.* 59:92-97.

63   Chesnut, C.H. 1991. Theoretical overview: Bone development, peak bone mass, bone loss, and fracture risk. *Am. J. Medicine* 91(Suppl 5B):2-4.

64   Heaney, R.P. 1991. Effect of calcium on skeletal development, bone loss, and risk of fractures. *Am. J. Medicine* 91(Suppl 5B):23-28.

65   Benardot, D. 1997. Unpublished data from USOC research project on national team gymnasts. Laboratory for Elite Athlete Performance.

66   Talbot, D., and Jamieson, J. 1977. An examination of the effect of vitamin E on the performance of highly trained swimmers. *Can. J. Appl. Sport Sci.* 2:67.

67   Bunnell, R.H., DeRitter, E., and Rubin, S.H. 1975. Effect of feeding polyunsaturated fatty acids with a low vitamin E diet on blood levels of tocopherol in men performing hard physical labor. *Am. J. Clin. Nutr.* 28:706.

68   Sharman, I.M., Down, M.G., and Sen, R.N. 1971. The effect of vitamin E and training on physiological function and athletic performance in adolescent swimmers. *Br. J. Nutr.* 26:265.

69   Sharman, I.M., Down, M.B., and Norgan, N.G. 1976. The effects of vitamin E on physiological function and athletic performance of trained swimmers. *J. Sports Med.* 16:215.

70   Brady, P.S., Brady, L.J., and Ullrey, D.E. 1979. Selenium, vitamin E, and the response to swimming stress in the rat. *J. Nutr.* 109:1103.

71   Dillard, C.J., Liton, R.E., Savin, W.M., Dumelin, E.E., and Tappel, A.L. 1978. Effects of exercise, vitamin E, and ozone on pulmonary function and lipid peroxidation. *J. Appl. Physiol.* 45:927.

72   Shephard, R.J., Campbell, R., Pimm, P., Stuart, D., and Wright, G.R. 1974. Vitamin E, exercise, and the recovery from physical activity. *J. Appl. Physiol.* 33:119-126.

73   Lukaski, H.C. 1995. Micronutrients (magnesium, zinc, and copper): Are mineral supplements needed for athletes? *Int. J. Sport Nutr.* 5:S74-S83.

74   Benardot, D. 1999. Nutrition for gymnasts. *The Athlete Wellness Book*, ed. Marshall, N.T. Indianapolis, IN: USA Gymnastics, 12-13.

75   Lotz, M., Zisman, E., and Bartter, F.C. 1968. Evidence for a phosphorus-depletion syndrome in man. *New Engl. J. Med.* 278:409-415.

76   National Research Council. 1989. *Recommended Dietary Allowances*, 10th ed. Washington, DC: National Academy of Sciences.

77   Bucci, L. 1993. *Nutrients as ergogenic aids for sports and exercise*. Boca Raton, FL: CRC Press.

78   Keller, W.D., and Kraut, H.A. 1959. Work and nutrition. *World Rev. Nutr. Diet* 3:65.

79   Cade, R., Conte, M., Zauner, C., Mars, D., Peterson, J., Lunne, D., Hommen, N., and Packer, D. 1984. Effects of phosphate loading on 2,3-diphosphoglycerate and maximal oxygen uptake. *Med. Sci. Sports Exerc.* 12:263.

80   Duffy, D.J., and Conlee, R.K. 1986. Effects of phosphate loading on leg power and high intensity treadmill exercise. *Med. Sci. Sports Exerc.* 18:674.

81   Shils, M.E. Magnesium. 1993. *Modern nutrition in health and disease*, 8th ed., ed. Shils, M.E., Olson, J.A., and Shike, M., Philadelphia: Lea & Febiger, 164-184.

82   Steinacker, J.M., Grunert-Fuchs, M., Steininger, K., and Wodick, R.E. 1987. Effects of long-time administration of magnesium on physical capacity. *Int. J. Sports Med.* 8:151.

83   Golf, S.W., Bohmer, D., and Nowacki, P.E. 1993. Is magnesium a limiting factor in competitive exercise? A summary of relevant scientific data. In *Magnesium*, ed. Golf, S., Dralle, D., and Vecchiet, L., 209-220. London: John Libbey.

84   Brilla, L.R., and Haley, T.F. 1992. Effect of magnesium supplementation on strength training in humans. *J. Am. Coll. Nutr.* 11:326-329.

85   Hickson, J.F., Schrader, J., and Trischler, L.C. 1986. Dietary intake of female basketall and gymnastics athletes. *J. Am. Diet. Assoc.* 86:251-254.

86   Lukaski, H.C. 1995. Prevention and treatment of magnesium deficiency in athletes. In *Magnesium and physical activity*, ed. Vecchiet, L., 211-226. Carnforth, UK: Parthenon.

87   National Research Council. 1989. *Recommended Dietary Allowances*, 10th ed. Washington, DC: National Academy of Sciences.

88   Pivarnik, J.M. Water and electrolytes during exercise 1989. In *Nutrition in exercise and sport*, ed. Hickson, J.F., and Wolinsky, I. Boca Raton, FL: CRC Press, 185-200.

89   National Research Council. 1989. *Recommended Dietary Allowances*, 10th ed. Washington, DC: National Academy of Sciences.

90   National Research Council. 1989. *Recommended Dietary Allowances*, 10th ed. Washington, DC: National Academy of Sciences.

91   National Research Council. 1989. *Recommended Dietary Allowances*, 10th ed. Washington, DC: National Academy of Sciences.

92   Pivarnik, J.M. 1989. Water and electrolytes during exercise. In *Nutrition in exercise and sport*, ed. Hickson J.F., and Wolinsky, I. Boca Raton: CRC Press. 185-200.87   Clarkson, P. 1991. Vitamins, iron, and trace minerals. In *Ergogenics: Enhancement of performance in exercise and sport*, ed. Lamb, D., and Williams, M. Indianapolis, IN: Benchmark Press.

93   Clarkson, P. 1991. Vitamins, iron, and trace minerals. In *Ergogenics Enhancement of performance in exercise and sport*, ed. Lamb, D., and Williams, M. Indianapolis, IN: Benchmark Press.

94   Aruoma, O.I., Reilly, T., MacLauren, D., and Halliwell, B. 1988. Iron, copper, and zinc concentrations in human sweat and plasma: The effect of exercise. *Clinic. Chim. Acta* 177: 81-87.
95   Wolinsky, I., and Driskell, J.A. 1997. *Sports nutrition: Vitamins and trace elements*. Boca Raton, FL: CRC Press, 148.
96   Bucci, L. 1993. *Nutrients as ergogenic aids for sports and exercise*. Boca Raton, FL: CRC Press.
97   Stephenson, L.S. 1995. Possible new developments in community control of iron-deficiency anemia. *Nutrition Reviews* 53(2):23-30.
98   Dressendorfer, R.H., and Sockolov, R. 1980. Hypozincemia in runners. *Physician Sports Med.* 8:97-100.
99   Haralambie, G. 1981. Serum zinc in athletes during training. *Int. J. Sports Med.* 2:135-138.
100 Singh, A., Deuster, P.A., and Moser, P.B. 1990. Zinc and copper status of women by physical activity and menstrual status. *J. Sports Med. Phys. Fitness* 30:29-35.
101 Krotkiewski, M., Gudmundsson, M., Backstrom, P., and Mandroukas, K. 1982. Zinc and muscle strength and endurance. *Acta Physiol. Scand.* 116:309-311.
102 Fischer, P.W.F., Giroux, A. and L'Abbe, M.R. 1984. Effect of zinc supplementation on copper status in adult man. *Am. J. Clin. Nutr.* 40:743-746.
103 Hooper, P.L., Visconti, L., Garry, P.J., and Johnson, G.E. 1980. Zinc lowers high-density lipoprotein cholesterol levels. *JAMA* 244:1960-1961.
104 Spencer, H. 1986. Minerals and mineral interactions in human beings. *J. Am. Diet. Assoc.* 86:864-867.
105 Zamora, A.J., Tessier, F., Marconnet, P., Margaritis, I., and Marini, J.F. Mitochondria changes in human muscle after prolonged exercise, endurance training, and selenium supplementation. *Eur. J. Appl. Physiol.* 71(6):505-511.
106 Bucci, L. 1993. *Nutrients as ergogenic aids for sports and exercise*. Boca Raton, FL: CRC Press.
107 Tessier, F., Margaritis, I., Richard, M.-J., Moynot, C., and Marconnet, P. 1995. Selenium and training effects on the glutathione system and aerobic performance. *Med. Sci. Sports Exerc.* 27 (3):390-396.
108 Lukaski, H.C. 1995. Micronutrients (magnesium, zinc, and copper): Are mineral supplements needed for athletes? *Int. J. Sports Med.* 5:S74-S83.
109 Lukaski, H.C., Hoverson, B.S., Gallagher, S.K., and Bolonchuk, W.W. 1990. Physical training and copper, iron, and zinc status of swimmers. *Am. J. Clin. Nutr.* 53:1093-1099.
110 Wolinsky, I., and Driskell, J.A. 1997. *Sports nutrition: Vitamins and trace elements*. Boca Raton, FL: CRC Press.
111 Wolinsky, I., and Driskell, J.A. 1997. *Sports nutrition: Vitamins and trace elements*. Boca Raton, FL: CRC Press.
112 Evans, G.W. 1989. The effect of chromium picolinate on insulin controlled parameters in humans. *Int. J. Biosocial Res.* 11:163.
113 Clancy, S.P., Clarkson, P.M., DeCheke, M.E., Nosaka, K., Freedson, P.S., Cunningham, J.J., and Valentine, J.J. 1994. Effects of chromium picolinate supplementation on body composition, strength, and urinary chromium loss in football players. *Int. J. Sport Nutr.* 4:142.
114 Hasten, D.L., Rome, E.P., Franks, B.D., and Hegsted, M. 1992. Effects of chromium picolinate on beginning weight training students. *Int. J. Sport Nutr.* 2:343.
115 Stearns, D., Wise, J., Paterno, S., and Wetterhahn. 1995. Chromium (III) picolinate produces chromosome damage in Chinese hamster ovary cells. *FASEB J* 9:1643-8.

Chapter 2

1   Williams, M.H. 1999. *Nutrition for health, fitness and sport*, 5th ed. New York, NY: WCB McGraw-Hill, 276-277; 285-287; 292-293; 317-318.
2   Rehrer, N.J. 1996. Factors influencing fluid bioavailability. *Aust. J. Nutr. Diet* 53 (4 Suppl):S8-S12.
3   Hubbard, R.W., Szlyk, P.C., and Armstrong, L.E. 1990. Influence of thirst and fluid palatability on fluid ingestion during exercise. In *Fluid homeostasis during exercise*, ed. Gisolfi, C.V., Lamb, D.R., 39-95. Carmel, IN: Benchmark Press.

4   Davis, J.M., Burgess, W.A., Slentz, C.A., Bartoli, W.P., and Pate, R.R. 1988. Effects of ingesting 6% and 12% glucose-electrolyte beverages during prolonged intermittent cycling in the heat. *Eur. J. Appl. Physiol.* 57:563-569.

5   Rehrer, J.N., Beckers, E.J., Brouns, F., ten Hoor, F., and Saris, W.H.M. 1989. Exercise and training effects on gastric emptying of carbohydrate beverages. *Med. Sci. Sports Exerc.* 21:540-549.

6   Rehrer, J.N., Brouns, F., Beckers, E.J., and Saris, W.H.M. 1994. The influence of beverage composition and gastrointestinal function on fluid and nutrient availability during exercise. *Scand. J. Med. Sci. Sports* 4:159-172.

7   Noakes, T.D., Rehrer, N.J., and Maughan, R.J. 1991. The importance of volume-regulating gastric emptying. *Med. Sci. Sports Exerc.* 23:307-313.

8   Sun, W.M., Houghton, L.A., Read, N.W., Grundy, D.G., and Johnson, A.G. 1988. Effect of meal temperature on gastric emptying of liquids in man. *Gut* 29:302-305.

9   Costill, D.L., and Saltin, B. 1974. Factors limiting gastric emptying. *J. Appl. Physiol.* 37:679-683.

10   Ryan, A.J., Navarne, A.E., and Gisolfi, C.V. 1991. Consumption of carbonated and noncarbonated sports drinks during prolonged treadmill exercise in the heat. *Int. J. Sport Nutr.* 1:225-239.

11   Lambert, G.P., Bleiter, T.L., Chang, R., Johnson, A.K., and Gisolf, C.V. 1993. Effects of carbonated and noncarbonated beverages at specific intervals during treadmill running in the heat. *Int. J. Sport Nutr.* 3:177-193.

12   Rehrer, J.N., Brouns, F., Beckers, E.J., and Saris, W.H.M. 1994. The influence of beverage composition and gastrointestinal function on fluid and nutrient availability during exercise. *Scand. J. Med. Sci. Sports* 4:159-172.

13   Wolf, S. The psyche and the stomach. 1981. *Gastroenterology* 80:605-614.

14   Rehrer, N.J. 1996. Factors influencing fluid bioavailability. *Aust. J. Nutr. Diet* 53 (4 Suppl):S8-S12.

15   Rehrer, N.J. 1996. Factors influencing fluid bioavailability. *Aust. J. Nutr. Diet* 53 (4 Suppl):S8-S12.

16   Gisolfi, C.V., Summers, R., and Schedl, H. 1990. Intestinal absorption of fluids during rest and exercise. In *Fluid homeostasis during exercise,* ed. Gisolfi, C.V., Lamb, D.R., 39-95. Carmel, IN: Benchmark Press.

17   Maughan, R.J., and Noakes, T.D. 1991. Fluid replacement and exercise stress. A brief review of studies on fluid replacement and some guidelines for the athlete. *Sports Med.* 12:16-31.

18   Hargreaves, M. 1996. Physiological benefits of fluid and energy replacement during exercise. *Aust. J. Nutr. Diet* 53 (4 Suppl):S3-S7.

19   Burke, L.M. 1996. Rehydration strategies before and after exercise. *Aust. J. Nutr. Diet* 53 (4 Suppl): S22-S26.

20   Nadel, E.R., Mack, G.W., and Nose, H. 1990. Influence of fluid replacement beverages on body fluid homeostasis during exercise and recovery. In *Fluid homeostasis during exercise,* ed. Gisolfi, C.V., and Lamb, D.R., vol. 3, *Perspectives in exercise science and sports med.,* 181-205. Carmel, IN: Benchmark Press.

21   Kristal-Boneh, E., Glusman, J.G., Shitrit, R., Chaemovitz, C., and Cassuto, Y. 1995. Physical performance and heat tolerance after chronic water loading and heat acclimation. *Aviat. Space Environ. Med.* 66:733-738.

22   Burke, L.M. 1996. Rehydration strategies before and after exercise. *Aust. J. Nutr. Diet* 53 (4 Suppl):S22-S26.

23   Lyons, T.P., Riedesel, M.L., Meuli, L.E., and Chick, T.W. 1990. Effects of glycerol-induced hyperhydration prior to exercise in the heat on sweating and core temperatures. *Med. Sci. Sports Exerc.* 22:477-483.

24   Burke, L.M. 1996. Rehydration strategies before and after exercise. *Aust. J. Nutr. Diet* 53 (4 Suppl):S22-S26.

25   Montner, P., Stark, D.M., Riedesel, M.L., Murata, G., Robergs, R., Timms, M., and Chick, T.W. 1996. Pre-exercise glycerol hydration improves cycling endurance time. *Int. J. Sports Med.* 17:27-33.

26   Lyle, D.M., Lewis, P.R., Richards, D.A.B., Richards, R., Bauman, A.E., Sutton, J.R., and Cameron, I.D. 1994. Heat exhaustion in the Sun-Herald city-to-surf fun run. *Med. J. Aust.* 161:361-365.

27   McConnell, G., Burge, C.M., Skinner, S.L., and Hargreaves, M. 1995. Ingested fluid volume and physiological responses during prolonged exercise in a mild environment [abstract]. *Med. Sci. Sports Exerc.* 27:S19.

28   Walsh, R.M., Noakes, T.D., Hawley, J.A., and Dennis, S.C. 1994. Impaired high-intensity cycling performance time at low levels of dehydration. *Int. J. Sports Med.* 15:392-398.

29   Maughan, R.J., Fenn, C.E., and Leiper, J.B. 1989. Effects of fluid, electrolyte and substrate ingestion on endurance capacity. *Eur. J. Appl. Physiol.* 58:481-486.

30   Mitchell, J.B., Costill, D.L., Houmard, J.A., Fink, W.J., Pascoe, D.D., and Pearson, D.R. 1989. Influence of carbohydrate dosage on exercise performance and glycogen metabolism. *J. Appl. Physiol.* 67:1843-1849.

31   Tsintzas, O.K., Liu, R., Williams, C., Campbell, I., and Gaitanos, G. 1993. The effect of carbohydrate ingestion on performance during a 30-km race. *Int. J. Sport Nutr.* 3:127-139.

32   Coggan, A.R., and Coyle, E.F. 1987. Reversal of fatigue during prolonged exercise by carbohydrate infusion or ingestion. *J. Appl. Physiol.* 63:2388-2395.

33   Coyle, E.F., Hagberg, J.M., Hurley, B.F., Martin, W.H., Ehami, A.A., and Holloszy, J.O. 1983. Carbohydrate feeding during prolonged strenuous exercise can delay fatigue. *J. Appl. Physiol.* 55:230-235.

34   Coyle, E.F., Coggan, A.R., Hemmert, M.K., and Ivy, J.L. 1986. Muscle glycogen utilization during prolonged, strenuous exercise when fed carbohydrate. *J. Appl. Physiol.* 61:165-172.

35   Tsintzas, O.K., Williams, C., Boobis, L., and Greenhaff, P. 1995. Carbohydrate ingestion and glycogen utilization in different muscle fiber types in man. *J. Physiol.* 489:243-250.

36   Hargreaves, M., Costill, D.L., Coggan, A.R., Fink, W.J., and Nishibata, I. 1984. Effect of carbohydrate feedings on muscle glycogen utilization and exercise performance. *Med. Sci. Sports Exerc.* 16:219-222.

37   Yaspelkis, B.B., Patterson, J.G., Anderla, P.A., Ding, Z., and Ivy, J.L. 1993. Carbohydrate supplementation spares muscle glycogen during variable-intensity exercise. *J. Appl. Physiol.* 75:1477-1485.

38   Below, P.R., Mora-Rodriguez, R., Gonzalez-Alonso, J., and Coyle, E.F. 1995. Fluid and carbohydrate ingestion independently improves performance during one hour of intense exercise. *Med. Sci. Sports Exerc.* 27: 200-210.

39   Below, P.R., Mora-Rodriquez, R., Gonzalez-Alonso, J., and Coyle, E.F. 1995. Fluid and carbohydrate ingestion independently improve performance during 1 h of intense exercise. *Med. Sci. Sports Exerc.* 27:200-210.

40   Nicholas, C.W., Williams, C., Lakomy, H.K.A., Phillips, G., and Nowitz, A. 1995. Influence of ingesting a carbohydrate-electrolyte solution on endurance capacity during intermittent, high intensity shuttle running. *J. Sports Sci.* 13:283-290.

41   Simard, C., Tremblay, A., and Jobin, M. 1988. Effects of carbohydrate intake before and during an ice hockey match on blood and muscle energy substrates. *Res. Q. Exerc. Sport* 59:144-147.

42   Coyle, E.F., Coggan, A.R., Hemmert, M.K., and Ivy, J.L. 1986. Muscle glycogen utilization during prolonged, strenuous exercise when fed carbohydrate. *J. Appl. Physiol.* 61:165-172.

43   Murray, R., Paul, G.L., Seifert, J.G., Eddy, D.E., and Halaby, G.A. 1989. The effects of glucose, fructose, and sucrose ingestion during exercise. *Med. Sci. Sports Exerc.* 21:275-282.

44   Owen, M.D., Kregel, K.C., Wall, P.T., and Gisolfi, C.V. 1986. Effects of ingesting carbohydrate beverages during exercise in the heat. *Med. Sci. Sports Exerc.* 18:568-575.

45 Murray, R., Paul, G.L., Seifert, J.G., Eddy, D.E., and Halaby, G.A. 1989. The effects of glucose, fructose, and sucrose ingestion during exercise. *Med. Sci. Sports Exerc.* 21:275-282.

46 Bjorkman, O., Sahlin, K., Hagenfeldt, L., and Wahren, J. 1984. Influence of glucose and fructose ingestion on the capacity for long-term exercise in well-trained men. *Clin. Physiol.* 4:483-494.

47 Hargreaves, M. 1996. Physiological benefits of fluid and energy replacement during exercise. *Aust. J. Nutr. Diet* 53 (4 Suppl):S3-S7.

48 Mason, W.L., McConell, G.K., and Hargreaves, M. 1993. Carbohydrate ingestion during exercise: Liquid vs. solid feedings. *Med. Sci. Sports Exerc.* 25:966-969.

49 Coggan, A.R., and Coyle, E.F. 1987. Reversal of fatigue during prolonged exercise by carbohydrate infusion or ingestion. *J. Appl. Physiol.* 63:2388-2395.

50 Coyle, E.F., and Montain, S.J. 1992. Benefits of fluid replacement with carbohydrate during exercise. *Med. Sci. Sports Exerc.* 24 (suppl):324S-330S.

51 Wagenmakers, A.J.M., Brouns, F., Saris, W.H.M., and Halliday, D. 1993. Oxidation rates of orally ingested carbohydrates during prolonged exercise in men. *J. Appl. Physiol.* 75:2774-2780.

52 Broad, E.M., Burke, L.M., Gox, G.R., Heeley, P., and Riley, M. 1996. Body-weight changes and voluntary fluid intakes during training and competition sessions in team sports. *Int. J. Sport Nutr.* 6:307-320.

53 Noakes, T.D., Adams, B.A., Myburgh, K.H., Greff, C., Lotz, T., and Nathan, M. 1988. The danger of inadequate water intake during prolonged exercise. *Eur. J. Appl. Physiol.* 57:210-219.

54 Rothstein, A., Adolph, E.F., and Wills, J.H. 1947. Voluntary dehydration. In *Physiology of man in the desert*, ed. Adolph, E.F., 254-270. New York: Interscience.

55 Carter, J.E., and Gisolfi, C.V. 1989. Fluid replacement during and after exercise in the heat. *Med. Sci. Sports Exerc.* 21:532-539.

56 Gonzalez-Alonso, J., Heaps, C.L., and Coyle, E.F. 1992. Rehydration after exercise with common beverages and water. *Int. J. Sports Med.* 3:399-406.

57 Maughan, R.J., and Leiper, J.,B. 1995. Sodium intake and post-exercise rehydration in man. *Eur. J. Appl. Physiol.* 71:311-319.

58 Maughan, R.J., Leiper, J.B., and Shirreffs, S.M. 1996. Restoration of fluid balance after exercise-induced dehydration: Effects of food and fluid intake. *Eur. J. Appl. Physiol.* 73:317-325.

59 Burke, L.M. 1996. Rehydration strategies before and after exercise. *Aust. J. Nutr. Diet* 53 (4 Suppl):S22-S26.

Chapter 3

1 Williams, M.H. 1992. *Nutrition for fitness and sport.* (Dubuque, IO: William C. Brown Publishers). 224-225.

2 Katch, F.I., and McArdle, W.D. 1993. *Introduction to nutrition, exercise, and health.* 4th ed. Philadelphia: Lea & Febinger.

3 Williams, M.H. 1999. *Nutrition for health, fitness, and sport.* (New York: WCB McGraw-Hill). 317-318.

4 Archimedes was a Greek mathematician, engineer, and physicist. He discovered formulas for determining the area and volume of different shapes the principal of buoyancy.

5 Grediagan, M.A., Cody, M., Rupp, J., Benardot, D., and Shern, R. 1995. Exercise intensity does not effect body composition change in untrained. Moderately overfat women. *J. Am. Dietetics Ass.* 95 (6): 661-665.

6 Saltzman, E., and Roberts, S.B. 1995. The role of energy expenditure in energy regulation: findings of a decade of research. *Nutr. Rev.* 53(8): 209-220.

7 Forbes, G.F., Brown, M.R., Welle, S.L., and Lipinski, B.A. 1986. Deliberate overfeeding in women and men: energy cost and composition of the weight gain. *Brit. J. of Nutr.* 56: 1-9.

8   Roberts, S.B., Young, V.R., Fuss, P., et al. 1990. Energy expenditure and subsequent nutrient intakes in overfed young men. *Am. J. Clin. Nutr.* 259: R461-9.

9   Diaz, E.O., Prentice, A.M., Goldberg, G.R., Murgatroyd, P.R., and Coward, W.A. 1992. Metabolic response to experimental overfeeding in lean and overweight healthy volunteers. *Am. J. Clin. Nutr.* 56: 641-55.

10   Leibel, R.L., Rosenbaum, M., and Hirsch, J. 1995. Changes in energy expenditure resulting from altered body weight. *New Eng. J. Med.* 332: 621-8.

Chapter 4

1   Greenhaff, P.L., Casey, A., Short, A.H., Harris, R., Soderlund, K., and Hultman, E. 1993. Influence of oral creatine supplementation of muscle torque during repeated bouts of maximal voluntary exercise in man. *Clin. Sci.* 84:565-571.

2   Harris, R.C., Soderlund, K., and Hultman, E. 1992. Elevation of creatine in resting and exercised muscle of normal subjects by creatine supplementation. *Clin. Sci.* 83:367-374.

3   Maughan, R.J. 1995. Creatine supplementation and exercise performance. *Intl. J. Sport Nutr.* 5:94-101.

4   Walker, J.B. 1979. Creatine biosynthesis, regulation, and function. *Adv. Enzmmol.* 50:117-142.

5   Butterfield, G., Cady, C., and Moynihan, S. 1992. Effect of increasing protein intake on nitrogen balance in recreational weight lifters. *Med. Sci. Sports Exerc.* 24:S71.

6   Nagle, F.J., and Bassett, D.R. 1989. Energy metabolism. In *Nutrition in exercise and sport*, ed. Hickson, J.F., and Wolinsky, I. Boca Raton, FL: CRC Press, 87-106.

7   Costill, D.L., and Hargreaves, M. 1992. Carbohydrate nutrition and fatigue. *Sports Med.* 13 (2):86

8   Valeriani, A. 1991. The need for carbohydrate intake during endurance exercise. *Sports Med.* 12 (6):349.

9   Williams, M.H. 1992. *Nutrition for fitness and sport.* New York: WCB/McGraw-Hill, 58-64.

10   Bergstrom, J., Hermansen, L., Hultman, E., and Saltin, B. 1967. Diet, muscle glycogen, and physical performance. *Acta. Physiol. Scand.* 71:140.

11   Costill, D.L., and Hargreaves, M. 1992. Carbohydrate nutrition and fatigue. *Sports Med.* 13 (2):86.

12   Nagle, F.J., and Bassett, D.R. 1989. Energy metabolism. In *Nutrition in exercise and sport*, ed. Hickson, J.F., and Wolinsky, I. Boca Raton, FL: CRC Press, 87-106.

13   Coyle, E.F. 1983. Effects of glucose polymer feedings on fatigability and the metabolic response to prolonged strenuous exercise. In *Ross symposium on nutrient utilization during exercise*, ed. Fox, E.L. Columbus, OH: Ross Laboratories, 4-11.

14   Nagle, F.J., and Bassett, D.R. 1989. Energy metabolism. In *Nutrition in exercise and sport*, ed. Hickson, J.F., and Wolinsky, I. Boca Raton, FL: CRC Press, 87-106.

15   Greenhaff, P.L. 1995. Creatine and its application as an ergogenic aid. *Int. J. Sport Nutr.* 5:S100-S110.

16   Greenhaff, P.L., Casey, A., Short, A.H., Harris, R., Soderlund, K., and Hultman, E. 1993. Influence of oral creatine supplementation on muscle torque during repeated bouts of maximal voluntary exercise in man. *Clin. Sci.* 84:565-571.

17   Maughan, R.J. 1995. Creatine supplementation and exercise performance. *Intl. J. Sport Nutr.* 5:94-101.

18   Kozak, C.J., Benardot, D., Cody, M., Doyle, J.A., and Thompson, W.R. 1996. The effect of creatine monohydrate supplementation on anaerobic power and anaerobic endurance in elite female gymnasts. Master's thesis, Georgia State University.

19   Harris, R.C., Soderlund, K., and Hultman, E. 1992. Elevation of creatine in resting and exercised muscle of normal subjects by creatine supplementation. *Clin. Sci.* 83:367-374.

20   Maughan, R.J. 1995. Creatine supplementation and exercise performance. *Intl. J. Sport Nutr.* 5:94-101.

21   Walker, J.B. 1979. Creatine biosynthesis, regulation, and function. *Adv. Enzmmol.* 50:117-142.

22   Pritchard, N.R., and Kalra, P.A. 1998. Creatine supplements linked to renal damage. *The Lancet* 351:1252-1253.

23   Maughan, R.J. 1995. Creatine supplementation and exercise performance. *Intl. J. Sport Nutr.* 5:94-101.

24   Lyons, T.P., Riedesel, M.L., Meuli, L.E., and Chick, T.W. 1990. Effects of glycerol-induced hyperhydration prior to exercise in the heat on sweating and core temperature. *Med. Sci. Sports Exerc.* 22(4):477-483.

25   Montgomery, D.L, and Beaudin, P.A. 1982. Blood lactate and heart rate response of young females during gymnastic routines. *J. Sports Med.* 22:358-365.

26   Butterfield, G., Cady, C., and Moynihan, S. 1992. Effect of increasing protein intake on nitrogen balance in recreational weight lifters. *Med. Sci. Sports Exerc.* 24:S71.

27   Tarnopolsky, M.A., MacDougall, J.D., and Atkinson, S.A. 1988. Influence of protein intake and training status on nitrogen balance and lean body mass. *J. Appl. Physiol.* 64 (1):187-193.

28   Spriet, L.L. 1995. Caffeine and performance. *Int. J. Sport Nutr.* 5:S84-S99.

29   Bucci, L. 1993. *Nutrients as ergogenic aids for sports and exercise.* Boca Raton, FL: CRC Press.

30   Kanter, M.M., and Williams, M.H. 1995. Antioxidants, carnitine, and choline as putative ergogenic aids. *Int. J. Sport Nutr.* 5:S120-S131.

31   Bucci, L. 1993. *Nutrients as ergogenic aids for sports and exercise.* Boca Raton, FL: CRC Press, 6; 20.

32   Babayan, V.K. 1967. Medium-chain triglycerides: Their composition, preparation, and application. *J. Am. Oil Chem. Soc.* 45:23.

33   Bach, A.S., and Babayan, V.K. 1982. Medium-chain triglycerides: An update. *Am. J. Clin. Nutr.* 36:950.

34   Avakian, E.V., and Sugimoto, B.R. 1980. Effect of Panax ginseng extract on blood energy substrates during exercise. *Fed. Proc.* 39:287.

Chapter 5

1   Horswill, C.A. 1993. Weight loss and weight cycling in amateur wrestlers: Implications for performance and resting metabolic rate. *Int. J. Sport Nutr.* 3:245-260.

2   Strauss, R.H., Lanese, R.R., and Leizman, D.J. 1988. Illness and absence among wrestlers, swimmers, and gymnasts at a large university. *Am. J. Sports Med.* 16:653-655.

3   Ryan, A.J. 1981. Anabolic steroids are fool's gold. *Fed. Proc.* 40:2682-2688.

4   Kleiner, S.M. 1995. The role of meat in the athlete's diet: It's effect on key macro- and micronutrients. *Gatorade Sports Sci. Inst.: Sports Sci. Exch.* 8 (5).

5   Bar-Or, O., Clarkson, P., Coyle, E., Davis, J.M., Ekblom, B., Gisolfi, C., Hagerman, F., Horswill, C., Kanter, M., Kraemer, W., Lamb, D., Maughan, R., Murray, R., and Spriet, L. 1993. *Gatorade Sports Sci. Inst.: Sports Sci. Exch. Roundtable* 4 (4).

6   Gregory, J., Greene, S., Thompson, J., Scrimgeour, C., and Rennie, M. 1992. Effects of oral testosterone undecanoate on growth, body composition, strength and energy expenditure of adolescent boys. *Clin. Endocr.* 37:207-213.

7   Binnerts, A., Swart, G., Wilson, J., Hoogerbrugge, N., Pols, H., Birkenhager, J., and Lamberts, S. 1992. The effect of growth hormone administration in growth hormone deficient adults on bone, protein, carbohydrate, and lipid homeostasis, as well as on body composition. *Clin. Endocr.* 37:79-87.

8   Deyssig, R., Frisch, H., Blum, W., and Waldhor, T. 1993. Effect of growth hormone treatment on hormonal parameters, body composition, and strength in athletes. *Acta. Endocr.* 128:313-318.

9   Yarasheki, K., Campbell, J., Smith, K., Rennie, M., Holloszy, J., and Bier, D. 1992. Effect of growth hormone and resistance exercise on muscle growth in young men. *Am. J. Phys.* E261-E267.

10   Williams, M.H. 1993. Nutritional supplements for strength-trained athletes. *Gatorade Sports Sci. Inst.: Sports Sci. Exch.* 6 (6).

11   Bucci, L., Hickson, J., Pivarnik, J., Wolinsky, I., McMahon, J., and Turner, S. 1990. Ornithine ingestion and growth hormone release in bodybuilders. *Nutr. Res.* 10:239-245.

12 Fogelholm, M., Naveri, H., Kiilavuori, K., and Harkonen, M. 1993. Low-dose amino acid supplementation: No effects on serum human growth hormone and insulin in male weightlifters. *Int. J. Sport Nutr.* 3:290-297.

13 Lambert, M., Hefer, J., Millar, R., and Macfarlane, P. 1993. Failure of commercial oral amino acid supplements to increase serum growth hormone concentrations in male bodybuilders. *Int. J. Sport Nutr.* 3:298-305.

14 Bucci, L., Hickson, J., Wolinksy, I., and Pivarnik, J. 1992. Ornithine supplementation and insulin release in bodybuilders. *Int. J. Sport Nutr.* 2:287-291.

15 Summinski, R., Robertson, R., Goss, E., Robinson, A., DaSilva, S., Kane, J., Utter, A., and Metz, K. 1993. The effect of amino acid ingestion and resistance exercise on growth hormone responses in young males [Abstract]. *Med. Sci. Sports Exer.* 25:S77.

16 Fry, A., Kraemer, W., Stone, M., Warren, B., Kearney, J., Maresh, C., Weseman, C., and Fleck, S. 1993. Endocrine and performance responses to high volume training and amino acid supplementation in elite junior weightlifters. *Int. J. Sport Nutr.* 3:306-322.

17 Elam, R. 1988. Morphological changes in adult males from resistance exercise and amino acid supplementation. *J. Sports Med. Phys. Fitness* 28:35-39.

18 Elam, R., Hardin, D., Sutton, R., and Hagen, L. 1989. Effects of arginine and ornithine on strength, lean body mass, and urinary hydroxyproline in adult males. *J. Sports Med. Phys. Fitness* 29:52-56.

19 Barron, R., and Vanscoy, G. 1993. Natural products and the athlete: Facts and folklore. *Ann. Pharmacother.* 27:607-615.

20 Williams, M. 1992. *Nutrition for fitness and sport.* Dubuque, IA: Brown and Benchmark.

21 Hawkins, C.J., Walberg-Rankin, J., and Sebolt, D. 1991. Oral arginine does not affect body composition or muscle function in male weightlifters. *Med. Sci. Sports Exer.* 23:S15.

22 Cynober, H., Vaubourolle, M., Dore, A., and Giboudeau, J. 1984. Kinetics and metabolic effects of orally administered ornithine alphaketoglutarate in healthy subjects. *Am. J. Clin. Nutr.* 39:514-519.

23 Williams, M.H. 1993. Nutritional supplements for strength-trained athletes. *Gatorade Sports Sci. Inst.: Sports Sci. Exch.* 47 6(6).

24 Bar-Or, O., Clarkson, P., Coyle, E., Davis, J.M., Ekblom, B., Gisolfi, C., Hagerman, F., Horswill, C., Kanter, M., Kraemer, W., Lamb, D., Maughan, R., Murray, R., and Spriet, L. 1993. Physiology and nutrition for competitive sport. *Gatorade Sports Sci. Inst.: Sports Sci. Exch. Roundtable* 14 4(4).

25 Geil, P.B., and Anderson, J.W. 1994. Nutrition and health implications of dry beans: A review. *J. Am. Coll. Nutr.* 13:549-558.

26 Mares-Perlman, J.A., Subar, A.F., Block, G., Greger, J.L., and Luby, M.H. 1995. Zinc intake and sources in the U.S. adult population: 1976-1980. *J. Am. Coll. Nutr.* 14:349-357.

27 Pate, R.R., Miller, B.J., Davis, J.M., Slentz, C.A., and Klingshirn, L.A. 1993. Iron status of female runners. *Int. J. Sport Nutr.* 3:222-231.

28 Telford, R.D., Bunney, C.J., Catchpole, E.A., Catchpole, W.R., Deakin, V., Gray, B., Hahn, A.G., and Kerr, D.A. 1992. Plasma ferritin concentration and physical work capacity in athletes. *Int. J. Sport Nutr.* 2:335-342.

29 Singh, A., Moses, E., and Deuster, P. 1992. Chronic multivitamin-mineral supplementation does not enhance physical performance. *Med. Sci. Sports Exer.* 24:726-732.

30 Telford, R., Catchpole, E., Deakin, V., Hahn, A., and Plank, A. 1992. The effect of 7-8 months of vitamin/mineral supplementation on athletic performance. *Int. J. Sport Nutr.* 2:135-153.

31 Clancy, S., Clarkson, P., DeCheke, M., Nasaka, K., Cunningham, J., and Feedson, P. 1993. Chromium supplementation in football players [Abstract]. *Med. Sci. Sports Exer.* 24:S194.

32 Hallmark, M., Reynolds, T., DeSouza, C., Dotson, C., Anderson, R., and Rogers, M. 1993. Effects of chromium supplementation and resistive training on muscle strength and lean body mass in untrained men [Abstract]. *Med. Sci. Sports Exer.* 25:S101.

33 Nielsen, E. 1992. Facts and fallacies about boron. *Nutr. Today* 27:6-12.

34 Ferrando, A., and Green, N. 1993. The effect of boron supplementation on lean body mass, plasma testosterone levels, and strength in bodybuilders. *Int. J. Sport Nutr.* 3:140-149.

35   Brilla, L., and Haley, T. 1992. Effect of magnesium supplementation on strength training in humans. *J. Am. Coll. Nutr.* 11:326-329.
36   Williams, M.H. 1993. Nutritional supplements for strength trained athletes. *Gatorade Sports Sci. Inst.: Sports Sci. Exch.* 47 6(6).

Chapter 6

1   Ekblom, B., and Bergh, U. 1994. Physiology and nutrition for cross-country skiing. In *Perspectives in exercise science and sports medicine: Physiology and nutrition for competitive sport,* ed. Lamb, D., Knuttgen, H., and Murray, R., 373. Indianapolis, IN: Benchmark Press.
2   Economos, C.D., Bortz, S.S., and Nelson, M.E. 1993. Nutritional practices of elite athletes. *Sports Med.* 16:383.
3   Burke, L., Gollan, R., and Read, R. 1991. Dietary intakes and food use of groups of elite Australian male athletes. *Int. J. Sport Nutr.* 1:378.
4   Murray, R., and Horswill, C.A. 1998. Nutrient requirements for competitive sports. In *Nutrition in exercise and sport,* 3rd ed., ed. Wolinsky, I., Boca Raton, FL: CRC Press. 521-558.
5   Pate, R.R., and Branch, J.D. 1992. Training for endurance sport. *Med. Sci. Sports Exer.* 24:S340.
6   Armstrong, L. 1991. Considerations for replacement beverages: Fluid-electrolyte balance and heat illness. In *Fluid replacement and heat stress,* ed. Marriott, B. and Rosemont, C. Washington, DC: National Academy Press.
7   Sawka, M.N., and Wenger, C.B. 1988. Physiological responses to acute exercise-heat stress. In *Human performance physiology and environmental medicine at terrestrial extremes,* ed. Pandolf, K.B., Sawka, M.N., and Gonzalez, R.R. Benchmark Press: Indianapolis, IN.
7a   Williams, M.H. 1999. Nutrition for health, fitness and sport, 5th ed. New York, NY: WCB McGraw-Hill, 76.
8   Hargreaves, M., Dillo, P., Angus, D., and Febbraio, M. 1996. Effect of fluid ingestion on muscle metabolism during prolonged exercise. *J. Appl. Physiol.* 80 (1): 363-6.
9   Armstrong, L.E., Costill, D.L., and Fink, W.J. 1985. Influence of diuretic-induced dehydration on competitive running performance. *Med. Sci. Sports Exerc.* 17:456.
10   Walsh, R.M., Noakes, T.D., Hawley, J.A., and Dennis, S.C. 1994. Impaired high-intensity cycling performance time at low levels of dehydration. *Int. J. Sport Nutr.* 15:392.
11   Maughan, R. 1991. Carbohydrate-electrolyte solutions during prolonged exercise. In *Perspectives in exercise science and sports medicine: Ergogenics—enhancement of performance in exercise and sport,* ed. Lamb, D., and Williams, M. Indianapolis, IN: Brown and Benchmark. 35-50.
12   Coyle, E.F., Coggan, A.R., Hemmert, M.K., and Ivy, J.L. 1986. Muscle glycogen utilization during prolonged strenuous exercise when fed carbohydrate. *J. Appl. Physiol.* 61:165-172.
13   Costill, D.L. 1985. Carbohydrates nutrition before, during, and after exercise. *Fed. Proc.* 44:364.
14   Williams, C., Wilson, W., and Burrin, J. 1996. Influence of carbohydrate supplementation early in exercise on endurance running capacity. *Med. Sci. Sports Exerc.* 28:1373-1379.
15   Tsintzas, O.K., Williams, C., Singh, R., Wilson, W., and Burrin, J. 1995. Influence of carbohydrate-electrolyte drinks on marathon running performance. *Eur. J. Appl. Physiol.* 70:154-160.
16   Murray, R., Paul, G.L., Seifert, J.G., Eddy, D.E., and Halaby, G.A. 1989. The effects of glucose, fructose, and sucrose ingestion during exercise. *Med. Sci. Sports Exerc.* 21:275-282.
17   Davis, J.M., Cokkinides, V.E., Burgess, W.A., and Bartoli, W.P. 1989. Effects of a carbohydrate/electrolyte drink or water on the stress hormone response to prolonged intense cycling: Renin, angiotestin-I, aldosterone, ACTH, and cortisol. In *Hormones and Sport,* vol. 55, *Serono symposia publication,* ed. Laron, Z., and Rogo, A.D., 193-204. New York: Raven Press.
18   Costill, D.L., and Hargreaves, M. 1992. Carbohydrate nutrition and fatigue. *Sports Med.* 13:86.

19   Coyle, E.F., and Coyle, E. 1993. Carbohydrates that speed recovery from training. *Physician Sports Med.* 21:111.

20   Sherman, W.M. 1995. Metabolism of sugars and physical performance. *Am. J. Clin. Nutr.* 62:228S.

21   Coggan, A.R., and Swanson, S.C. 1992. Nutritional manipulations before and during endurance exercise: Effects on performance. *Med. Sci. Sports Exerc.* 24:S331.

22   American College of Sports Medicine. 1996. Position stand on exercise and fluid replacement. *Med. Sci. Sports Exerc.* 28:i.

23   Broad, E.M., Burke, L.M., Cox, G.R., Heeley, P., and Riley, M. 1996. Body weight changes and voluntary fluid intakes during training and competition sessions in team sports. *Int. J. Sport Nutr.* 6:307.

24   Eichner, E.R., Laird, R., Nadel, E., and Noakes, T. 1994. Hyponatremia in sport: Symptoms and prevention. *Gatorade Sports Sci. Inst.: Sports Sci. Exch. Roundtable* 12: 5(1).

25   Lambert, G.P., Bleiler, T.L., Change, R.T., Johnson, A.K., and Gisolfi, C.V. 1993. Effects of carbonated and non-carbonated beverages at specific intervals during treadmill running in the heat. *Int. J. Sport Nutr.* 3:177-193.

26   Lugo, M., Sherman, W.M., Wimer, G.S., and Garleb, K. 1993. Metabolic responses when different forms of carbohydrate energy are consumed during cycling. *Int. J. Sport Nutr.* 3:398.

27   Sherman, W.M., and Lamb, D.R. 1988. Nutrition and prolonged exercise. In *Perspectives in exercise science and sports medicine: Prolonged exercise,* ed. Lamb, D.R., and Murray, R., 213. Indianapolis, IN: Benchmark Press.

28   Coyle, E.F., and Coyle, E. 1993. Carbohydrates that speed recovery from training. *Physician Sports Med.* 21:111.

29   Tarnopolsky, M., MacDugall, J., and Atkinson, S. 1988. Influence of protein intake and training status on nitrogen balance and lean body mass. *J. Appl. Physiol.* 66:187.

30   Grandjean, A. 1989. Macronutrient intake of U.S. athletes compared with the general population and recommendations made for athletes. *Am. J. Clin. Nutr.* 49:1070.

31   Murray, R., Bartoli, W.P., Eddy, D.E., and Horn, M.K. 1995. Physiological and performance responses to nicotinic-acid digestion during exercise. *Med. Sci. Sports Exerc.* 27 (7):1057-1062.

Chapter 8

1   Maughan, R.J., and Shirreffs, S.M. 1997. Preparing athletes for competition in the heat: Developing an effective acclimatization strategy. *Gatorade Sports Sci. Inst.: Sports Sci. Exch.* 2: 65(10).

2   Gatorade Sports Nutrition Advisory Board. 1996. *Eating on the road.* Chicago, IL: Gatorade Sports Science Institute.

3   Mielcarek, J., and Kleiner, S. 1993. Time zone changes. In *Sports nutrition: A guide for the professional working with active people,* ed. Benardot, D. Chicago: American Dietetic Association.

4   Loat, E.R., and Rhodes, E.C. 1989. Jet lag and human performance. *Sports Med.* 8:226-238.

Chapter 9

1   Grivetti, L.E., and Applegate, E.A. 1997. From Olympia to Atlanta: A cultural-historical perspective on diet and athletic training. *J. Nutr.* 127 (5):860S-868S.

2   Recht, L.D., Lew, R.A., and Schwartz, W.J. 1995. Baseball teams beaten by jet lag. *Nature* 377 (6550):583.

3   Whitley, J.D., and Terrio, T. 1998. Changes in peak torque arm-shoulder strength of high school baseball pitchers during the season. *Percept. Motor Skills* 86:1361-1362.

4   MacWilliams, B.A., Choi, T., Perezous, M.K., Chao, E.Y., and McFarland, E.G. 1998. Characteristic ground-reaction forces in baseball pitching. *Am. J. Sports Med.* 26:66-71.

5   Yoshida, T., Nakai, S., Yorimoto, A., Kawabata, T., and Morimoto, T. 1995. Effect of aerobic capacity on sweat rate and fluid intake during outdoor exercise in the heat. *Eur. J. Appl. Physiol.* 71:235-239.

6   Bast, S.C., Perry, J.R., Poppiti, R., Vangsness, C.T., and Weaver, F.A. 1996. Upper extremity blood flow in collegiate and high school baseball pitchers: A preliminary report. *Am. J. Sports Med.* 24 (6):847-851.

7   Schulz, R., and Curnow, C. 1988. Peak performance and age among superathletes: Track and field, swimming, baseball, tennis, and golf. *J. Gerontology* 43 (5):113-120.

8   Hickson, J.F., Johnson, T.E., Lee, W., and Sidor, R.J. 1990. Nutrition and the precontent preparations of a male bodybuilder. *J. Am. Diet. Assoc.* 90 (2):264-267.

9   Britschgi, F., and Zund, G. 1991. Bodybuilding: Hypokalemia and hypophosphatemia. *Schweiz Med. Wochenschr.* 121 (33):1163-1165.

10   Hickson, J.F., Johnson, T.E., Lee, W., and Sidor, R.J. 1990. Nutrition and the precontent preparations of a male bodybuilder. *J. Am. Diet. Assoc.* 90 (2):264-267.

11   Barron, R.L., and Vanscoy, G.J. 1993. Natural products and the athlete: Facts and folklore. *Ann. Pharmacother.* 27 (5):607-615.

12   Kleiner, S.M., Bazzarre, T.L., and Litchford, M.D. 1990. Metabolic profiles, diet, and health practices of championship male and female bodybuilders. *J. Am. Diet. Assoc.* 90 (7):962-967.

13   Bosselaers, I., Buemann, B., Victor, O.J., and Astrup, A. 1994. Twenty-four hour energy expenditure and substrate utilization in body builders. *Am. J. Clin. Nutr.* 59:10-12.

14   Andersen, R.E., Barlett, S.J., Morgan, G.D., and Brownell, K.D. 1995. Weight loss, psychological, and nutritional patterns in competitive male body builders. *Int. J. Eat. Disord.* 181 (1):49-57.

15   Kreider, R.B., Ferreira, M., Wilson, M., Grindstaff, P., Plisk, S., Reinardy, J., Cantler, E., and Almada, A.L. 1998. Effects of creatine supplementation on body composition, strength, and sprint performance. *Med. Sci. Sports Exerc.* 30 (1):73-82.

16   Clancy, S.P., Clarkson, P.M., DeCheke, M.E., Nosaka, K., Freedson, P.S., Cunningham, J.J., and Valentine, B. 1994. Effects of chromium picolinate supplementation on body composition, strength, and urinary chromium loss in football players. *Int. J. Sport Nutr.* 4 (2):142-153.

17   Burke, L.M., and Hawley, J.A. 1997. Fluid balance in team sports: Guidelines for optimal practices. *Sports Med.* 24 (1):38-54.

18   Criswell, D., Powers, D., Lawler, J., Tew, J., Dodd, S., Iryiboz, Y., Tulley, R., and Wheeler, K. 1991. Influence of a carbohydrate-electrolyte beverage on performance and blood homeostasis during recovery from football. *Int. J. Sport Nutr.* 1 (2):178-191.

19   Parks, P.S., and Read, M.H. 1997. Adolescent male athletes: Body image, diet, and exercise. *Adolescence* 32 (127):593-602.

20   Wang, M.Q., Downey, G.S., Perko, M.A., and Yesalis, C.E. 1993. Changes in body size of elite high school football players: 1963-1989. *Percept. Motor Skills* 76 (2):379-383.

21   Gomez, J.E., Ross, S.K., Calmbach, W.L., Kimmel, R.B., Schmidt, D.R., and Dhanda, R. 1998. Body fatness and increased injury rates in high school football linemen. *Clin. J. Sport Med.* 8 (2):115-120.

22   Kaplan, T.A., Digel, S.L., Scavo, V.A., and Arellana, S.B. 1995. Effect of obesity on injury risk in high school football players. *Clin. J. Sport Med.* 5 (1):43-47.

23   Huddy, D.C., Nieman, D.C., and Johnson, R.L. 1993. Relationship between body image and percent body fat among college male varsity athletes and nonathletes. *Percept. Motor Skills* 77 (3):851-857.

24   DePalma, M.T., Koszewski, W.M., Case, J.G., Barile, R.J., DePalma, B.F., and Oliaro, S.M. 1993. Weight control practices of lightweight football players. *Med. Sci. Sports Exerc.* 25 (6):694-701.

25   Hickson, J.F., Jr., Duke, M.A., Risser, W.L., Johnson, C.W., Palmer, R., and Stockton, J.E. 1987. Nutritional intake from food sources of high school football athletes. *J. Am. Diet. Assoc.* 87 (12):1656-1659.

26   Jehue, R., Street, D., and Huizenga, R. 1993. Effect of time zone and game time changes on team performance: National Football League. *Med. Sci. Sports Exerc.* 25 (1):127-131.

27   Maddux, G.T. 1970. *Men's gymnastics.* Pacific Palisades, CA: Goodyear Publishing, 9.

28   Houtkooper, L.B., and Going, S.B. 1994. Body composition: How should it be measured? Does it affect sport performance? *Gatorade Sports Sci. Inst.: Sports Sci. Exch.* 52: 7 (5s).

29   Bortz, S., Schoonen, J.C., Kanter, M., Kosharek, S., and Benardot, D. 1993. *Physiology of anaerobic and aerobic exercise.* In *Sports nutrition: A guide for the professional working with active people,* ed. Benardot, D., 2-10. Chicago, IL: American Dietetic Association.

30   Benardot, D., and Czerwinski, C. 1991. Selected body composition and growth measures of junior elite gymnasts. *J. Am. Diet. Assoc.* 91 (1):29-33.

31   Benardot, D., Schwarz, M., and Heller, D.W. 1989. Nutrient intake in young, highly competitive gymnasts. *J. Am. Diet. Assoc.* 89:401-403.

32   Benardot, D. 1996. Working with young athletes: Views of a nutritionist on the Sports Medicine team. *Int. J. Sport Nutr.* 6 (2):110-120.

33   Loosli, A.R. 1993. Reversing sports-related iron and zinc deficiencies. *Phys. Sportsmed.* 21 (6):70-78.

34   Benardot, D., and Czerwinski,.C. 1991. Selected body composition and growth measures of junior elite gymnasts. *J. Am. Diet. Assoc.* 91 (1):29-33.

35   Burns, J., and Dugan, L. 1994. Working with professional athletes in the rink: The evolution of a nutrition program for an NHL team. *Int. J. Sport Nutr.* 4 (2):132-134.

36   Akermark, C., Jacobs, I., Rasmussen, M., and Karlsson, J. 1996. Diet and muscle glycogen concentration in relation to physical performance in Swedish elite ice hockey players. *Int. J. Sport Nutr.* 6 (3):272-284.

37   Houston, M.E. 1979. Nutrition and ice hockey performance. *Can. J. Appl. Sport Sci.* 4 (1):98-99.

38   Tegelman, R., Aberg, T., Pousette, A., and Carlstrom, K. 1992. Effects of a diet regimen on pituitary and steroid hormones in male ice hockey players. *Int. J. Sports Med.* 13 (5):424-430.

39   Horswill, C.A., Hickner, R.C., Scott, J.R., Costill, D.L., and Gould, D. 1990. Weight loss, dietary carbohydrate modifications, and high intensity, physical performance. *Med. Sci. Sports Exerc.* 22 (4):470-476.

40   Grediagin, M.A., Cody, M., Rupp, J., Benardot, D., and Shern, R. 1995. Exercise intensity does not effect body composition change in untrained, moderately overfat women. *J. Am. Diet. Assoc.* (95) 6:661-665.

41   Kreider, R.B., Ferreira, M., Wilson, M., Grindstaff, P., Plisk, S., Reinardy, J., Cantler, E., and Almada, A.L. 1998. Effects of creatine supplementation on body composition, strength, and sprint performance. *Med. Sci. Sports Exerc.* 30 (1):73-82.

42   Nevill, M.E., Williams, C., Roper, D., Slater, C., and Nevill, A.M. 1993. Effect of diet on performance during recovery from intermittent sprint exercise. *J. Sports Sci.* 11 (2):119-126.

43   Sherman, W.M., Doyle, J.A., Lamb, D.R., and Strauss, R.H. 1993. Dietary carbohydrate, muscle glycogen, and exercise performance during seven days of training. *Am. J. Clin. Nutr.* 57 (1):27-31.

44   Berning, J.R., Troup, J.P., VanHandel, P.J., Daniels, J., and Daniels, N. 1991. The nutritional habits of young adolescent swimmers. *Int. J. Sport Nutr.* 1(3): 240-248.

45   Guinard, J.X., Seador, K., Beard, J.L., and Brown, P.L. 1995. Sensory acceptability of meat and dairy products and dietary fat in male collegiate swimmers. *Int. J. Sport Nutr.* 5(4): 315-328.

46   Lamb, D.R. Basic principles for improving sport performance. 1995. *Gatorade Sports Science Exchange* (#55) 8(2).

47   Microsoft. 1993-1996. "Wrestling." *Encarta 97 Encyclopedia.* CD-ROM: Microsoft Corporation.

48   Sossin, K., Gizis, F., Marquart, L.F., and Sobal, J. 1997. Nutrition beliefs, attitudes, and resource use of high school wrestling coaches. *Int. J. Sport Nutr.* 7 (3):219-228.

49   Oppliger, R.A., Case, H.S., Horswill, C.A., Landry, G.L., and Shelter, A.C. 1996. American College of Sports Medicine position stand: Weight loss in wrestlers. *Med. Sci. Sports Exerc.* 28 (6):ix-xii.

50   Wroble, R.R., and Moxley, D.P. 1998. Weight loss patterns and success rates in high school wrestlers. *Med. Sci. Sports Exerc.* 30 (4):625-628.

51   Wroble, R.R., and Moxley, D.P. 1998. Acute weight gain and its relationship to success in high school wrestlers. *Med. Sci. Sports Exerc.* 30 (6):949-951.

52   Roemmich, J.N., and Sinning, W.E. 1997. Weight loss and wrestling training: Effects on growth-related hormones. *J. Appl. Physiol.* 82 (6):1760-1764.

53   Roemmich, J.N., and Sinning, W.E. 1997. Weight loss and wrestling training: Effects on nutrition, growth, maturation, body composition, and strength. *J. Appl. Physiol.* 82 (6):1751-1759.

54   Rankin, J.W., Ocel, J.V., and Craft, L.L. 1996. Effect of weight loss and refeeding diet composition on anaerobic performance in wrestlers. *Med. Sci. Sports Exerc.* 28 (10):1292-1299.

55   Choma, C.W., Sforzo, G.A., and Keller, B.A. 1998. Impact of rapid weight loss on cognitive function in collegiate wrestlers. *Med. Sci. Sports Exerc.* 30 (5):746-749.

56   Horswill, C.A. 1993. Weight loss and weight cycling in amateur wrestlers: Implications for performance and resting metabolic rate. *Int. J. Sport Nutr.* (3):245-260.

57   Oppliger, R.A., Harms, R.D., Herrmann, D.E., Streich, C.M., and Clark, R.R. 1995. The Wisconsin wrestling minimum weight project: A model for weight control among high school wrestlers. *Med. Sci. Sports Exerc.* 27 (8):1220-1224.

Chapter 10

1   Sizer, F., and Whitney, E. 1997. *Nutrition: Concepts and controversies* (7th ed.). Albany, NY: West/Wadsworth: 383.

2   American College of Sports Medicine. 1999. Overtraining: Consensus statement. *Sports Medicine Bulletin* 31 (1): 29.

3   American College of Sports Medicine. 1999. Overtraining: Consensus statement. *Sports Medicine Bulletin* 31 (1): 29.

4   Asp, S., Rohde, T., and Richter, E.A. 1997. Impaired muscle glycogen resynthesis after a marathon is not caused by decreased muscle GLUT-4 content. *J. Appl. Physiol.* 83 (5):1482-1485.

5   Farber, H.W., Schaefer, E.J., Franey, R., Grimaldi, R., and Hill, N.S. The endurance triathlon: Metabolic changes after each event and during recovery. *Med. Sci. Sports Exerc.* 23 (8):959-965.

6   Dressendorfer, R.H., and Wade, C.E. 1991. Effects of a 15-d race on plasma steroid levels and leg muscle fitness in runners. *Med. Sci. Sports Exerc.* 23 (8):954-958.

7   Sherman, W.M., and Maglischo, E.W. 1991. Minimizing chronic athletic fatigue among swimmers: Special emphasis on nutrition. *Sports Sci. Exch.* 4(35).

8   Niekamp, R.A., and Baer, J.T. 1995. In-season dietary adequacy of trained male cross-country runners. *Int. J. Sport Nutr.* 5:45-55.

9   Butterworth, D.E., Nieman, D.C., Butler, J.V., and Herring, J.L. 1994. Food intake patterns of marathon runners. *Int. J. Sport Nutr.* 4 (1):1-7.

10   Houtkooper, L. 1992. Food selection for endurance sports. *Med. Sci. Sports Exerc.* 24 (9):S349-S359.

11   Hickner, R.C., Fisher, J.S., Hansen, P.A., Racette, S.B., Mier, C.M., Turner, M.J., and Holloszy, J.O. 1997. Muscle glycogen accumulation after endurance exercise in trained and untrained individuals. *J. Appl. Physiol.* 83 (3):897-903.

12   Helmich, P., Christensen, S.W., Darre, E., Jahnsen, F., and Hartvig, T. 1989. Non-elite marathon runners: Health, training, and injuries. *Br. J. Sports Med.* 23 (3):177-178.

13   Fogelholm, M., Tikkanen, H., Naveri, H., and Harkonen, M. 1989. High-carbohydrate diet for long distance runners: A practical view-point. *Br. J. Sports Med.* 23 (2):94-96.

14   Nieman, D.C., Gates, J.R., Butler, J.V., Pollett, L.M., Dietrich, S.J., and Lutz, R.D. 1989. Supplementation patterns in marathon runners. *J. Am. Diet. Assoc.* 89 (11):1615-1619.

15   Rokitzki, L., Hinkel, S., Klemp, C., Cufi, D., and Keul, J. 1994. Dietary, serum, and urine ascorbic acid status in male athletes. *Int. J. Sports Med.* 15 (7):435-440.

16   Rokitzki, L., Sagredos, A.N., Reuss, F., Buchner, M., and Keul, J. 1994. Acute changes in vitamin B6 status in endurance athletes before and after a marathon. *Int. J. Sport Nutr.* 4 (2):154-165.

17   Terblanche, S., Noakes, T.D., Dennis, S.C., Marais, D., and Eckert, M. 1992. Failure of magnesium supplementation to influence marathon running performance or recovery in magnesium-replete subjects. *Int. J. Sport Nutr.* 2 (2):154-164.

18   Barnett, D.W., and Conlee, R.K 1984. The effects of a commercial dietary supplement on human performance. *Am. J. Clin. Nutr.* 40 (3):586-590.

19   Davies, K.J.A., Quintanilha, A.T., Brooks, G.A., and Packer, L. 1982. Free radicals and tissue damage produced by exercise. *Biochim. Biophys. Res. Commun.* 107:1198-1205.

20   Wolinsky, I., and Driskell, J.A. 1997. *Sports nutrition: Vitamins and trace elements.* New York: CRC Press.

21   Margaritis, I., Tessier, F., Richard, M.J., and Marconnet, P. 1997. No evidence of oxidative stress after a triathlon race in highly trained competitors. *Int. J. Sports Med.* 18 (3):186-190.

22   Rokitzki, L., Logemann, E., Sagredos, A.N., Murphy, M., Wetzel-Roth, W., and Keul, J. 1994. Lipid peroxidation and antioxidative vitamins under extreme endurance stress. *Acta. Physiol. Scan.* 4(2):149-158.

23   Sloniger, M.A., Cureton, K.J., and O'Bannon, P.J. 1997. One-mile run-walk performance in young men and women: Role of anaerobic metabolism. *Can. J. Appl. Physiol.* 22 (4):337-350.

24   Penn, I.W., Wang, Z.M., Buhl, K.M., Allison, D.B., Burastero, S.E., Heymsfield, S.B. 1994. Body composition and two-compartment model assumptions in male long-distance runners. *Med. Sci. Sports Exerc.* 26:392-397.

25   Reeder, M.T., Dick, B.H., Atkins, J.K., Pribis, A.B., and Martinez, J.M. 1996. Stress fractures: Current concepts of diagnosis and treatment. *Sports Med.* 22 (3):198-212.

26   Deuster, P.A., Kyle, S.B., Moser, P.B., Vigersky, R.A., Singh, A., and Schoomaker, E.B. 1986. Nutritional intakes and status of highly trained amenorrheic and eumenorrheic women runners. *Fertil. Steril.* 46 (4):636-643.

27   Houmard, J.A., Scott, B.K., Justice, C.L., and Chenier, T.C. 1994. The effects of taper on performance in distance runners. *Med. Sci. Sports Exerc.* 26 (5):624-631.

28   Beidleman, B.A., Puhl, J.L., and DeSouza, M.J. 1995. Energy balance in female distance runners. *Am. J. Clin. Nutr.* 61:303-311.

29   Rontoyannis, G.P., Skoulis, T., and Pavlou, K.N. 1989. Energy balance in ultramarathon running. *Am. J. Clin. Nutr.* 49:976-979.

30   Eden, B.D., and Abernethy, P.J. 1994. Nutritional intake during an ultraendurance running race. *Int. J. Sport Nutr.* 4:166-174.

31   Millard-Stafford, M.L., Sparling, P.B., Rosskopf, L.B., and DiCarlo, L.J. 1992. Carbohydrate-electrolyte replacement improves distance running performance in the heat. *Med. Sci. Sports Exerc.* 24 (8):934-940.

32   Noakes, T.D., Adams, B.A., Myburgh, K.H., Greeff, C., Lotz, T., and Nathan, M. 1988. The danger of an inadequate water intake during prolonged exercise: A novel concept revisited. *Eur. J. Appl. Physiol.* 57 (2):210-219.

33   Dennis, S.C., and Noakes, T.D. 1999. Advantages of a smaller body mass in humans when distance-running in warm, humid conditions. *Eur. J. Appl. Physiol.* 79 (3):280-284.

34   Bentley, D.J., Wilson, G.J., Davie, A.J., and Zhou, S. 1998. Correlations between peak power output, muscular strength, and cycle time trial performance in triathletes. *J. Sports Med. Phys. Fitness* 38 (3):201-207.

35   Laurenson, N.M., Fulcher, K.Y., and Korkia, P. 1993. Physiological characteristics of elite and club level female triathletes during running. *Int. J. Sports Med.* 14 (8):455-459.

36   Gulbin, J.P., and Gaffney, P.T. 1999. Ultraendurance triathlon participation: Typical race preparation of lower-level triathletes. *J. Sports Med. Phys. Fitness* 39 (1):12-15.

37   Banister, E.W., Carter, J.B., and Zarkadas, P.C. 1999. Training theory and taper: Validation in triathlon athletes. *Eur. J. Appl. Physiol.* 79 (2)182-191.

38   Guezennec, C.Y., Chalabi, H., Bernard, J., Fardellone, P., Krentowski, R., Zerath, E., and Meunier, P.J. 1998. Is there a relationship between physical activity and dietary calcium intake? A survey in 10,373 young French subjects. *Med. Sci. Sports Exerc.* 30 (5):732-739.

39   Kerr, C.G., Trappe, T.A., Starling, R.D., and Trappe, S.W. 1998. Hyperthermia during Olympic triathlon: Influence of body heat storage during the swimming stage. *Med. Sci. Sports Exerc.* 30 (1):99-104.

40   Rogers, G., Goodman, C., and Rosen, C. 1997. Water budget during ultra-endurance exercise. *Med. Sci. Sports Exerc.* 29 (11):1477-1481.

41   O'Toole, M.L., Douglas, P.S., Laird, R.H., and Hiller, D.B. 1995. Fluid and electrolyte status in athletes receiving medical care at an ultradistance triathlon. *Clin. J. Sport Med.* 5 (2):116-122

42   Speedy, D.B., Faris, J.G., Hamlin, M., Gallagher, P.G., and Campbell, R.G. 1997. Hyponatremia and weight changes in an ultradistance triathlon. *Clin. J. Sport Med.* 7 (3):180-184.

43   Rehrer, N.J., van Kemenade, M., Meester, W., Brouns, F., and Saris, W.H. 1992. Gastrointestinal complaints in relation to dietary intake in triathletes. *Int. J. Sport Nutr.* 2 (1):48-59.

44   Clark, N., Tobin, J., Jr., and Ellis, C. 1992. Feeding the ultraendurance athlete: Practical tips and a case study. *J. Am. Diet. Assoc.* 92 (10):1258-1262.

45   Frentsos, J.A., and Baer, J.T. 1997. Increased energy and nutrient intake during training and competition improves elite triathletes' endurance performance. *Int. J. Sport Nutr.* 7 (1):61-71.

46   Ribeiro, J.P., Cadavid, E., Baena, J., Monsalvete, E., Barna, A., and DeRose, E.H. 1990. Metabolic predictors of middle-distance swimming performance. *Br. J. Sports Med.* 24 (3):196-200.

47   Lee, E.J., Long, K.A., Risser, W.L., Poindexter, H.B., Gibbons, W.E., and Goldzieher, J. 1995. Variations in bone status of contralateral and regional sites in young athletic women. *Med. Sci. Sports Exerc.* 27 (10):1354-1361.

48   Berning, J.R., Troup, J.P., VanHandel, P.J., Daniels, J., and Daniels, N. 1991. The nutritional habits of young adolescent swimmers. *Int. J. Sport Nutr.* 1 (3):240-248.

49   Saris, W.H., Schrijver, J., van Erp Baart, M.A., and Brouns, F. 1989. Adequacy of vitamin supply under maximal sustained workloads: The Tour de France. *Int. J. Vitam. Nutr. Res. Suppl.* 30:205-212.

50   Brouns, F., Saris, W.H., Stroecken, J., Beckers, E., Thijssen, R., Rehrer, J.N., and ten Hoor, F. 1989. Eating, drinking, and cycling: A controlled Tour de France simulation study, Part II. Effect of diet manipulation. *Int. J. Sports Med.* 10 (S1):S41-S48.

51   Weiler, J.M., Layton, T., and Hunt, M. 1998. Asthma in United States Olympic athletes who participated in the 1996 Summer Games. *J. Allergy Clin. Immunol.* 102 (5):722-726.

Chapter 11

1   Davis, M. 1995. Repeated sprint work is enhanced with consumption of a carbohydrate-electrolyte beverage. *Med. Sci. Sports Exerc.* 27:S223.

2   Nicholas, C.W., Williams, C., Phillips, G., and Nowitz, A. 1995. Influence of ingesting a carbohydrate-electrolyte solution on endurance capacity during intermittent, high intensity shuttle running. *J. Appl. Sports Sci. Res.* 13:282-290.

3   Below, P.R., Mora-Rodrigues, R., Gonzalez-Alonso, J., and Coyle, E.F. 1995. Fluid and carbohydrate ingestion independently improve performance during one hour of intense exercise. *Med. Sci. Sports Exerc.* 27 (2):200-210.

4   Murray, R., Paul, G.L., Seifert, J.G., and Eddy, D.E. 1991. Responses to varying rates of carbohydrate ingestion during exercise. *Med. Sci. Sports Exerc.* 23 (6):713-718.

5   Gisolfi, C.V., Summers, R.W., Schedl, H.P., and Bleiler, T.L. 1992. Intestinal water absorption from select carbohydrate solutions in humans. *J. Appl. Physiol.* 73:2142-2150.

6   Lambert, C.P. 1991. Effects of carbohydrate feeding on multiple-bout resistance exercise. *J. Appl. Sports Sci. Res.* 5:129-197.

7   Ryan, A.J., Lambert, G.P., Shi, X., Chang, R.T., Summers, R.W., and Gisolfi, C.V. 1998. Effect of hypohydration on gastric emptying and intestinal absorption during exercise. *J. Appl. Physiol.* 84 (5):1581-1588.

8   Horswill, C.A. 1998. Effective fluid replacement. *Int. J. Sport Nutr.* 8:175-195.

9   American College of Sports Medicine. 1996. Position stand on exercise and fluid replacement. *Med. Sci. Sports Exerc.* 28:i-vii.

10   Corley, G., Demarest-Litchford, M., and Bazzarre, T.L. 1990. Nutrition knowledge and dietary practices of college coaches. *J. Am. Diet. Assoc.* 90 (5):705-709.

11   Nowak, R.K., Knudsen, K.S., and Schulz, L.O. 1988. Body composition and nutrient intakes of college men and women basketball players. *J. Am. Diet. Assoc.* 88 (5):575-578.

12   Mannix, E.T., Healy, A., and Farber, M.O. 1996. Aerobic power and supramaximal endurance of competitive figure skaters. *J. Sports Med. Phys. Fitness* 36 (3):161-168.

13   Delistraty, D.A., Reisman, E.J., and Snipes, M. 1992. A physiological and nutritional profile of young female figure skaters. *J. Sports Med. Phys. Fitness* 32 (2):149-155.

14   Ziegler, P., Hensley, S., Roepke, J.B., Whitaker, S.H., Craig, B.W., and Drewnowski, A. 1998. Eating attitudes and energy intakes of female skaters. *Med. Sci. Sports Exerc.* 30 (4):583-586.

15   Smith, A.D., and Ludington, R. 1989. Injuries in elite pair skaters and ice dancers. *Am. J. Sports Med.* 17 (4):482-488.

16   Kjaer, M., and Larsson, B. 1992. Physiological profile and incidence of injuries among elite figure skaters. *J. Sports Sci.* 10 (1):29-36.

17   Tumilty, D. 1993. Physiological characteristics of elite soccer players. *Sports Med.* 16 (2):80-96.

18   Wittich, A., Mautalen, C.A., Oliveri, M.B., Bagur, A., Somoza, F., and Rotemberg, E. 1998. Professional football (soccer) players have a markedly greater skeletal mineral content, density, and size than age- and BMI-matched controls. *Calcif. Tissue Int.* 63 (2):112-117.

19   Duppe, H., Gardsell, P., Johnell, O., and Ornstein, E. 1996. Bone mineral density in female junior, senior, and former football players. *Osteoporos. Int.* 6 (6):437-441.

20   Tumilty, D. 1993. Physiological characteristics of elite soccer players. *Sports Med.* 16 (2):80-96.

21   Rico-Sanz, J. 1998. Body composition and nutritional assessments in soccer. *Int. J. Sport Nutr.* 8 (2):113-123.

22   Maughan, R.J. 1997. Energy and macronutrient intakes of professional football (soccer) players. *Br. J. Sports Med.* 31 (1):45-47.

23   Clark, K. 1994. Nutritional guidance to soccer players for training and competition. *J. Sports Sci.* 12:S43-S50.

24   Kirkendall, D.T. 1993. Effects of nutrition on performance in soccer. *Med. Sci. Sports Exerc.* 25 (12):1370-1374.

25   Hargreaves, M. 1994. Carbohydrate and lipid requirements of soccer. *J. Sports Sci.* 12:S13-S16.

26   Groppel, J.L., and Roetert, E.P. 1992. Applied physiology of tennis. *Sports Med.* 14 (4):260-268.

27   Bergeron, M.F., Maresh, C.M., Kraemer, W.J., Abraham, A., Conroy, B., and Gabaree, C. 1991. Tennis: A physiological profile during match play. *Int. J. Sports Med.* 12 (5):474-479.

28   Vergauwen, L., Brouns, F., and Hespel, P. 1998. Carbohydrate supplementation improves stroke performance in tennis. *Med. Sci. Sports Exerc.* 30 (8):1289-1295.

29   Bergeron, M.F., Maresh, C.M., Armstrong, L.E., Signorile, J.F., Castellani, J.W., Kenefick, R.W., LaGasse, K.E., and Riebe, D.A. 1995. Fluid-electrolyte balance associated with tennis match play in a hot environment. *Int. J. Sport Nutr.* 5 (3):180-193.

30   Baxter-Jones, A.D., Helms, P., Baines-Preece, J., and Preece, M. 1994. Menarche in intensively trained gymnasts, swimmers, and tennis players. *Ann. Hum. Biol.* 21 (5):407-415.

Index

About the Author

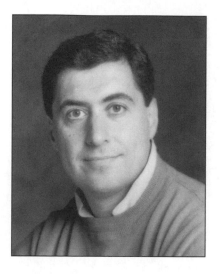

Dan Benardot, PhD, RD, is an associate dean for research and is on the faculty of the departments of nutrition and kinesiology and health at Georgia State University and has been involved in sports nutrition research since 1981. He is the codirector of the Laboratory for Elite Athlete Performance at GSU, which provides training and nutrition plans that help athletes in their pursuit of excellence.

As the national team nutritionist and chair of the Athlete Wellness Program for USA Gymnastics, Benardot worked with the gold-medal winning women's gymnastics team at the 1996 Atlanta Olympic Games. He has been funded by the United States Olympic Committee to do research with elite athletes and has also worked with top athletes from a variety of team and individual sports.

Benardot served as editor in chief of *Sports Nutrition: A Guide for Professionals Working with Active People* and has earned numerous awards for outstanding service from the American Dietetic Association. Born in Greece, Benardot gained his love for sport while growing up in the Lake Placid region of northern New York State. He now lives with his wife and two children in Atlanta, Georgia, where he enjoys tennis, skiing, and photography.

*You'll find
other outstanding
nutrition resources at*

www.humankinetics.com

In the U.S. call

1-800-747-4457

Australia 08 8277 1555
Canada 1-800-465-7301
Europe .... +44 (0) 113 278 1708
New Zealand 09-523-3462